THE CHANGING
MEDICAL
PROFESSION

THE CHANGING MEDICAL PROFESSION

An International Perspective

EDITED BY

Frederic W. Hafferty
John B. McKinlay

New York   Oxford
OXFORD UNIVERSITY PRESS
1993

Oxford University Press

Oxford   New York   Toronto
Delhi   Bombay   Calcutta   Madras   Karachi
Kuala Lumpur   Singapore   Hong Kong   Tokyo
Nairobi   Dar es Salaam   Cape Town
Melbourne   Auckland   Madrid

and associated companies in
Berlin   Ibadan

Published by Oxford University Press, Inc.,
200 Madison Avenue, New York, New York 10016

Oxford is a registered trademark of Oxford University Press

Library of Congress Cataloging-in-Publication Data
The Changing medical profession
[edited by] Frederic W. Hafferty, John B. McKinlay.
p.   cm.
Includes bibliographical references and index.
ISBN 0-19-507592-7
1. Social medicine.
2. Medicine.
3. Physician and patient.
I. Hafferty, Fredric W., 1947– .
II. McKinlay, John B.
[DNLM: 1. Medicine. 2. Physicians—trends.
W 21 C4558 1993]
RA418.C59   1993
362. 1' 72—dc20   DNLM/DLC   for Library of Congress
92-48382

2 4 6 8 9 7 5 3 1

Printed in the United States of America
on acid-free paper

For M. D. C.

ACKNOWLEDGMENTS

First and foremost we thank the contributors to this book, who have so unselfishly given their time and talents to this project. Recognizing that one strength of this book was its ability to provide readers with a multiplicity of viewpoints, all contributors agreed to craft their chapters under rather severe page limitations. In addition, a few of these individuals went far beyond the call of normal duty and produced their contributions under extremely short deadlines. If *fun* can be considered an operative word in any such a joint undertaking, then this is what they helped to make this project.

Several people played key roles in the evolution of this book. David Willis, former editor of the *Milbank Quarterly,* played an important role in developing the original Milbank Supplemental Issue and in facilitating its migration to Oxford University Press. James House, and then Valerie Aubry, both of Oxford University Press, provided the initial entrée for this book and gave it a home. Aubry's considerable efforts on our behalf recently have been supplemented by David Roll, the current sociology editor at the Press. Others, both "outsiders" and contributing authors, have graciously donated their special talents and time in discussing both individual chapters and the broader themes with us: Eliot Freidson, Donald Light, David Sciulli, John Stoeckle, David Wilsford, and Irving Zola.

Finally, Fred would like to express his appreciation to Tracy Kemp for her unselfish help in the preparation of various parts of this book and to Bonnie Briest for her unsurpassed editorial expertise. As always, I am eternally grateful to my wife, Cindy, for her unflagging support, to our son David, age two, who was conceived, born, and is growing up in the partial shadow of this book, and to Philip, age five, who in asking me for a personal copy said, "I won't mind that there aren't any pictures; I can just dream the words."

CONTENTS

III   Discussion

THE CHANGING
MEDICAL
PROFESSION

Introduction

Frederic W. Hafferty and John B. McKinlay

For those seeking to understand the structure, organization, and texture of health care, the least that can be said is that we live in analytically challenging times. The pace of change is both ominous and relentless. The profession of medicine, an organizational infant a mere hundred years ago, continues to evolve. Today, those who aspire to become physicians face a future practice environment fundamentally different from that which they might have envisioned upon first deciding to don the healer's mantle. In this respect, today's doctors in the making face a realm of uncertainties quite different from those faced by their predecessors.

Accompanying this change within medicine has been a series of revolutions in science, technology, politics, and society. Over the past century we have moved from the dunes of Kitty Hawk to the moon and beyond, from a single wireless transatlantic station to a global communications network, from distance measured in hoofbeats to a distance rendered strange by air travel exceeding the speed of sound. Nation-states have crumbled, new ones have emerged, and old ones are being reborn. We have moved from news about that which has happened to news in real time, from the serenity of the familiar to a world that announces its presence on our doorstep with punishing regularity. We have witnessed the shrinking of political and economic boundaries, the growth of a global economy, the emergence of a global village, and the continuing evolution of governments as sources of power and influence.

In the face of these massive changes, important issues are being raised about the future of medicine as a profession. These include the evolving nature of physician autonomy, changes in the structure and dynamics of the physician-patient relationship, the transformation of collegial relations, and an ongoing debate about what constitutes quality in health care—how it should be assessed and the role medicine can and should play in its delivery. Observers have become more aware of the rather modest contributions made by medicine to the decline in mortality in the twentieth century, relative to the impact of improved housing, hygiene, and diet (McKinlay and McKinlay 1977; McKinlay, McKinlay, and Beaglehole 1989). Correspondingly, we have witnessed an explosion of public interest in alternative therapies, including those considered as addenda to traditional medicine and those considered to be external or even in conflict with allopathic practices (Wallis 1991;

3

Murray and Rubel 1992). Ultimately we are witnessing a reconceptualization of medicine's role in society and its relationship to the state and other centers of power and influence, including corporations.

Within social science circles, medicine has long been considered the prototypic profession. In turn, the concept "profession" has provided social scientists with an important tool for understanding medicine as a special type of occupation. From the writings of Talcott Parsons (1951), who presented an idealized model of the physician-patient relationship, we have come to be increasingly sensitive to the dimensions of authority, power, and exploitation that may exist within this dyad. We are examining how the practice of medicine is being shaped by the relationships that exist among professions (Abbott 1988), as well as those between professions and state, public, and corporate interests.

Over the past few decades, the most influential framework for viewing professions as a particular organizational form has been professional dominance theory. This approach had its origins in the Chicago school of sociology with the writings of Everett C. Hughes, Howard Becker, and, most recently, Eliot Freidson. In analyzing medicine's rise to a position of occupational dominance and autonomy, Freidson eschewed Parsons's normative vision and argued that medicine had achieved the legally sanctioned status of a special occupation whose control over the work of others was paralled by its own immunity from external review.

Freidson's early work was formulated during a time that many (including Freidson) now refer to as the golden age of medicine. By the mid- to late 1970s, the forces that long had promoted medicine's influence and prestige no longer appeared to be as decisive or clear-cut, and alternatives to Freidson's theory of professional dominance began to emerge. The two most notable were deprofessionalization (often associated with the writings of Marie Haug) and proletarianization (associated with the writings of John McKinlay, Magali Larson, and Martin Oppenheimer). A debate of sorts followed in which readers were treated to a series of articles and book chapters detailing the relative merits and deficiencies of these different viewpoints (Hafferty 1988; Hafferty and Light 1989; Hafferty and Wolinsky 1991). In several of Freidson's rebuttal pieces (1983*b*, 1984, 1986*a*, 1986*b*, 1987, 1989*e*), he acknowledged the presence of significant change in medicine but continued to argue that the changes evident were not sufficient to weaken medicine's professional powers.

Although Freidson has continued to insist that medicine is not becoming deprofessionalized or proletarianized, it would be a mistake to characterize his writings as static or ensnared by tradition. In this book, for example, Freidson (Chapter 4) appears to echo earlier calls by McKinlay (1982) and Haug (1988) in suggesting that questions about medicine's continued professional dominance are best left to history or are impossible to ascertain except within the most specific contexts. Although we certainly agree with Freidson's basic methodological point that forces appearing notable today will probably not proceed unscathed or unaltered into the future, we also believe that it is analytically unsatisfactory to jettison efforts to anticipate the future of medicine. As argued much more persuasively by David Frankford in Chapter 3, it is not just morally desirable but phenomenologically quite important that we continue to focus critical attention on this dynamic and thus the relationship between matters of personal and societal health and issues of control, professional discretion, and individual autonomy.

Roots

This book assesses the current status of medicine as a profession in both the United States and abroad. It has its origins in a special supplemental issue of the *Milbank Quarterly* (Volume 66, Supplement 2, 1988), guest edited by one of this book's editors (McKinlay), and entitled "The Changing Character of the Medical Profession." The issue was enthusiastically received, prompting a recommendation by the general editor, David P. Willis, that a revised and extended edition be published. The original *Milbank* issue was organized around four sections: chapters covering background and theoretical perspectives, an essay written from an insider's (M.D.) point of view, several papers covering medicine in countries other than the United States (the bulk of these focusing on Western industrialized nations), and a discussion chapter integrating all of these materials.

This book differs from its parent in several respects. First, it is organized into three broad parts. Part I contains chapters covering issues of theoretical and conceptual importance. Chapter 1, "The Professional Dominance, Deprofessionalization, Proletarianization, and Corporatization Perspectives: An Overview and Synthesis," by Fredric Wolinsky, provides a broad overview of the three major analytical perspectives in what has been characterized as the professional dominance-deprofessionalization-proletarianization debate. Although Wolinsky draws (and rightly so) some rather definite conclusions as to the most viable and empirically supportable position within this trilogy, the main purpose of this chapter is to provide readers with an overview of the major arguments advanced by these perspectives as they attempt to wrestle with the issue of professional dynamics. Chapter 2, "The Medical Profession and the State," is co-authored by Julio Frenk and Luis Durán-Arenas. This chapter provides readers with conceptual tools for understanding the dynamics of the relationship between the state and professions, as well as with an overview of some of the issues highlighting critical state theory. Chapter 3, "Professions and the Law," by David Frankford, was included to challenge readers about assumptions they might have concerning the nature of the law as an instrument of state policy and its use as a tool for the advancement of professional interests. Within the professions literature, one recent trend has been to highlight the nature of state-supported prerogatives and how professions function as a quasi-monopoly, enjoying the protection of legally sanctioned licensure and practice act entitlements. This chapter holds some of these notions up to critical scrutiny. Chapter 4, "How Dominant Are the Professions?" by Eliot Freidson extends his influential and extensive work on professions in new and provocative directions, particularly with respect to the dynamics of internal stratification and the role of professional expertise in the future of professional dominance.

Part II is the heart of this book. It contains eleven case studies, each allowing readers to explore the changing character of the medical profession from a different political, social, cultural, and historical context. It substantially updates six of the original seven case studies that appeared in the *Milbank* Supplemental Issue and adds almost as many (five) case studies from new countries. It seeks to build upon one point made in the Supplemental Issue: an adequate understanding of medicine as a profession is highly dependent on a variety of factors, not the least of which is the evolving character of professional-state relations (Hafferty 1988). Thus, although important similarities may be observed across any number of countries, particularly with respect to medicine's control over the clinical core of its work, there also exist tremendous differences among countries in terms of the organization and financing of medical care. Less clear, but exquisitely provocative, is the possibility that factors related to the control of clinical work are not altogether immune from such organizational and financial contingencies. We will return to this last point shortly.

The additional five case studies selected for this book were arrived at through a mixture of purpose and serendipity. The United States was added as a separate and distinct case study to allow for an explicit rather than implicit treatment of this nation. New Zealand was added to the original contingent of Great Britain, Canada, and Australia to provide readers with an opportunity to explore how countries with common political and cultural roots might evolve differently in terms of health policy. France, with its state structure almost a polar opposite of that of the United States (see Krause 1991; Wilsford 1991; and Freidson, Frenk and Durán-Arenas, and Wilsford in this book), was added as an obvious omission to the original block of Western industrialized nations. Czechoslovakia and China were added not only to promote comparisons between socialist and capitalist countries but also to allow for some additional comparisons among China, Czechoslovakia, Sweden (and other Nordic countries), and the former Soviet Union. In addition, it was anticipated that the inclusion of countries undergoing marked political, social, and economic change (e.g., Czechoslovakia and the Commonwealth of Independent States) would shed some prognostic light on how medicine as a profession might fare under such circumstances.

These purposeful additions aside, there remain some obvious omissions: Germany (Light and Schuller 1986; Light, Liebfried, and Tennstedt 1986; Stone 1991), countries in Africa, Central or South America, and the Third World (e.g., Cuba or Mexico [see Cleaves 1987 for an example of the latter]). In some cases a particular omission was due to an inability to identify an expert willing to author such a chapter. In other instances the reason was more ethnocentric, with arguments raised as to whether a detailing of medicine in this or that country would add to an understanding of how health care can and could be shaped in the United States or other Western industrialized nations. Finally, there was the reality of page limitations. In the end, not all countries would or could be represented. As it was, the authors contributing to this book graciously labored under restrictive page limitations, allowing for the inclusion of more case studies but at the cost of their ability to develop their own arguments more fully. As such, any glaring omissions are almost certainly the fault of the book editors.

Part III contains three discussion chapters. The two "outside" authors, Rudolf Klein and Sol Levine, bring considerable expertise to this project in the areas of occupations and professions in general, and health care organization and financing in particular. Both were provided with working drafts of the individual chapters and asked, based on this material, to address issues they considered important in understanding the changing character of medicine as a profession from an international perspective. It was anticipated that Sol Levine would approach the issues of professional dynamics and the changing status of the medical profession from the top down, stressing issues of humanism and values in medicine, and that Rudolf Klein would draw upon his considerable cross-national experience and develop his ideas with the international perspective of this book in mind. In each case our expectations were fulfilled. The final discussion chapter, which we wrote, is our attempt to raise some final issues and questions. These three chapters are intended to provide readers with a plethora of ideas and perspectives to encourage them to reexplore the case studies from a different vantage point.

In summary, the structure of this book is intended to provide readers with some conceptual materials up front, facilitating their exploration of the case studies individually and collectively. The discussion chapters are intended to serve not so much as a summary of the preceding chapters but as a stimulus inviting the reader to explore anew or reexamine these case materials. In both of these ways we hope that readers might be drawn more fully into the book as a whole.

I

THEORETICAL AND CONCEPTUAL OVERVIEW

1

The Professional Dominance, Deprofessionalization, Proletarianization, and Corporatization Perspectives: An Overview and Synthesis

Fredric D. Wolinsky

This chapter begins by advancing a theoretical perspective about professional dominance in medicine and then moves on to a discussion concerning whether that perspective has ever or currently applies to medicine and how it might be changing. The chapter thus provides an overview of both the perspective and the discussion, as well as some additional thoughts about antitrust law and the role of imputed trust.

The Professional Dominance Perspective

In a series of provocative works, Eliot Freidson developed what has come to be known as the professional dominance perspective (see especially 1970*a*, 1970*b*, 1977, 1980, 1983*b*, 1984, 1985, 1986*a*, 1986*b*, 1987). It begins with the argument that the word *profession* has two meanings: a special kind of occupation and an avowal or promise. For Freidson, the study of the profession of medicine, and hence the professional dominance perspective, requires emphasis on both meanings (1970*a*:xvii):

> [I]t is useful to think of a profession as an occupation which has assumed a dominant position in a division of labor, so that it gains control over the determination of the substance of its own work. Unlike most occupations, it is autonomous or self-directing. The occupation sustains this special status by its persuasive profession of the extraordinary trustworthiness of its members. The trustworthiness it professes naturally includes ethicality and also knowledgeable skill. In fact, the profession claims to be the most reliable authority on the nature of the reality it deals with.

Thus, a profession is defined as an occupation that has achieved autonomy or self-direction based on the dual characteristics of its specialness and promise.

There must also be formal institutions that exist for the sole purpose of serving to protect the profession from external "competition, intervention, evaluation, and direction by others" (Freidson 1970*b*). These formal institutions separate and stabilize the organized autonomy of medicine from that of occupations that by default are left to their own devices because the nature of their work is not of sufficient public concern, not dependent on a functional division of labor, and not sufficiently observable to warrant attempts at formal external intervention into the manner in which they perform their duties (such as cab drivers or lighthouse workers; see Freidson 1970*b*:136). Furthermore, the scope of the profession's autonomy extends beyond itself, including all other occupations within its segment (industrial cluster) of the division of labor.

Within any labor segment, only one occupation may achieve such organized autonomy. Freidson (1970*b*:136) writes that within the health care industry:

> [W]e find that . . . the only occupation that is truly autonomous is medicine itself. It has the authority to direct and evaluate the work of others without in turn being subject for formal direction and evaluation by them. Paradoxically, its autonomy is sustained by the *dominance* of its expertise in the division of labor.

Although other occupations within the health care industry may claim to be professions, they uniformly lack either organized autonomy or dominance, a critical distinction for Freidson (1970*b*:137):

> While the members of all [health care occupations] may be committed to their work, may be dedicated to service, and may be specially educated, the dominant profession stands in an entirely different structural relationship to the division of labor than does the subordinate profession. To ignore that difference is to ignore something major. One might call many occupations "professions" if one so chooses, but there is a difference between the dominant profession and the others.

The difference is that the true profession has achieved autonomy.

Achieving autonomy, says Freidson (1970*a*), is a two-stage process. The first stage consists primarily of demonstrating that the occupation does reliable and valuable work, a criterion that is often facilitated and demonstrated by the establishment of educational requirements, licensing procedures, a code of ethics, the formation of a professional association, and some element of peer control. An occupation can achieve most of these on its own. Frequently, the possession of such traits is used to distinguish the paraprofessions (e.g., nursing and physician extenders) from the less prestigious occupations (e.g., nursing aides and transporters).

The second stage of the process involves the conferral of autonomy. It results from the critical interaction of political and economic power, and occupational representation. Although it may be facilitated by educational institutions and the other forces that help to differentiate the paraprofessions from the less prestigious occupations, autonomy is always a granted, legal process. The occupation cannot obtain it on its own. The conferral of autonomy occurs only if the public recognizes that the occupation (now a profession) has an extensive collectivity and service orientation (i.e., that it professes to adhere to an ethical code, as exemplified for medicine in the Hippocratic Oath or the Prayer of Maimonides). Whether the profession actually has such an orientation is irrelevant. All that really matters is whether the public has imputed that such a service orientation exists. If society has been persuaded to make that imputation, then autonomy is granted and supported.

If society grants the profession its autonomy, the profession must be self-regulating, providing its own quality control or self-management. This requirement represents a significant departure from the formal, hierarchical control by lay individuals to which mere occupations are subject (Freidson 1984). The reason for this departure is that after the profession has been granted autonomy, no one else has the power to regulate it. The self-regulation is especially important inasmuch as the profession of medicine dominates the rest of the health care industry. The conferral of professional autonomy may seem rather straightforward, but it has potentially staggering implications. If the autonomous profession so chooses, it can be lax on the issue of self-regulation, leaving its members to practice as they please. Because there is no other social control over the profession, the possibility arises for the profession to misuse its autonomy and abuse its clientele—both the public and the other workers in the health care industry. To avoid such misuse and abuse, the profession must have and employ formal and informal ways of collegially regulating the performance of its members.

This potential for failure to self-regulate represents the flaw of professional autonomy, and ultimately of professional dominance. Freidson (1970*a*:370) notes that the flaw allows and encourages

> the development of self-sufficient institutions, it develops and maintains a self-deceiving vision of the objectivity and reliability of its knowledge and the virtues of its members. . . . [Medicine's] very autonomy has led to insularity and a mistaken arrogance about its mission in the world.

In essence, Freidson argues, medicine has deceived itself to the point where it believes that it truly is self-regulating, deserving of professional autonomy, and acting in the public interest. Freidson is quick to point out, however, that the flaws he describes stem not from the men and women recruited to the profession of medicine but from the structural characteristics—such as autonomy—inherent in professions themselves.

Although there are somewhat different interpretations of how professional autonomy actually came about (Anderson 1985; Havighurst 1990; Starr 1982; Stevens 1971; Wolinsky 1980, 1988*a*), there is a general consensus that it was conferred on American medicine around 1910, when the Flexner Report, documenting the existence of a gap between the level of medical knowledge and its practical application, was published. In essence, organized medicine, primarily represented by the American Medical Association (AMA) was granted broad, monopolist-like powers over the health care industry (such as it was at the time), in exchange for its promise to provide quality medical care and eliminate the sad state of affairs that Flexner described. From that point on, medicine and the health care industry have never been the same.

The Ensuing Discussion

In the more than two decades since Freidson (1970*a*, 1970*b*) first presented the professional dominance perspective, much has changed in the United States in general and in the American health care delivery system in particular. Indeed, a number of scholars have argued that the traditional autonomy of the profession of medicine has eroded as medicine has become subject to the same kind of formalized and hierarchical controls from outside the profession that other occupations routinely face. The two most well-known schools of criticism focus on the notions of deprofessionalization and proletarianization.

Marie Haug (1973, 1975, 1977, 1988; see also Haug and Lavin 1978, 1981, 1983), the primary force behind the deprofessionalization argument, argues that the profession of medicine has been losing its prestigious societal position and the trust that goes with it. She cites five principal reasons for this loss. The first two are related. One is that medicine's monopoly over access to its defined body of knowledge has been eroded by the increased use of automated retrieval systems, such as computerized algorithms for symptom assessment. The other is that marked increases in educational attainment have made the public less likely to view medical knowledge as mysterious. As a result, people are more likely to challenge physicians' authority today than ever before.

The third reason involves the increasing specialization within medicine. This has made doctors more dependent on each other but also on nonphysician experts, especially engineers. Dependence on the former diffuses the power of any single physician, inasmuch as he or she must rely on the advice and expertise of colleagues. Dependence on the latter diffuses the power of all physicians, inasmuch as they must rely on advice and expertise from outside the profession. Thus, both individual and professional dominance (autonomy) have been reduced.

As her fourth reason, Haug cites the growth of consumer self-help groups coupled with the emergence of a variety of allied health care workers, which has increased the reliance on the lay, or at least the nonprofessional, referral systems. For many people the experiential information exchanged in these lay (or nonprofessional) encounters poses a rather attractive alternative to the physicians' academic knowledge. Thus, the profession's magnetic field is no longer as unopposed as it once was. The final reason is that the physicians' altruistic image has not weathered well the recent storms over the rising cost of health care. Indeed, she notes that physicians are now being held far more accountable for their role in cost containment. These continuing increases in medical care costs, which are viewed as excessive, serve to deflate the confidence of the public about medicine's commitment toward the common good.

In concluding the article that first presented the deprofessionalization argument, Haug (1973:209) wrote that her predictions for the declining dominance of medicine were "only a hypothesis. The thrust of this paper is that it [the deprofessionalization argument] is as viable as the professionalization [professional dominance] hypothesis. Both will be tested by history." Looking back some fifteen years later, Haug (1988) implied that history had not been as kind to her hypothesis as she had hoped. Indeed, although she noted that evidence favoring her view could be found, it was not sufficient to "retain it with 95 percent confidence." She also noted that there was not sufficient evidence to reject it either. More to the point, she concluded by taking a more reflective view of the evidence:

I once argued that technology could destroy the monopolization of knowledge and lead to the obsolescence of the concept of profession (Haug, 1976). That has not come to pass, at least not so far. We do know that the old authority-based super-ordinate role of physicians vis-à-vis patients no longer holds as widely as it once did. Finally, new government regulations and organizational forms hedge physician autonomy in many aspects of their work, as a result of what Starr (1982) warns is a far-reaching transformation and corporatization of the delivery of medical care. (pp. 54–55)

Haug chose not to elaborate on these statements, nor has she come back to them since. Nonetheless, based on the corpus of her work, one can infer that she has, in fact, stepped back from her original position. To be sure, the element of trust and its role in professional dominance apparently remains (evident in her comment about "the old authority-based superordinate role"). She seems to have shifted, however, from the argument that deprofessionalization will be the means to bring about the end of professional dominance to a view that corporatization will transform the context in which the profession is dominant.

John McKinlay (1973, 1977, 1986, 1988; see also McKinlay and Arches 1985; McKinlay and Stoeckle 1988) has been the most eloquent spokesperson for the proletarianization argument. He builds on Marx's theory of history, emphasizing the inevitability of all workers in capitalistic societies like the United States to be stripped eventually of their control over their work. This occurs when individuals are reduced to selling their services rather than producing finished goods. McKinlay argues that the growing corporatization and bureaucratization of medicine has re-sulted in eliminating the self-employment and autonomy of physicians. As the number and extent of intermediaries between patients and their doctors increases, physicians become more like other laborers. Moreover, as the medical workplace becomes more bureaucratized, physicians increasingly are subject to rules and other hierarchical structures that are not of their own making. As a result, the ability of doctors to govern themselves, especially by using their preferred informal methods of self-regulation, declines. Thus, the proletarianization argument seeks to explain (McKinlay and Stoeckle 1988:200)

the process by which an occupational category is divested of control over certain prerogatives relating to the location, content, and essentiality of its task activities, thereby subordinating it to the broader requirements of production under advanced capitalism.

Specifically what is lost are seven traditional professional prerogatives: control over entrance criteria, training content, autonomy, and the object, tools, means, and remuneration of labor.

McKinlay and Stoeckle (1988; see also McKinlay, 1988) demonstrate support for this thesis by contrasting physicians in small-scale fee-for-service practices at the turn of the century with physicians currently practicing in bureaucratic settings on these seven profession prerogatives. They conclude that

every single prerogative listed has changed, many changes occurring over the last decade. The net effect of the erosion of these prerogatives is the reduction of the

members of a professional group to some common level in the service of the broader
interests of capital accumulation. (p. 201)

Specifically, the federal government and other outside interests now affect the
content of medical school curricula, medical work has become segmented, patients
have become clients of the organizational entity rather than the individual doctor,
technological tools and the physical plant are now owned by the corporation rather
than the individual doctor, and physicians have become employees of the corporation. Under these circumstances, McKinlay and Stoeckle argue, physicians can
no longer be considered professionally dominant.

The changes associated with the proletarianization process, however, are occurring so gradually that it is difficult for many to recognize. This unawareness is
especially problematic for physicians (McKinlay and Stoeckle 1988:201):

> For doctors who are increasingly subject to this process, it is masked both by their
> false consciousness concerning the significance of their everyday activities and by
> an elitist conception of their role, so that even if the process is recognized, doctors
> are quite reluctant to admit it.

Even for nonphysicians, however, the gradual nature of the trend toward proletarianization may not be discernible until the twenty-first century (McKinlay and
Stoeckle 1988). Indeed, noting how much has happened between 1970, when
Freidson (1970*a*, 1970*b*) first advanced the professional dominance perspective,
and 1988, McKinlay and Stoeckle write that "if what occurs . . . is anything like
the dramatic transformation we have witnessed . . . doctoring will bear little resemblance to what is being discussed today."

Freidson does not find much evidence for either of the critical appraisals of his
analysis of medicine's privileged professional status. His dismissal of the deprofessionalization thesis asserts that although some specifics may have changed in the
absolute, the overall situation remains relatively the same:

> The professions . . . continue to possess a monopoly over at least some important
> segment of formal knowledge that does not shrink over time, even though both
> competitors and rising levels of lay knowledge may nibble away at its edges. New
> knowledge is constantly acquired that takes the place of what has been lost and
> thereby maintains the knowledge gap. Similarly, while the power of computer tech-
> nology in storing codified knowledge cannot be ignored, it is the members of each
> profession who determine what is to be stored and how it is to be done, and who
> are equipped to interpret and employ what is retrieved effectively. With a continual
> knowledge gap, potentially universal access to stored data is meaningless. (Freidson
> 1981:8)

Thus, although Freidson readily acknowledges the changing events that Haug identified, he nonetheless refuses to accept them as evidence for the deprofessionalization
argument. He dismisses outright the notions that the profession of medicine has
lost its relative position of prestige and respect, expertise, or monopoly over that
expertise.

With regard to the proletarianization thesis, Freidson (1984) takes a different
tack. He emphasizes that although the autonomy of individual physicians may have

been reduced, the autonomy of the profession as a whole remains intact. Freidson readily admits that individual physicians may now have to take orders from other physicians, much like blue-collar or clerical workers must take orders from others. The difference, however, is that the orders come from other physicians, and only from other physicians. In essence, although he recognizes many of the same changes that McKinlay identified, Freidson (1985:26) views them as occurring within medicine rather than outside it, a critical distinction for him:

> [T]hese changes might be interpreted as bureaucratization in Weber's ideal-typical sense, for they are accompanied by an increase in hierarchical positions as health care organizations grow in size, records become more elaborate, specific standards govern the formal evaluation of more and more work, supervision in the form of evaluation of work becomes more widespread, and hierarchical positions of responsibility increase in number and variety. However, ... those changes do not affect the position of the profession as a corporate body in the social as well as institutional division of labor so much as they affect the *internal* organization of the profession, in the relations among physicians. In essence, I suggest, they are creating more distinct and formal patterns of stratification within the profession than have existed in the past, with the position of the rank and file practitioner changing most markedly.

Freidson believes that the stage is not set for the profession of medicine to have its advantaged position wrested away from the outside. Rather, he believes, a variety of modifications will occur within the profession.

There are two key points in Freidson's response to his critics. Both relate to a clarification, but not a modification, of the scope conditions for the theory of professional dominance. The first point is that the theory of professional dominance is, and always has been, cast in relative, not absolute, terms. That is, relative to any other occupation in the health care or related industries, medicine has been and always will be in a position of professional dominance. No other health-related occupation will ever come to dominate medicine. Even Vicente Navarro (1988), one of the best-known Marxian critics of capitalistic health care delivery systems and professional dominance theory, acknowledges this fact.

The second point in Freidson's response is that the theory of professional dominance is, and always has been, cast in terms of the profession, not in terms of the individual physician. That is, the professional dominance of medicine is a collective or, to use Freidson's albeit connotatively troubling term, a corporate property. Thus, the emergence of a vertical stratification system, as opposed to the horizontal divisions that exist in a company of equals, within the profession itself does not alter the profession's relations (i.e., dominance) with (i.e., over) its external environment (i.e., the health care industry).

Essentially, then, Freidson's response to his critics has been threefold. He has (1) agreed that the events that they have identified are important but disallowed that they circumvent his theory, (2) clarified but not changed two important aspects concerning the scope of his theory, and (3) described the emergence of, or "the magnification and formalization of these [previously informal] relationships [between doctors] into" (Freidson 1985), a vertical stratification system within the profession itself. Thus, he has effectively refused to yield any ground, either empirically or conceptually.

The discussion surrounding the deprofessionalization and proletarianization alternatives and Freidson's response to them has two troubling aspects. The first is that at least three intriguing questions have not been raised: (1) When does a physician-administrator cease being a colleague to physicians? (2) Under what circumstances could nonphysician participation in or dominance of the reimbursement structure threaten medicine's organized autonomy? and (3) Is organized medicine (the AMA) all powerful, or was it just at the right place at the right time? The salience of the first question derives from Freidson's (1985) identification and acceptance of the emergence of a vertical stratification dimension within medicine. If the hierarchical gap between physician-administrators and physicians (or between any two hierarchical layers within the profession) becomes too great, will a new dominant profession of physician-administrators emerge? This would happen only if the physician-administrators as a class fully and permanently divest themselves of all actual medical practice. The likelihood of this possibility seems small. The traditional (and current) career path for physician-administrators is that of rising through the practice ranks within the organization, much like the career path of academic department heads and deans, who generally retain their professorial heritage, including the norms to which they have become socialized. On the other hand, in the future, the rapid expansion of the physician-administrator stratum may begin to strain the capacity of traditional career development paths. If such circumstances produce physician-administrators whose experiences with doctoring are only vicarious, a new dominant profession might emerge. Further exploration of this issue appears warranted.

The salience of the second question arises from the increasing role of nonphysicians in the utilization review aspects of the reimbursement process. Utilization review nurses are already the principal line of defense for third-party payers trying to contain costs. Freidson (1985) argues that this is irrelevant because nurses merely follow algorithms established by physicians. Thus, the guidelines that are being imposed on physicians were developed by physicians. But to the extent that these utilization review guidelines leave the nurse with any discretion in determining whether the procedures provided by the physician were appropriate and justified, the profession's right to self-regulation is diminished. Moreover, the role of nonphysicians in establishing what is effective medical therapy and should therefore be practiced and reimbursed in the first place is increasing. This includes, for example, the Agency for Health Care Policy Research's (AHCPR) Medical Treatment Effectiveness Program (MEDTEP), which houses the much-touted Patient Outcomes Research Team (PORT) grants (see Salive, Mayfield, and Weissman 1990). Further exploration of this issue seems warranted as well.

The salience of the third question lies in picking the latter answer to it. If the AMA was simply in the right place at the right time, then organized medicine's monolithic influence might not be fully durable. In particular, organized medicine's inappropriate influence in extramedical domains (that is, the medicalization of life; see Conrad and Schneider 1980; Illich 1976; Zola 1972) may have begun to deteriorate with the emergence of a postindustrial and service-oriented societal order. As a result, the changes that both Haug and McKinlay identify may actually be the reduction to, and restriction of, medicine's professional dominance to legitimately medical matters. That would represent a process, which might be called shrinkage, quite different from either deprofessionalization or proletarianization. Although he approaches it from a somewhat different orientation, Navarro (1988) has made rather similar observations. Further consideration of this issue would also appear warranted.

The second troubling aspect of the discussion surrounding the deprofessionalization and proletarianization alternatives and Freidson's response to them is that there has been no real debate. Rather, what we have had is Haug presenting her views on how some of the changes in the role of medicine are more consistent with a deprofessionalization hypothesis, McKinlay presenting his views on how some of the other changes in the role of medicine are more consistent with a proletarianization trend, and Freidson's somewhat tardy and begrudging responses dismissing those collective changes as being unimportant for the professional dominance perspective. These three principals appear to be talking past rather than to one another. Moreover, by the late 1980s they appear to have stopped talking altogether. Freidson's last paper (actually a brief restatement) on this topic was published in 1987, and both McKinlay's and Haug's (the latter of which was merely a restatement of previous arguments with no additional data) appeared in 1988. Thus, in the four years since the publication of the special issue of the *Milbank Quarterly*, they have been silent.

Moreover, there has been an absence of testable hypotheses, especially on the part of the deprofessionalization and proletarianization alternatives. Haug at least implicitly recognized this when she equivocally stated (1988) that there was not enough evidence to accept or to reject her hypothesis. This cannot be. Scientific hypotheses must be refutable. What evidence is necessary to accept or refute her deprofessionalization, or, for that matter, McKinlay's proletarianization hypothesis? Neither Haug nor McKinlay has provided a list of the evidence necessary for either outcome.

In contrast, Freidson, at least implicitly, has identified the evidence necessary to support the professional dominance perspective. Professional autonomy is always a process that is legally conferred or granted, never taken. Moreover, the profession must maintain backing for its position from the political entity of the state. Thus, as long as the autonomy of the profession is legally maintained, professional dominance remains intact. The suggestion is that the end of professional dominance would be marked by legal strictures against the organized autonomy of medicine. For that reason, the field of antitrust law is the venue in which to examine the evidence, because the conferral of autonomy granted medicine monopolistic dominion over the health care industry. Monopolistic dominion constitutes a clear violation of the spirit, if not the letter, of the antitrust statutes.

Antitrust Law: Reaffirmation or Challenge

Perhaps the most appropriate legal case to consider is that of *Wilk v. AMA*, which pertains to organized medicine's violation of the nation's antitrust laws in its dealings with chiropractors. After a lengthy trial, U.S. district judge Susan Getzendanner in 1987 ruled that the AMA and its members had participated in a conspiracy against chiropractors that violated the Sherman Anti-Trust Act. The violation was based on Principle 3 of the AMA's Principles of Medical Ethics, which was in force until 1980. Principle 3 made it unethical for physicians to associate professionally with chiropractors. It is not, however, the finding of an antitrust violation in this case that is interesting. Rather, it is the remarkable opportunity that Judge Getzendanner provided to the AMA to justify its conspiratorial behavior that is intriguing. Judge Getzendanner (1988:81) wrote in the permanent injunction order against the AMA:

> Under the Sherman Act, every combination or conspiracy in restraint of trade is illegal. The court has held that the conduct of the AMA and its members constituted a conspiracy in restraint of trade based on the following facts: the purpose of the boycott was to eliminate chiropractic; chiropractors are in competition with some medical physicians; the boycott had substantial anti-competitive effects; and the plaintiffs were injured as a result of the conduct.

Nonetheless, she allowed the AMA to argue the "patient care defense" based on four elements:

> (1) that they genuinely entertained a concern for what they perceive as scientific method in the care of each person with whom they have entered into a doctor-patient relationship; (2) that this concern is objectively reasonable; (3) that this concern has been the dominant motivating factor in defendants' promulgation of Principle 3 and in the conduct intended to implement it; and (4) that this concern for scientific method in patient care could not have been adequately satisfied in a manner less restrictive of competition. (pp. 81–82)

Presumably, if the AMA had been able to make a convincing patient care defense, Judge Getzendanner would have ruled that their violation of the antitrust act was acceptable. However, because the AMA did not alter Principle 3 until 1980, even though there was clear evidence, accepted by the AMA itself in 1979, that some of what chiropractors did had therapeutic value, and the court felt that the AMA's legitimate concerns could have been addressed by something less than a "nationwide conspiracy to eliminate a licensed profession," Judge Getzendanner ruled that the AMA's violation of the antitrust act was wrong and required a permanent injunction.

The injunctive relief was relatively moot because the AMA had already modified its ethical code and eliminated the boycott. Judge Getzendanner did not award the chiropractors any monetary compensation, did not require the AMA to hold or support any joint seminars to extol the virtues of chiropractic, did not require the AMA to endorse chiropractic or defend its scientific validity, and did not restrain the AMA from speaking out against chiropractic in the future. Perhaps most important was Judge Getzendanner's refusal to order that the standards of the Joint Commission for the Accreditation of Health Care Organizations (JCAHCO), which require a majority of hospital board members to be physicians, constituted a conspiracy against nonphysician health care workers. This failure to declare the standards a conspiracy actually constitutes federal court approval of the principle of professional dominance. That is, Judge Getzendanner merely established the rules that organized medicine must adhere to if and when it ever violates antitrust laws in the future. As such, *Wilk v. AMA* may be viewed as remarkable testimony about the continued long-term viability of the professional dominance perspective.

Not everyone, however, shares that interpretation. In his 1990 Michael M. Davis Lecture, Clark C. Havighurst argues that there have been two approaches to antitrust law in the United States, reflected in the traditional and market paradigms. Havighurst (1990:4) notes that antitrust law traditionally

> embraced the professional paradigm of medical care for a long time by generally ignoring the "learned professions" and inviting the inference that they might be exempt. One theory—the currency of which was surprising in light of the lack of legal precedence for it—was that physicians were engaged in something more exalted than "trade or commerce" (the statutory terms) and were therefore beyond the reach of the Sherman Act. There were also hints that, even if the antitrust statutes applied, only special, softer rules would be appropriate for physicians.

In contrast, the more contemporary market paradigm is one "under which the industry is driven and shaped by consumer choice rather than professional fiat." (Notice the similarity of that argument with Haug's position; see especially Haug and Lavin 1983.)

According to Havighurst (1990), the shift toward the market paradigm, which increasingly discounted medicine's special status, was clearly observable as early as the 1950s. How does Havighurst reconcile that interpretation with Judge Getzendanner's 1987 ruling in *Wilk v. AMA*? Although he reluctantly recognizes *Wilk v. AMA* as "the most prominent modern dictum embracing the paradigm's view that professional organizations can safely be allowed to police the private sector with coercive sanctions as long as their motives remain strictly professional and pure" (p. 7), he views the decision in the matter as an isolated and aberrant judgment, one on which legal precedent is not likely to be established. He supports this view by two statements. First, he asserts that "it is most unlikely that lawyers today are counseling physician clients in reliance on the *Wilks* exception" (p. 7). Second, he argues that the decision in *Wilk v. AMA* represents the "only serious modern departure from rigorous judicial insistence that competitive effects alone, rather than alleged worthy purposes, govern antitrust cases against professionals" (p. 7). Furthermore, Havighurst foresees and even encourages increasing restraints on the circumstances under which such antitrust actions (like those defined in *Wilk v. AMA*) can be tolerated.

One arena in which Havighurst specifically advocates greater activism on the part of the enforcers of the antitrust statutes involves the information gap. He (1990:15) writes, "In my view, the antitrust laws should be used to discourage joint ventures in the production of information by professional bodies that are each capable of acting independently in the affected field." He is particularly concerned about developing antitrust standards "for appraising joint ventures in accrediting, certification, credentialing, technology assessment, and the development of practice guidelines." By logical extension, then, Havighurst would be opposed to the recent move toward consensus within organized medicine around plans for restructuring the health care delivery system (see American College of Physicians 1990, 1991; American Medical Association 1990; Lundberg 1991; Todd et al. 1991), for fear that such actions would deprive the public of an important opportunity to resolve the health care crisis economically.

Taking a clear activist stance, Havighurst (1990:21) concluded his lecture by laying bare his preferences:

> Perhaps we need to be more explicit about the goals of antitrust law in the health care industry. I see antitrust law as driving a peaceful revolution that is similar to the revolutions that have recently occurred in central and eastern Europe. The law's immediate object in the health care industry, like the object of reform in those previously oppressed nations, should be to put an end to one-party rule by a powerful, self-appointed elite.

From Havighurst's point of view, all that remains to be seen is *when* antitrust enforcers and the courts will bring a "charter of freedom" to the health care delivery system.

The Role of Imputed Trust

Under what circumstances might organized medicine be able to fend off the pressures of an activist antitrust or some other assault on its professional dominance? The answer involves the major problem facing the professional dominance perspective today. In the end, that perspective comes down to autonomy. All other characteristics of a profession flow from it. Autonomy is the acid test of professional status. It is granted, never taken, based on the avowed promise of the profession to self-regulate, thus living up to its ethical code. It should follow, then, that the only way in which a profession may lose its autonomy is to have it taken away because it failed to keep its promissory house in order. Therefore, the issue is not which forces external to medicine will wrest away its professional dominance but whether medicine will lose that professional dominance by the benign neglect of its avowed promise.

According to Freidson's (1970*a*, 1970*b*) theory on the emergence of the profession and its dominance, the conferral of autonomy was based on the public imputation of medicine's extraordinary trustworthiness. Therefore, it should follow that the potential revocation of that autonomy may occur at any point at which the public imputes that the profession has not lived up to its side of the bargain. Such an imputation may be based entirely on perceptions, making moot the issue of who (or what) is in reality to blame for the current crisis in the health care delivery system. Thus, the future of medicine's professional dominance may actually ride on the outcome of the manipulation of public opinion, that is, the maintenance (or support, to use Freidson's term) of the public imputation that medicine warrants professional autonomy.

If that is the case, then in order for medicine to retain its professional dominance, it must exchange its traditionally combative style for one far more cooperative. In particular, it must return to a fiduciary agency (Parsons 1975) from which it has wandered over the past three decades. That includes significantly greater stewardship of the limited resources available for the provision of health care. And as the profession becomes more conscientious about the way in which it allocates and consumes health care resources, it must also become more cognizant of how it has been so disproportionately rewarded for its services in the past.

When the special issue of the *Milbank Quarterly* was published in 1988, the ultimate question was what the future would hold for the professional dominance of medicine. For the most part, I said that it was up to medicine. If the profession maintained its current posture, it might just lose its dominant position. But that loss would not be due to deprofessionalization, as described by Haug, or to proletarianization, as described by McKinlay. Rather, the loss of professional dominance would accrue from the benign neglect of maintaining the public's imputation of medicine's original avowed promise. Indeed, I argued that what we were witnessing then as the monopsonistic intervention of and regulation by the federal government (and in similar ways by other third-party payers) was actually a growing attempt to stimulate self-regulation among physicians and their return to stewardship and their role as a fiduciary agency. If medicine failed to heed the call, I argued, its privileged status and professional dominance might well go the way of the dinosaur.

Since 1988, organized medicine has begun to respond. There are two clear features of that response. First, the response has been specifically structured around the notion of trust. Second, there has been a marked shift from reactive to proactive efforts. Basically, organized medicine finally has recognized that it must make the appearance of stepping to center stage to restore trust and direct the restructuring of the health care delivery system, or it will survive as a less dominant profession within an externally dictated environment.

Supporting evidence for this interpretation comes from two sources. First, there is the blatantly self-serving and multimillion dollar advertising campaign currently underway in which the AMA showcases five ideal-typical physicians dedicated to the principles of fiduciary agency, stewardship, and commitment to the public good (AMA 1991). The first two vignettes in this campaign involve relatively young doctors (implying the continuation of the long white line) with extraordinarily committed practices devoted to the care of babies with AIDS and poor inner-city individuals who would otherwise have no access to quality medical care. Noting that more money could be made and made easier in affluent suburbs, the protagonist from the latter vignette simply states that this would neither be "right" nor why he went into medicine. Implicit, if not explicit, in the AMA's advertising campaign is the notion that these showcased physicians are representative of its membership and the profession at large.

The second source of evidence involves organized medicine's recent forays into the debate on national health insurance. Although the American College of Physicians (1990) arguably got there first, the AMA has officially presented its own proposal, known as Health Access America, which is designed "to improve access to affordable, high-quality health care" (see Todd et al. 1991). Moreover, the AMA devoted its entire May 15, 1991, issue of the *Journal of the American Medical Association* to the topic "Caring for the Uninsured and the Underinsured." The fact that both the six principles and sixteen key points in the AMA's Health Access America, as well as the American College of Physicians' (1991) current draft of its Universal Health Care blueprints for change, are blatantly self-serving is irrelevant. The issue is whether this campaign (coupled with the advertising campaign just described, as well as other strategies) will be sufficient to restore the public's imputed trust of medicine. All are well-crafted attempts to manipulate public opin-

ion, as *JAMA* editor George Lundberg's (1991:2567) concluding paragraph introducing the special issue illustrates:

> An aura of inevitability is upon us. It is no longer acceptable morally, ethically, or
> economically for so many of our people to be medically uninsured or seriously
> underinsured. We can solve this problem. We have the knowledge and the resources,
> the skills, the time, and the moral prescience. We need only clear-cut objectives
> and proper organization of our resources. Have we now the national will and
> leadership?

To paraphrase Haug and McKinlay, only time will tell.

Acknowledgment

Partial support for the preparation of this chapter was provided by a grant from the National
Institutes of Health (R37 AG 09692). The opinions expressed herein are those of the author
and should not be construed as representing the official position or policy of either the
National Institutes of Health or the Indiana University School of Medicine.

2

The Medical Profession
and the State

Julio Frenk and Luis Durán-Arenas

In the course of its development, the social institution of medicine has experienced a series of changes—some slow and silent, others visible and rapid, all pervasive and far reaching. The scope of medical activities has expanded to growing numbers of people and spheres of human life. As the problem-solving capacity of medicine has increased, most societies have constructed an order of discourse that regards health as a basic human need and medical care as a social right. But at the same time there has been a widespread adoption of rationalizing rules and procedures, which may constrain the direct relationship between client and provider. A conspicuous change has been the concentration of the production of both knowledge and services in increasingly complex organizations, with an elaborate division of labor and a diversification in the forms of economic interaction among the key actors. There is today an expansive and expensive health care industry, operating on a global scale. As costs escalate, pressure has mounted to demonstrate the effectiveness of interventions. Adding another critical dimension are the wide inequalities among and within countries, in both levels of health and access to services. Such inequalities persist despite the almost universal growth in the supply of physicians, which has led to a recomposition of the medical labor market. On the political side, physicians have become organized into formal associations as they struggle to control the content, conditions, and terms of their own work.

This chapter focuses on one of the major changes that has deeply affected all the others: the involvement of the state in the regulation, financing, and delivery of medical care. In order to place this process in its broader context, it is first necessary to develop a conceptual framework. The chapter thus begins with an attempt to delimit the major analytic categories that are useful to elucidate the professional status of medicine. This framework will then serve to orient the analysis of the modalities, determinants, and consequences of state intervention. We conclude by pointing out some implications for the debate about the future of the medical profession.

Conceptual Framework

Much of the social sciences literature on the professions has treated medicine as the exemplary expression of professional autonomy. Recent theoretical elaborations and empirical findings, however, suggest that the notion of a medical profession vested with the authority and autonomy to control every dimension of its work is no longer operative in many settings. Instead, the realities of employment by complex organizations, growing intervention by third parties, cleavages among different professional segments, and imbalanced labor markets seem to be defining the conditions of medical practice beyond the preferences of physicians or the ideology of professionalism.

In order to comprehend the implications of emerging trends for the medical profession, it is necessary to propose an explicit frame of reference. Ours has been inspired by Zald's (1970) conceptual work on the political economy of complex organizations. This model draws on analogies to the nation-state so as to analyze organizations in terms of polity structures and systems of economic exchange. Political and economic relations are examined at two levels: those that occur within a given organization and those that refer to the broader environment external to a particular organization. Table 2.1 presents our analytical framework. The entries in each cell contain the processes that define, at a given historical moment, the basic aspects of the social organization of a profession. As such, they represent some of the main objects of a theory of professionalization.

The internal/external and political/economic distinctions are always problematic. In many instances they become blurred in the flow of real-life events. For conceptual purposes, however, it seems valid to differentiate between those processes that, in the case of medical care, take place within given establishments, such as hospitals, and those that are external to any individual organization, involving the health system as a whole. Further, regardless of what the causal connections between the polity and the economy are assumed to be, it is usually possible to distinguish relationships that involve production and markets from those that are centered around interests and power. The intersection of the two dichotomies yields a fourfold classification, which attempts to integrate various concepts that have been proposed in the sociological literature on the professions. Although in their original usages these concepts often overlap each other, we believe that they define distinct aspects of the social organization of a profession.

In Table 2.1, the concepts of dominance and autonomy are derived from the work of Eliot Freidson (1970a, 1970b). These concepts characterize processes that take place within organizations where professionals work. Although the concept of autonomy has been given wider meaning by other authors, the restricted usage proposed here is basically consistent with what Freidson (1970a:45) calls "core autonomy," that is, control over the technical content of work. This narrow definition of autonomy also corresponds to what Larson (1977) calls discretion. Whether the broader social and economic terms of work are also controlled by a profession is, according to Freidson, secondary to both the central meaning of autonomy and indeed the definition of an occupation as a profession.

For Freidson (1970b:136), dominance is restricted to that aspect of the social

Table 2.1. Political-economic framework for the analysis of the social organization of professions

	Type of relationship	
Dimension of analysis	Internal	External
Political	Power relations to other occupations: **Dominance**	Relations to the state; corporatist representation: **Sovereignty**
Economic	Degree of control over the process of producing services: **Autonomy**	Structure of the markets for services and for manpower: **Independence**

organization of a profession that defines its relationships with other occupations in the division of labor. Clearly, many of these relationships are of an economic character, dealing with the direct production of services. In the case of medicine, this is what Robb (1975) calls clinical communication among the various occupational groups in a hospital, such as doctors, nurses, and administrators. In our usage, however, dominance refers exclusively to the power relationships among those groups, although we recognize that such power is mobilized mainly to guide the production of services. This restricted usage is very close to Robb's concept of organizational communication, which represents the level at which "questions of relative power become crucial" (Robb 1975:377). It also agrees with Freidson's (1985) critique of broader interpretations of the concept of medical dominance, which identify it with ideological or cultural hegemony.

Turning next to the external environment, a major area of theoretical and practical concern refers to the forms in which the profession is collectively organized in order to negotiate its interests with the state. Here we follow the common practice of adopting the narrow definition of the state as the institutions of government providing the administrative, legislative, and judicial vehicles for the actual exercise of public authority and power rather than the broad definition of the state as the total political organization of a society (Frenk 1990). In Table 2.1, the political relationship of the profession with the state is called sovereignty. This term is taken from Starr's (1978) work, although his usage seems to be considerably wider than ours, encompassing certain aspects of the cultural authority of physicians and what we label independence in Table 2.1. This latter term is intended to reflect some basic structural elements of the market for services, such as the level of demand and the presence of a monopsonist, and of the professional labor market, such as the degree of control over the supply of professionals and the potential for migration. Some of these elements are mentioned by Wilensky (1964), in connection with the extent of freedom from dependence of various occupational groups. Analysis of markets also figures prominently in Larson's study (1977) and in Starr's work (1982).

Two additional phenomena, technology and ideology, are frequently included in conceptual discussions about the professions. Although they are not explicitly incorporated into Table 2.1, they interact in dynamic ways with its elements. Technology determines to a large extent the complexity of medical work, and it thereby delimits the structural possibilities for autonomy. Within those limits, however, it is possible to observe important variations across time and space in the degree of actual control by physicians over the production of services. Insofar as they influence the effectiveness of diagnostic and therapeutic interventions, technological advances also underlie the level of demand for medical services and the potential definition of those services as public goods, the production and distribution of which is to be guaranteed by the state. Yet even when the quantity and quality of technological resources are similar, the modalities of state intervention in medical care can vary substantially across countries.

Just as technology sets some broad structural limits, so ideology seems to demarcate superstructural bounds for the social organization of professions. Included here are the claims that occupational groups make about their specialized knowledge and their service orientation, as part of the ideology of professionalism. Also included among the ideological processes that surround professional work is what Starr (1982:13–15) calls cultural authority. This is to be distinguished from social authority, which essentially corresponds to our concept of dominance. In contrast, cultural authority refers to the ability of the profession to define and judge the experience and needs of clients. According to Johnson (1972:45), one of the conditions for professionalization is the definition of consumers' needs by producers. A final ideological factor refers to the prevailing definitions about rational ways in which services should be provided. As Zald (1978) points out, ideological definitions of rational organization constitute a basic part of the control environment of industries, including those that are involved in the production of professional services.

In this way, technology and ideology help to delineate, in historically specific terms, the material and cultural matrices in which the various elements of the political economy of the professions interact. One of the useful applications of the framework presented in Table 2.1 is that it makes it possible to dissect those elements, so that they can be interrelated through concrete hypotheses. Indeed, a basic component of a general theory of professionalization should be the specification of the causal relationships among the processes of dominance, autonomy, sovereignty, and independence. However, even in the absence of a fully developed theory, the political-economy framework can help to describe and analyze the particular position of a profession at a given historical moment.

In this respect, the literature on the professions has been adversely affected by a lack of general agreement on the meaning of the concepts presented in Table 2.1 and by a tendency to conceive of professionalization as a unidimensional phenomenon. It is reasonable to assume that at least part of the discrepancies among authors regarding both the existing and the future status of professions may be due to these sources of conceptual confusion. We suggest that the four processes depicted in Table 2.1 need to be kept analytically distinct, since the specific social condition of a profession in a particular country at a particular time depends on their configuration. For instance, medicine can lose a substantial amount of control to the state regarding external economic conditions but still retain control over the internal process of production. A situation like this, which seems to be the case in Great Britain, would be characterized as one of high autonomy with low independence.

In many developing countries, where the world ideology of modernity (Meyer 1980:115) and the scarcity of private resources have compelled the state to be the major driving force in the expansion of medicine, physicians may have very little sovereignty but retain dominance within specific medical care establishments, as seems to be the case in Mexico (Frenk 1990).

These examples illustrate the manner in which the political-economy approach can guide cross-national inquiries into the social organization of the medical profession. In fact, it is possible to compare the relative positions of the cases described in this book along the four dimensions. We will use the framework only to provide the constructs for the remainder of our analysis. Lack of space prevents us from a detailed examination of the intraorganizational relationships of autonomy and dominance, which Fredric D. Wolinsky discussed in Chapter 1. Also, these are the dimensions that the literature has analyzed most often, whereas considerably less attention has been paid to the external economic and political processes. Hence, we will concentrate on the extraorganizational relationships and, more specifically, on the relations of the medical profession to the state. However, because of the close connection between the twin processes of state intervention and bureaucratization, we will first examine briefly the relationship between the profession and bureaucracy, although many aspects of this relation have to do with the intraorganizational dimension. Finally, we will sketch the major effects of state intervention on the remaining dimensions that define the professional status of medicine.

State, Bureaucracy, and Professions

The direct, undisturbed interaction between professionals and their clients is no longer the predominant form of medical work in modern societies. Complex organizations of all types now mediate such interaction. Physicians receive training, obtain a license to practice, see patients, are evaluated, and get paid in or by complex organizations. The state occupies a key position in this network of mediated relationships. Hence, bureaucracy, the state, and the profession form a triangle that needs to be dissected. A strategy to do so consists in examining each pair of relationships.

The Relationship between Bureaucracy and Professions

In this analysis, we use the term *bureaucracy* to mean complex organizations in general and not exclusively the ideal type Weber (1946a) proposed. There are two major traditions in sociology regarding the relationship between bureaucracy and professions. The first, which could be termed the compatibility perspective, was originally formulated by Weber (1947a, 1947b). Indeed, Weber saw both bureaucracy and professionalization as two expressions of a single process of increased rationalization in Western societies. For Weber, bureaucracy and expertise are intimately linked, each reinforcing the other. In his analysis, bureaucracy is administration through expertise.

One of the first challenges to this position came from Parsons (1947:58–60), who, in the introduction to his translation of Weber's work, criticized the latter for having failed to recognize the basic differences between two principles of authority: one, based on the authority of the office, which is characteristic of rational-legal structures; the other, based on the authority of expertise, which characterizes professional work. For Parsons these two principles of authority are neutrally incompatible, with no indication as to whether one could dominate the other. Similar arguments were made by Stinchcombe (1959), who held that craft and bureaucratic administration of work should be kept analytically distinct.

More recent authors following the tradition of this incompatibility perspective have looked into the potential for conflict between bureaucracy and professionals. How such conflict is resolved serves to identify two major subgroups within this tradition. The first view, exemplified most clearly by Freidson's work (1970*a*, 1970*b*), suggests that professionals prevail in their conflict with bureaucracy. For instance, by virtue of their autonomy and self-regulation, physicians assume a dominant position in the division of labor. The second view posits that bureaucracy inevitably dominates professions. This is the position of writers on deprofessionalization (Haug 1973; Toren 1975) and on professional proletarianization (Oppenheimer 1973; McKinlay 1977; McKinlay and Arches 1985).

In contrast to the incompatibility perspective, a number of authors, including Larson (1977) and Benson (1973), have pointed to the necessary concomitance between bureaucracy and professions. This tradition can be subdivided into two groups according to the perceived consequences of such concomitance. C. Wright Mills (1956) and Illich (1976), among others, suggest an alliance between bureaucrats and professionals that has given rise to a powerful nucleus of technical experts who in fact have become a new ruling class. Others, like Carr-Saunders and Wilson (1933) and Halmos (1970), see the professionalization of bureaucracies as a humanizing mechanism that will infuse complex organizations with an ethic of service.

In our opinion, both the compatibility and the incompatibility perspectives have the shortcoming of analyzing the relationship between bureaucracy and professions without incorporating the mediating effect of the state. In terms of our conceptual framework, most of the literature has focused on the intraorganizational dimension, without paying sufficient attention to the external environment. This makes it necessary to examine the links between bureaucracy and the state.

The Relationship between State and Bureaucracy

An almost obvious relationship is found in the fact that the state itself is largely organized as a bureaucracy. This is particularly true of the administrative branch of government. In fact, state administration was the main model that inspired Weber's elaboration of the ideal-typical bureaucracy. Since the state represents one of the most conspicuous clusters of complex organizations in modern societies, we are faced with a critical issue: What kind of organizations are these? Are they essentially the same as private organizations by virtue of sharing some structural characteristics? Or does the fact that an organization belongs to the public sector mark it as something different from its private counterparts?

A difficulty in answering these questions lies in the great heterogeneity of the state apparatus. Indeed, the state contains a number of quite different organizations—some involved in functions of social control and order maintenance, others in the direct production of goods and services. Yet the state apparatus has an organic unity that allows us to identify it as an object of analysis. It is precisely this dual character of the state—its diversity and its concomitant unity—that provides two different levels of analysis at which we can attempt to address the issue of the type of organization represented by the state.

Let us first consider the most general level: the state as an organic unity. In this respect, Weber (1946*b*:78) made a fundamental contribution when he defined the state as a type of organization whose essential characteristic is its "monopoly of the legitimate use of physical force." As such, the state differs in a radical way from other organizations because it is structured not around the attainment of a **goal** but around its monopoly over the **means** of legitimate violence. Thus, Weber (1946*b*) argued (and in this he differs both from classical economists and from Marxists) that there is no goal that states have not assumed and, conversely, that there is no state that has assumed all possible goals. The crucial point is that by being structured around specific means rather than specific goals, the state as an organization has the plasticity to mobilize its resources so as to accomplish a changing set of goals.

Given this capacity, we can move to the analysis of specific organizations within the state apparatus. Once a state has decided to pursue a specific goal, it may create an organization or set of organizations for that purpose. It may be that, given the technological requirements for the production of a specific good or service, structures are not very different between privately and publicly owned organizations. These kinds of comparisons, and the conclusions that derive from them, are totally valid but only at this level of analysis. Indeed, although it is entirely possible to analyze the internal structure of concrete state bureaucracies, it is necessary to link such analysis to the macro level of the state as a totality that is beyond any particular organizational structure and therefore constitutes a "metabureaucracy." Only at this broader level can one discern, amid the diversity of state organizations, their unity in a differentiated institution whose distinctive characteristic is its monopoly over the means of violence. This defining characteristic of the state establishes the institutional matrix in which specific state bureaucracies function. No matter how similar such bureaucracies are to their private counterparts in their internal structures and processes, they are set apart by the linkage to a wider apparatus with a distinctive form of power at its command.

In sum, we have argued for a conception of the state as a relatively autonomous totality of complex organizations. The notion of the relative autonomy of the state, which is consistent with the Weberian tradition, emerges as a necessary result of the way that the state is structured around its specificity of means and its goal plasticity. Such a conception attempts to avoid both the normative definitions of what the goals of the state ought to be, as proposed by neoclassical economic theory, and the material determinism by which certain schools of Marxist thought reduce the state to an instrument of the ruling class. By historically comparing variations in the modalities of state intervention in medical care, we may begin to understand the mechanisms through which state action affects the institutionalization of goal attainment in a visible sphere of social life.

The State and the Profession

There is an inherent tension in the triangular relationship of state, bureaucracy, and profession. The state creates the structural possibility for professional associations to obtain practice monopoly and thereby control professional work. In this sense, the state introduces an element of differentiation between bureaucracy and profession, since it provides the latter with the capacity for autonomous self-regulation. However, this is an inherently unstable arrangement. When the state grants monopoly to an occupation like medicine, it creates the conditions for pricing some segments of the population out of the market or, if the state itself is involved in financing medical care, for a continuous draining of state resources. Under those conditions, the state is likely to intervene in order to impose a rationality on the production of health services that is compatible with bureaucratic forms of control. As Johnson (1972) puts it, the state intervenes to mediate the relationship between providers and clients.

The notion of the state as a collective mediator allows us better to understand professionalization in terms of a specific form of relationship between the members of an occupation and the population of clients. In his classical work, Johnson (1972) suggested that a major consequence of the social division of labor is the reduction in the amount of shared experience among people. This leads to increased social distance, which has two major consequences: it creates a potential for autonomy, since practitioners can claim expert knowledge, and it introduces an irreducible amount of uncertainty in the relationship between client and practitioner. There is a basic tension between autonomy and uncertainty, which is solved through power relationships leading to various institutional forms of occupational control. One such form is professionalization, by which the occupation controls both the needs of the clientele and the manner in which those needs are catered for.

Johnson specifies the conditions under which professionalization as a mechanism for control can emerge: that there be a heterogeneous and large clientele facing a relatively homogeneous occupation. This kind of arrangement is unstable, however, since client choice tends to favor certain practitioners over others through the channeling of fees. In this way, the profession experiences important cleavages, which tend to undermine a basic condition for professional control: homogeneity among practitioners.

This line of relational reasoning is also present in Freidson's (1970a) analysis of the instabilities of solo practice. According to Freidson, there is an inherent tension in the fact that medicine has been **granted** autonomy by the state, which may, at least in principle, withdraw such autonomy. This tension is compounded in the case of consulting professions like medicine. In contrast with what Freidson calls scholarly professions, which do not have direct contact with clients, consulting professions not only require the favor of the ruling elite but also depend on client choice.

In order to protect themselves from such dependence on clients, practitioners develop a series of organizational arrangements, which tend to become increasingly formalized. A new kind of dependence is thus created, but now with respect to other colleagues. Ironically, this process also introduces cleavages among professionals. Indeed, in his more recent reflection about the professional status of medicine, Freidson (1985) pays great attention to internal stratification, particularly between everyday practitioners and physician-administrators who are charged with managing the growing complexity of medical practice.

Beyond the initial granting of autonomy, the major effect of subsequent forms of state intervention has been to increase the degree of heterogeneity among physicians, thereby undermining their professional status. However, not all modalities of state intervention produce this effect to the same extent. It is therefore necessary to analyze briefly what those different modalities might be.

Modalities of State Intervention in Medical Care

A common form of state intervention has been the concession of practice monopoly through licensure and other regulatory mechanisms. However, such a concession tends to generate the tensions that we have already analyzed. As a result, in practically all countries (Donnangelo 1975:4) the state has moved beyond simple regulation to become involved in the direct financing and delivery of health care.

The notion of the state as a mediator between producers and consumers is useful to classify the major intervention modalities related to the financing and delivery of services. In a previous work (Frenk and Donabedian 1987), one of us proposed a typology of state intervention based on two dimensions. The first reflects the relationship of the state to providers and can be characterized by the degree of **state control** over the production of medical care services. The second dimension indicates the relationship of the state with respect to consumers and can be characterized by the **basis for eligibility** to health care benefits.

State control has two major expressions: ownership, which refers to whether the state restricts its role only to financing services, with providers serving as private contractors, or whether it assumes the direct ownership of facilities and acts as employer of providers, and administrative arrangements, which indicates whether the administrative instrumentalities for exercising control are concentrated in a single state agency or are dispersed among several agencies. Four graded possibilities of state control thus emerge: concentrated ownership, dispersed ownership, concentrated financing, and dispersed financing. In general, direct ownership and administrative concentration imply a higher degree of state control than simple financing and administrative dispersion.

Eligibility of the population historically has been based on three major principles, poverty, contribution/privilege, and citizenship, which refer to services provided or financed by the state. In addition, many countries preserve a purely private set of services, in which access is based only on purchasing power (Soberón, Frenk, and Sepulveda 1986). The first two principles of eligibility to state programs are selective because they do not include all the population. Under the poverty principle, the state provides or finances medical services as a form of assistance to the least privileged groups of society, out of an ideology of solidarity, a need for political legitimacy, or a requirement to protect the rest of society from communicable diseases. The contribution/privilege principle is based on the selection of groups perceived to have strategic importance (e.g., the military, civil servants, industrial workers, members of the ruling party); hence, the state selects them as the beneficiaries of health insurance or other types of programs, to which they make a prior financial contribution. Finally, under modern definitions of citizenship, this principle extends eligibility to the whole population.

The combination of four levels of state control and three principles for eligibility defines twelve possible modalities of state intervention in medical care. They include conventional categories, such as national health service, national health insurance, and public assistance (Terris 1978; Roemer 1976). In addition, focusing on modalities rather than entire health systems allows for a deeper analysis of the various forms of state intervention that usually coexist in à country. For example, most Latin American countries exhibit two modalities: public assistance, whereby eligibility is based on poverty and services are directly delivered by the ministry of health through concentrated ownership, and social security, whereby state control typically is exerted through dispersed or concentrated ownership of facilities and eligibility is determined by the principle of contribution/privilege. Great Britain also exhibits two modalities of state intervention; they are not divided by the population served, as in Latin America, but by the type of service. In the case of ambulatory care, the state limits its role to financing, whereas it exercises direct ownership in the case of hospital care. For both types of services, state control is concentrated in the National Health Service and eligibility is based on the citizenship principle. The configuration of the British system could change as a result of its recent reforms, which aim at introducing selective market elements into service delivery, such as increased competition among providers, greater managerial autonomy for hospitals, and more private-sector involvement (Secretaries of State for Health—Wales, Northern Ireland, and Scotland 1989).

As the examples illustrate, the proposed typology makes it possible to characterize the patterns of state intervention within countries, as well as to carry out cross-national comparisons of the extent and nature of variation in those patterns. Understanding such variation leads to the critical question of its determinants.

The Determinants of State Intervention

The literature on national development has recorded an intense debate regarding the predominance of convergence or divergence among different countries (Meyer, Boli-Bennett, and Chase-Dunn 1975). The debate has also permeated the cross-national comparison of health care systems (Field 1973; Mechanic 1975; Anderson 1977; Elling 1980). In our view, this is a false dilemma, since both convergence and divergence forces seem to operate simultaneously but at two different levels. Indeed, the development of contemporary nation-states has been affected by both the internal circumstances characteristic to each of them and by their insertion in a world system (Wallerstein 1974) that defines relationships of dependence constraining the autonomy of domestic processes. Thus, on the one hand is a set of variables that seems to push different nations toward a convergent trend of increased state control and greater population coverage. These forces operate at the level of the world system. On the other hand are variables that make different countries remain unique or even diverge. These divergence factors operate at the internal level of each nation-state.

The joint analysis of the two levels defines a particular set of modalities of state intervention in a given country at a given time. Because our interest lies in the relationship of the state to the medical profession rather than in state intervention *per se,* we will not offer here a detailed examination of each determinant, a task that has been attempted elsewhere (Frenk and Donabedian 1987). Instead, we will merely mention their main mechanisms.

World System Determinants. Three major forces operate at the level of the world system to produce growing similarities among countries in the extent and form of state intervention. The first refers to the process of industrialization and urbanization (Mechanic 1975). Industrialization creates the requirement for a healthy and productive labor force while providing the means for the expression of trade union demands and for the financing of special sickness funds. In addition, urbanization has had a direct impact on the extension of coverage since increased population densities offer the conditions for developing an organized network of medical care facilities. The converging effect of this variable is mostly clearly seen in the similarities among social insurance schemes worldwide (Sigerist 1943).

The second variable is the emergence of a medical world economy, which includes the diffusion of knowledge, the transfer of technology, and the migration of medical personnel (Mechanic 1975). In this context, the state is often the only actor with enough economic resources or power to control the multinational medical-industrial complex.

Besides economic and technological factors, there is a third factor represented by the diffusion of a world ideology of modernity, which creates a shared set of rules defining the state as the legitimate agent of rational progress. These rules are highly institutionalized into a world polity (Meyer 1980). International organizations are important components of the world polity. They act on every aspect of medical care and have been very influential in the diffusion of the dominant health care paradigms.

Internal Nation-State Determinants. The variables operating at this level include ideological definitions, economic factors, and political forces, all of which account for differences among countries.

Salient among the ideological factors are the prevailing norms about the legitimacy of auspices and ownership (Zald and Hair 1972; Zald 1978), which define who may legitimately own, operate, or employ the resources required for the production of medical services. Although certain technical characteristics of a product may generate market imperfections and thereby call for the involvement of the state, it is also possible, as Steiner (1977) indicates, that a state may intervene purely as a response to broad normative concerns about what a society should provide to its members. Current attempts at reforming the role of the state offer an opportunity to assess the potential effects of ideological definitions on the modalities of state intervention in medical care.

Economic variables refer to the structure of the medical care market, specifically

Table 2.2. Attributes of medical associations according to state power and modes of interest representation

State power Organization of civil society	Representation of physicians Corporatist	Noncorporatist
Strong		
Corporatist State corporatism	Moderately weak and heterogeneous professional association (e.g., Spain under Franco, possibly Greece)	Very weak or nonexistent professional association (e.g., Mexico)
Societal corporatism	Moderately powerful and homogeneous professional association (e.g., Scandinavian countries)	Contradictory position
Noncorporatist State centralism	Transitional positions (possibly Eastern European countries)	Moderately weak professional association, possibly shared with nonmedical health workers (e.g., former Soviet Union, China)
Weak Pluralism	Powerful but potentially unstable professional association (e.g., United States, Great Britain, Canada, Australia, New Zealand, France)	Weak and heterogeneous professional associations (e.g., nineteenth-century United States)

to the availability of private resources, which include both insurance funds and providers of services. In general, the existence of private resources tends to limit the participation of the state, with more emphasis on regulation than on direct provision. In contrast, the scarcity of such resources has been a major force driving the state into greater control over the production of services. This is a very important source of divergence: given their availability of private resources, most developed countries have been able to extend coverage at a fast rate with lower levels of state control, whereas developing countries have generally extended coverage slowly, even with greater state intervention.

Finally, the major political variable concerns the system of interest representation that prevails in a country. This is a critical element in our analysis, since it directly refers to the political organization of the medical profession and to its degree of **sovereignty** with respect to the state, as defined by our conceptual model (Table 2.1). This is why we proceed next to a more detailed examination of its characteristics.

Professional Power and Corporatist Organization

The political organization of the medical profession exhibits great variation across countries. Table 2.2 offers a framework to analyze the sources of such variation, by developing the concept of sovereignty introduced in Table 2.1. A crucial factor is whether the mode of interest representation adopted by physicians is corporatist. The term *corporatism* is used here in a broad sense, to denote a system of interest representation characterized by hierarchical and noncompetitive occupational or functional associations, which represent their members' interests through direct negotiations with the state (Schmitter 1979; Jessop 1979; Frenk and Donabedian 1987; Frenk and González-Block 1992).

The organization of physicians cannot be analyzed in isolation. As shown in Table 2.2, it must be related to the organization of other groups in civil society with whom they deal (Starr 1982; Johnson 1972). In addition, the state mediates this relationship. Hence, the power of the state itself becomes a critical element because it shapes the organization of civil society and sets limits to the power of medical associations (Durán-Arenas and Kennedy 1991). Let us examine the elements presented in Table 2.2.

State Power. Power is a political concept. It answers questions such as: Who makes the decisions? Who has the ability to call others to account for what they do? Rokkan (in Tilly 1975:66) offers a model of a full-fledged nation-state and advances a number of phases in state building that shed light on the dimensions of state power. He defines four phases: penetration, standardization, participation, and redistribution. Although these phases do not follow a sequential order, their interaction defines three main dimensions of state power: degree of institutionalization, differentiation, and autonomy (Birnbaum 1988). In this sense, state power is related to Heidenheimer's (1989*b*) concept of stateness, which is defined by the degree to which "the instruments of government are differentiated from other organizations, centralized, autonomous and formally coordinated."

We define state power as the degree of control over decisional and implementation responsibilities on economic, social, and cultural functions. In accordance with Weber's (1946*b*) definition of the state, we postulate that the underlying force behind such control is state access to sanctions and penalties sufficient to dominate individual and group behavior (Tilly 1975:27; Schmitter 1979; Cleaves 1987). This definition includes two elements: the organizational and economic capacity of the state to exert control over social activity areas and the range of activities effectively under state control relative to the total range of activities in society (Boli-Bennet 1976). In this connection, Klein (1977*b*) addresses the equivalence of state power to the extension of the state sector and the increase in the scale of state activities, measured as the proportion of national income devoted to public expenditure. Greater state power means that more tasks and responsibilities are directed toward the political system and away from society. As shown in Table 2.2, we can define a taxonomy of strong and weak states based on the amount of power exerted by the state.

The manner in which each state intervenes varies widely. In some situations, the state controls medical care, the economy, and civil society; in others, it supports more autonomous intergroup relations. But in all cases, the state is the most influential actor determining the relative strength of physicians and other groups (Durán-Arenas and Kennedy 1991). For example, the degree of physicians' power in the United States depends not only on their capacity to organize along corporatist lines but also on the relative weakness of state intervention. In contrast, Swedish civil society has been more influential in controlling the medical profession through the state, so physicians' power is restricted (Korpi 1978).

Furthermore, when the state controls the organizations usually found in civil society (e.g., manufacturing enterprises, trade unions, professional associations), as in social regimes, it is most powerful. State power is greater when civil society is organized by the state than when the struggles within civil society shape state policy. That is the reason that physicians' power in the former Soviet Union was moderately weak: the state organized both physicians and other groups with which they interact.

In this way, a crucial determinant of professional power lies in the specific strategies that a state follows to deal with the organization of civil society.

State Strategies. To assess the effects of the state strategies, we will use Schmitter's (1979) definition of corporate intermediation as a particular arrangement for linking the organized interests of civil society with the decision-making structures of the state. We will expand this view to create a more complete taxonomy.

Schmitter (1979) advanced two types of corporatist intermediation: state corporatism and societal corporatism. Under the former, a dominant state organizes civil society by creating corporate bodies that are retained as its auxiliary and dependent organs. Two good examples are Spain under Franco's rule and Mexico. Societal corporatism is characterized by a more autonomous organization of civil society, in which there is a balance between the respective power of the state and of the various corporate entities. Sweden and other Scandinavian countries exemplify this type (Frenk and González-Block 1992).

To complete the taxonomy we have to add the noncorporatist forms of state intermediation. We propose two types. The first is pluralism, whereby an independent structure of civil society exists, defined by competition among multiple interest groups. Here the role of the state depends on the various conjunctions of interest groups within a network of pluralist representation (Jessop 1979). According to Heidenheimer (1989), Great Britain and the United States fit in this category, since the links of civil society to the state are loosely structured, adopting elite-dominated strategies of organization.

The second noncorporatist type is state centralism, in which the state structures civil society around a single corporate body (e.g., the communist party). This is the case of the former Soviet-type societies, where civil society was integrated to the structures sponsored by the state.

When one combines the level of state power (strong versus weak) with the form of organization of civil society and the representation of physicians (corporatist versus noncorporatist), it is possible to derive certain attributes of medical associations, as shown in Table 2.2. Let us briefly analyze some illustrative examples under each of the four strategies:

1. *State corporatism.* How civil society is structured by the state directly affects the capacity of the medical profession to organize politically. If civil society is organized under a state-corporatist structure, the chances of the medical profession's attaining much power are limited. If, in addition, physicians are not allowed to constitute their own association, then professional power will be at its lowest level. In Mexico political reasons led the state to fragment the medical profession

into trade unions. Because other occupational groups are organized in associations with representational monopoly, physicians are unable to counterbalance the interests of those other groups (Cleaves 1987; Frenk 1990).

2. *Societal corporatism.* When interest groups in civil society are able to influence the state, as through trade unions, they can achieve a balance with the corporate organization of professionals. Sweden represents this possibility (Roemer 1976; Durán-Arenas and Kennedy 1991; Frenk and González-Block 1992). The Swedish medical profession is moderately powerful because it deals with equally organized bodies of civil society. In the context of societal corporatism, the medical association tends to be homogeneous. In 1985, the dominant association represented 92 percent of physicians, strongly supported trade union philosophy, and spoke out in support of physicians on health policy issues (Garpenby 1989). Note in Table 2.2 that the combination of societal corporatism with noncorporatist representation of doctors represents a contradictory position, since it is unlikely that any group will be forcefully prevented from organizing its own association, as may be the case under the more authoritarian style of state corporatism.

3. *State centralism.* Another form of authoritarian co-optation of associations occurs in state centralist societies. In this case, co-optation is accompanied by homogenization. This was most apparent in socialist countries prior to 1990, where the authorities amalgamated different interest groups into one broad organization (the party) or its extensions (official trade unions). Although the state has more control, such a combination tends to be unstable (Durán-Arenas and Kennedy 1991). After the collapse of socialist regimes in Eastern Europe, physicians may begin to organize in a corporatist fashion as their countries undergo the transition to societal corporatism or to pluralism.

4. *Pluralism.* The most advantageous situation for physicians is one in which they have managed to achieve corporatist organization under a pluralist system in which the state plays a limited role. Since the beginning of the century and until recently, this was the situation in the United States. It also characterizes the other countries listed in the corresponding cell of Table 2.2. Such an arrangement, however, tends to be unstable, since competing interest groups are likely to negotiate their own demands with the state. Indeed, there is evidence that American physicians may be losing power to large health care organizations, industry conglomerates, and other interest groups (Relman 1980; Starr 1982; McKinlay and Stoeckle 1988).

Our analysis has illustrated the way in which the complex interaction among state power, civil society, and the organization of the medical profession results in differential levels of professional sovereignty.

Consequences of State Intervention

Having examined the major elements that define medical sovereignty, it is useful to come back to our conceptual framework (Table 2.1) in order to analyze the consequences of state intervention on the remaining dimensions of the social organization of the profession.

As a form of occupational control, professionalization faces many inherent instabilities, some of which we have already summarized. Such instabilities tend to be addressed by introducing a collective mediator in the direct relationship between clients and providers. In modern societies, the state has come to assume that mediating role. A major consequence of state mediation is that it disrupts the two necessary conditions for a professional form of control to exist (Johnson 1972): client heterogeneity and provider homogeneity. On the one hand, state intervention has tended to aggregate the interests of clients, who can act collectively as contributors to insurance funds, taxpayers, or beneficiaries of specific entitlements. On the other, state intervention tends to introduce several cleavages into the profession.

Many of the effects of state intervention are exerted through a substantial modification in the structure of the markets for medical services and personnel, through the dimension of independence (Table 2.1). For instance, a basic problem for the social organization of the profession refers to the existence of a monopsonist in the market for medical services. It could be argued that a major factor accounting for the privileged position of physicians in the United States has been the absence of such a monopsonist. Instead, there is a plurality of private insurance carriers, Blue Cross/Blue Shield plans, and public financing schemes, none of which has so far been able to concentrate enough market power to control physicians by itself. In contrast, the markets for medical services of many European countries with national health insurance programs have been dominated by the monopsonist role of the state. Even in the American case, the presence of large-scale buyers may limit professional autonomy and dominance in an attempt to control costs. Increasing competition in the market for services is also likely to undermine professional homogeneity.

In addition, the American medical profession, like that of most other countries (Kindig and Taylor 1985), may lose part of its independence as a result of the increased supply of physicians (Ginzberg et al. 1981; Rosenthal, Butler, and Field 1990). Although the initial granting of practice monopoly has limited the supply of doctors, the subsequent determinants of state intervention have generated pressures to expand the numbers of physicians. Such an expansion has produced many imbalances (Mejía 1987). For our purposes, we are interested on the way it has affected homogeneity among physicians, which is a necessary condition for a professional form of occupational control to exist.

There are many threats to this homogeneity (Frenk et al. 1991). It can be argued, for example, that an oversupply of physicians increases the probability of heterogeneity by the mere fact that the number of doctors is larger. Perhaps a more significant source of differentiation among practitioners is the tendency to specialize, because allegiance may then shift from the profession as a whole to specific specialties. Further, increased specialization in the context of a rising supply of physicians may lead to shrinking shares of the medical services market for each specialty and thereby to intensified turf wars among specialties. In addition, as more specialists attempt to expand their area of practice by providing primary care, conflicts with general practitioners may ensue.

Specialization occurs not only along technical lines. As Johnson (1972:54, 60) indicates, it can also take place along social lines, for example, when different segments of the profession provide services for clients from different social or ethnic groups. Just as technical specialization may shift allegiance and identity from the total profession to its subspecialties, so social specialization may subvert the solidarity of practitioners as they orient their loyalties toward particular organizations that may compete with each other for resources. Under those circumstances, the notion of medicine as a unitary profession, bound together by the community of interests of its practitioners and by their shared socialization experience, loses much of its connection to reality.

It seems that the process of internal stratification of the profession will continue growing, for this phenomenon is bound to structural features that promote inequalities in the general society (Frenk et al. 1991). Although this process originates in the extraorganizational dimensions of sovereignty and independence, it inevitably affects the intraorganizational dimensions of dominance and autonomy. A stratified profession implies that although physicians as a collectivity may still retain control over service production, individual practitioners are increasingly seeing their autonomy curtailed through formal review procedures. In addition, the presence of different classes of doctors charged with managerial, research, and practice roles creates a new constellation of positions in the division of labor. These new realities have been aptly summarized by Freidson (1985):

> The rules of the game have changed sufficiently in medicine to have introduced important changes in the relationship that members of the medical profession have with each other, both in the way they compete with each other in the marketplace and in the way they interact with each other at work, particularly in large, complex institutions subject to financing by the state.

Conclusions

We appear to need a revision—that is, a new vision—about the character of the medical profession. In a world in which rationalizing states, multinational companies, and international agencies ensure the diffusion of technologies, including those of medical care, and the transfer of ideologies, including those of modernization and professionalism, the striking variations across countries in the political and economic conditions of medical work pose a challenge for the development of innovative theories of professionalization.

According to Johnson (1972:38), professionalization as an institutionalized form of occupational control was the result of the specific historical conditions of Anglo-American culture in the course of industrialization. Such conditions have not been present in underdeveloped countries (Johnson 1973), nor are they prevalent any longer in developed societies. It is likely, therefore, that different forms of occupational control will become increasingly predominant. In those forms, the state and, more generally, large-scale bureaucratic organizations occupy central positions of control.

Even for some of the most established professions, like medicine, a growing body of sociological literature suggests an erosion of professional status. The nature, the extent, and even the existence of such erosion are far from settled (Light and

Levine 1988; Hafferty 1988; Freidson 1985). In fact, the sociology of professions presents the scientific and aesthetic appeal of a field that is rethinking its own premises, challenging its older descriptions, and offering new interpretations of social reality.

Acknowledgments

We thank Marilynn Rosenthal for her valuable suggestions and Kelly Scoggins for her editorial assistance.

3

Professions and the Law

David M. Frankford

Over the past twenty years the question of whether the medical profession is powerful has been the subject of intense scrutiny. In sociological literature this question of power has been debated by examining whether the medical profession is dominant or whether it is instead subject to a process of proletarianization or deprofessionalization. As this debate has evolved, various observers have attributed different significance to evidence regarding the structure and organization of health care and, particularly, the place of the medical profession within the health care industry. Additionally, each side has accused the other of failing to specify the meaning of its theoretical terms and of omitting empirical support (Freidson 1983a, 1984, 1985, 1986a, 1986b; Hafferty 1988; Haug 1988; McKinlay and Arches 1986; McKinlay and Stoeckle 1988; Mechanic 1991; Roemer 1986; Saks 1983). Recently law has been asked to provide evidence to confirm or disconfirm the different theories or to support phenomenological (or interactionist) description (Abbott 1988; Freidson 1983a, 1983b, 1984, 1985, 1986a, 1986b, 1989c, 1989d; Hafferty 1988; Havighurst 1983, 1986; Light 1991; Light and Levine 1988). This recourse to law, like much of the prior evidence, has continued to foster opposite conclusions, with one side claiming that law is dismantling professional power and the other side arguing the contrary (Hafferty 1988).

This chapter explores the reasons that such contradictory conclusions can be drawn. By focusing on the leading contenders in the field, McKinlay's theory of proletarianization and Freidson's description of professional dominance (Hafferty 1988), it examines whether law can vindicate such a theory or phenomenological description of professional power. It concludes that recourse to law cannot accomplish this task. The essential problem is the following: McKinlay's theory of power is premised on the existence of a historical process, and Freidson's phenomenological description presupposes the existence of a process for the construction of consciousness. Both must find a referent, external to their words, with which their words can correspond. For McKinlay, it is a historical process of events; for Freidson, it is a process for constructing consciousness. Both attempt to locate their respective referents in a body of law, which embodies either history (McKinlay) or phenomenological process (Freidson). Both regard law as a body of rules that lawyers produce and apply. Yet law is what lawyers do, what they practice; it is not something that they produce. The only "bodies of law" are those constructed by McKinlay and Freidson, and thus each points to his own construction to support his own theory or phenomenology. Furthermore, their characterizations of power suffer from an identical infirmity: each presupposes that power is immanent in law and that power lies behind the surface of legal practice, to be ferreted out by the appropriate theory or phenomenology. Each presumes a dichotomy between theories of power (language) and the object of theory (power). Yet once we abandon the metaphysical claim that our language pictures something that is distinct from our language, all we have left is our language; no human history, process, or system is intelligible apart from our use of words (Wittgenstein 1958). Therefore, when we debate power, we cannot meaningfully conceptualize this power as a being analogous to nature's power—as some sort of collective electricity, for example (Turner 1986: 107–60). Instead, power must be conceived as the significance that we attribute to our use of words (Foucault 1970, 1972, 1977). We can debate professional power, but we do not confirm, disconfirm, or describe power that exists outside our writing. Rather, when we debate such power, there is only the power of our words. We should view our power as an opportunity, for we can shape the power that McKinlay, Freidson, and others have been debating for many years.

My argument proceeds as follows. I first assert that both McKinlay and Freidson unify around two concepts of law: that law consists of a body of rules and that these rules embody relationships of power. I argue, however, that law is neither a body nor embodies anything; instead, law is a practice in which lawyers use language to justify practical judgments tied to particular contexts. It follows that McKinlay's and Freidson's recourse to a body of law ignores the distinctive character of law—legal justification and judgment in rich context—and that both posit a false picture of law that they then use to support their respective pictures of power. Finally, I argue that we can debate professional power, but because there is no power outside words, we must recognize that our work creates and deflates claims of justified power.

The Question of Professional Power: The Concepts of Law

Freidson and McKinlay rely, quite literally, on a body of law (Freidson 1983*b*:37 n.2) that each constructs to support a thesis concerning the power of the medical profession. McKinlay conceives of law as a system of rules that enables capitalist modes of production in medicine to exist through infusing capital into the medical industry and by maintaining the whole structure through legitimatizing the activities of powerful players in the medical game (McKinlay 1977; McKinlay and Arches 1985). Medicine itself plays an ambiguous role in this game, for it pathetically represents itself as powerful—and indeed it is often represented from the outside as powerful—while it nevertheless remains subject to the underlying logic of the game (McKinlay 1977). Law, as a system of rules, helps to maintain both faces of modern medicine. Legal rules relating to licensure and institutional credentialing give medical professionals the illusion that they are powerful (Derber 1982; Larson 1977, 1979; McKinlay 1977), but they also shove medical professionals into bureaucracies, swamp them with regulatory requirements, ensure their dependence on state financing, foster competition among them and against other professionals, and force them to treat patients as reified objects. In sum, legal rules rob professional labor of its power to control the object and material means of its work (McKinlay and Arches 1985; McKinlay and Stoeckle 1988).

Freidson points to the same particulars and effects of the legal system but attributes to legal rules a very different significance. For him, power neither derives from a historical process nor consists of disembodied formal knowledge. Instead, power derives from the employment of knowledge within social institutions (Freidson 1970*a*, 1970*b*, 1980, 1986*a*, 1986*b*, 1989*b*, 1989*c*, 1989*d*). There, in the workaday world and in the political economy, a carrier of formal knowledge interacts with clients, with the laity, and with other types of professionals, as well as with professional peers, equals who are nonetheless stratified by virtue of their different positions within an organizational or political hierarchy (Freidson 1983*a*, 1984, 1985, 1986*a*, 1986*b*, 1989*b*, 1989*c*). This process is stabilized and shaped by legal rules, for there are three ways by which law grants professionals a sheltered—albeit quite differentiated and stratified—place within our social division of labor (Freidson 1986*a*, 1986*b*, 1989*c*). First, occupational licensure and credentialing restrict work within institutions to specified occupations. Second, institutional credentialing specifies the types and characteristics of institutions that can service professional clients, and it places various professionals in stipulated, important institutional positions. Third, systems of accreditation of professional education ensure that the professions as an aggregate control the education of their members, while preserving a knowledge hierarchy both within and among the competing professional groups (Freidson 1986*a*, 1986*b*, 1989*b*, 1989*c*).

Given this rich institutional complex, Freidson (1986*a*) stresses that one cannot simply equate a profession's (or individual professional's) formal knowledge with power. Again legal rules play a significant role. Professionals maintain prominent positions within the heteronomous organizations that comprise the division of labor, and legal rules allow professionals to control the formal and technical content, standards, and day-to-day application and supervision of their knowledge (Freidson 1983*a*, 1984, 1985, 1986*a*, 1986*b*, 1989*b*, 1989*c*). Because these organizations are heteronomous, however, policies and goals are set by nonprofessionals, who sit either at the top of the organizational chart or outside, in the political economy (Freidson 1986*a*, 1986*b*, 1989*b*, 1989*c*). Therefore, the application of formal knowledge involves numerous interactions, and it is these interactions that constitute power, in either an individual or corporate sense (Freidson 1986*a*). Overall, then, because legal rules have both functional and symbolic importance (Freidson 1985:24, 1989*b*:66) and because they have been relatively stable (Freidson 1986*b*:71), power for Freidson depends on a complex system of political economy, including a system of law that maintains a system of power. Although "control over work is the key variable for Freidson" (Hafferty 1988:207), the medical profession's dominance at the workplace is ultimately maintained through ideas traded in the larger political economy, and, most saliently, in law (Larkin 1988:117–21; Navarro 1988:57–58).

In order to support his description of professional power, Freidson *has had* to make this move to a viewpoint or mechanism external to medicine. There is serious question whether Freidson's concept of professional dominance, developed in the

1960s and 1970s, could have hung together without recourse to some theory of political economy or system of professions (Abbott 1988; McKinlay 1977). And as Freidson's writings recount (Freidson 1983*a*, 1984, 1985, 1986*a*, 1986*b*), more recent events have clearly taken their toll on the notion that the medical profession is autonomous. As Hafferty has summarized, the internal components that make the medical profession cohere within Freidson's description have been rent asunder. To the extent there ever was, now there no longer is a common knowledge base, a socialized collective norm of collegiality, a collective consciousness of the medical profession as a singular distinctive group, and a common, collegial organizational structure (Hafferty 1988:207–16, 219–22). Therefore, even if we allowed both that Freidson's initial formulation captured a moment of reality and that changed social conditions have driven the alterations in his phenomenological description, it is now clear that in Freidson's writing, law has become the crucial component needed to stabilize the contemporaneous reality: the profession as a state within a state. Different writers from multiple countries have followed this step into law, albeit with different interpretations of the role of the state (Coburn 1988; Krause 1988*b*; Larkin 1988; Riska 1988; Willis 1988).

In sum, both McKinlay and Freidson recount the medical profession's power (or the loss thereof) and the legitimacy (or lack thereof) of such power, and each looks to a body of law for support. Despite their differences, their writings unify around two concepts of law. First is the significance of law. Law embodies something else—power, claims to legitimate power, underlying economic and techno-logical processes, or the process for the construction of social reality. For proletarianization, law is part of a historical process; it embodies both the underlying relations of production, driven by the logic of capitalist expansion, and the legit-imation of those relations (McKinlay 1977; McKinlay and Arches 1985; McKinlay and Stoeckle 1988). For professional dominance, law is part of a process that produces folk concepts; it helps formulate our ideas regarding the medical profession and its power, ideas that have a particularly important hold on us in the political economy, which includes law (Freidson 1986*a*:35–36, 1989*c*). Second, both use a single concept of the legal process: legal rules embodied within legal texts are used by legal professionals, the carriers of knowledge, to satisfy the needs and desires of their clients, with the latter conceptualized as individuals, private asso-ciations, or society. The legal process synthesizes these legal rules into a universal, unified, and coherent body of law, which—returning to the first concept—embodies underlying power, claims to legitimate power, economic relations, or phenome-nological process. My main argument is that with these two concepts, an idea of law is being imposed on law that does a violence to legal practice. By writing a theory or phenomenological description of law, McKinlay and Freidson attempt to "objectify" what is actually done, and in the process, they destroy the uniqueness of legal perspective (Bourdieu 1977:1–30).

Law as Practice

In law, lawyers practice the art of persuasion; they are the midwives to legal judgment. Their practices are arguments of justification: what ought to be done in the circumstance that must now be decided? The language of argument relies on legal concepts, just as all language must utilize meaningful concepts (Martin 1987). Yet just as the world cannot be reduced to a formula, as the French Enlightenment astronomer, mathematician, philosopher, and founder of modern probability theory Pierre Simon de Laplace had supposed (Mirowski 1989:70–73), no single concept or set of concepts is determinative in any particular situation (Oakes 1988; Weber 1977:98–143). Stated differently, no practical judgment can be compelled by prior texts—by what lawyers in the United States call the "authorities" that are listed (literally) in "tables of authorities." Judges exercise discretion in rendering judgment, and that is why we call them judges (Weber 1977:98–143). Without such an understanding, legal practice would be unintelligible. The process of argumentation and justification is often long and arduous precisely because legal judgment inexorably rests on judgment (Llewellyn 1960).

In their practices of justification, lawyers argue from texts that are authoritative within a community of practitioners, and they utilize a craft that is communally produced and intelligible within that community. Argument concerns the significance of these texts. These texts possess the magic of authority only because practices of rhetoric render such a quality unto them. No text embodies the authority of legal rules; rather, it is linguistic practices that are authoritative (Patterson 1989, 1990, 1991).

From the outside, lawyers' practices are often characterized as the individual application of knowledge to concrete situations (e.g., Parsons and Platt 1973:225–66), in which individual professionals are bound together in a system of trust (e.g., Barber 1983) formulated out of—or reflecting—socialized individual character and attitude (e.g., Freidson 1989*b*:66–75). Lawyers' practical knowledge, however, neither resembles such expertise nor relies on socialized individual qualities (Rosen 1989*a;* Sciulli and Jenkins 1990). Lawyers use neither disembodied formal knowledge nor embodied experiential knowledge, as has been supposed (Freidson 1984:4–5). There is no cognitive authority (e.g., Freidson 1986*b*) that reigns over practice, and there is no art separable from a science (e.g., Freidson 1970*a*). Rather, lawyers make their way in the law through their feel for the lay of the land. They use no cognitive and universal model as a map; it is the "outsider who has to find his way around in a foreign landscape and who compensates for his lack of practical mastery, the prerogative of the native, by the use of a model of all possible routes" (Bourdieu 1977:2). Like a child who has learned to ride a bicycle by doing it (as opposed to thinking about it), lawyers practice law—they make practical judgments—not by cogitating over some legal rules embodied in texts but by using tools constructed to get the job done (Rouse 1987). Lawyers' practices and existence cannot be ascribed to individual or social cognitive mastery—Descartes' *cogito ergo sum*— for no such theory can describe what lawyers do. They do what works, and they attain such accomplishments not by asking why or how it works but by learning through doing: "Law is something we do, not something we have as a consequence of something we do" (Bobbitt 1991:24).

An example will help clarify legal practices. Suppose that a legislature has enacted an occupational licensure provision: "No person other than a licensed medical professional shall engage in the practice of medicine." The statement is positively circular. What can it mean that the law permits only a "licensed medical professional" to practice medicine when the word *license* itself depends upon law? That is precisely my point: The statement *is* circular because its legal significance depends on its legal construction (Bobbitt 1991). Legal construction, in turn, depends on a community of practices. In our society's community of legal practitioners, lawyers must take statements of legislatures to be authoritative (Unger 1984, 1987). That practice means that they must take this legislative text seriously. Let us suppose that the context requiring practical judgment is like the one in *Wickline v. State of California* (California Court of Appeals 1986), a case that presents all the crucial variables for a theory or phenomenological description of professional power. A patient is hospitalized for the treatment of an obstructed aorta. The patient's insurer is the state of California, which exercises its authority under its Medi-Cal insurance plan. An employee of the state preauthorizes a ten-day length of stay for the patient. At the end of this stay, the patient is discharged. Unfortunately, the patient's leg is later amputated due to subsequent complications. The patient seeks compensation for her loss, and she comes before an authoritative decision maker: a court, a legislature, or an administrative agency. She claims that the "state" engaged in the unauthorized practice of medicine and that "it" should be held to account.

Look at the dilemma if the issue is phrased as one involving an abstract and universal question of legitimate authority: The legislative language derives from the authority of the state, but that authority is itself at issue in a legal contest in which the state's authority itself sets the rules for its own testing (e.g., Habermas 1988). If law is conceived as posing the abstract and universal question of legitimate authority, there is the most vicious of circles: the rules of the game are set by the rules of the game. As Wittgenstein might have put it, lawyers would be headed for a severe mental cramp; they would simply be frozen in place (Wittgenstein 1958, sec. 1, 10–14, 20–23, 54–55, 66–72, 320–26, 474, 607).

Lawyers' practices embody no such headache, for lawyers simply craft arguments to justify a particular outcome. The language in my statutory example includes the word *person*. Has a "person" acted in this situation such that the patient should obtain judgment? Let us suppose that in a prior case, judgment had been obtained against a private insurer like Aetna. Thus, the lawyer representing the injured patient argues that the word *person* has already been authoritatively defined. She argues that this prior authority sweeps in all institutional insurers, including Medi-Cal. The lawyer representing the state responds that California is not just "any institution" but is the state itself, which means that the prerogatives of the legislature are at issue. This lawyer, who seeks to justify a different result, argues that the prior case concerning Aetna does not "govern." He elucidates that although both California and Aetna can be described as institutions, the patient's usage sweeps too broadly. The word *person* in the legislation includes private actors like Aetna but not public ones like Medi-Cal. In surrebuttal, the patient's lawyer points to a case in which a county's public hospital had been held negligent for an injury occurring in its emergency room. The patient's lawyer uses this judgment to formulate "a rule" that public institutions are held liable for the negligence of their employees. The state's lawyer responds that the county hospital is just like a private actor because public hospitals compete with private ones. He argues that no one competes with Medi-Cal for there is only one sovereign, "universal" insurer and that the court must take this concern into account by rendering judgment for the state.

The language of the statute also includes the words *practice of medicine*. Did the state's employee here engage in the unauthorized practice of medicine? The lawyer for the patient answers strongly in the affirmative. It was as if a "fake doctor" had pushed the patient out the hospital door. The employee for Medi-Cal, she points out, had no medical degree. The lawyer for the state answers that the patient/litigant has formulated the word *license* incorrectly. The employee who engaged in utilization review for Medi-Cal was a registered nurse and thus had a nurse's license. The state's lawyer argues that this level of expertise is sufficient in this situation, given the need of an insurer, particularly one the size of Medi-Cal, to constrain costs. The lawyer representing the patient responds that a registered nurse might have sufficient expertise to handle a run-of-the-mill admission, but this case presents a demand for higher expertise. The lawyer for the patient thus argues that the nurse exceeded his authority. The lawyer for the state must then seek to justify an opposite conclusion. He argues that the Medi-Cal employee acted according to well-established and crystal clear rules and procedures. Because these procedures have been reviewed by Medi-Cal's supervising physicians, he claims, the legislature's words are satisfied: only a "licensed medical professional . . . engage[d] in the practice of medicine." He embellishes, "No rational insurance plan administered by the state in our times can be expected to do more."

Notice that in this to-and-fro, no concept of "person" or "practice of medicine" can be intelligible as the "plain language of the text" independent of a rich context (Southern California Law Review 1985). In a society in which justification comes not from arguments of justification but quite literally from the point of a gun—such as Pol Pot's Cambodia—our lawyers' arguments regarding the language of the text would be nonsense. Who would care about the problem of restraining the sovereign authority exercised under the Medi-Cal program? The arguments make sense—they are intelligible—only within a community of legal practitioners in which justification of sovereign authority through argumentation is taken seriously. The attempted justification is tied to a context that is rich in time and space, in which a particular practical judgment must be rendered: Does Wickline recover against the state of California on these "facts"?

Notice also that no concept of a "person" or of the "practice of medicine" determinately governs judgment (Weber 1977:98–143). Were it otherwise, the "problem" of the justification of sovereign authority would simply be moot: legal results could rest on a formula, the availability of which would mean that all lawyers could simply go away (Rosen 1989*b*). Isomorphically, if such an algorithm were available—if there were such determination—the debates concerning the power of the medical profession would themselves be unintelligible. Writings of professional dominance and proletarianization are calls for the justification of power (e.g., McKinlay 1973; Freidson 1970*a*, 1986*b*, 1989*b*:70). Therefore, each contains an underlying premise that power can be justified, that it can be called to account. Any understanding of law that separates it from practical judgment presupposes that legal results—power—are predetermined. If legal results are predetermined and if power is therefore, to that extent, predetermined, how can demands for justification be meaningful?

What stops the process of justification then? The practices of a community of lawyers do (Patterson 1993). Again, return to my crucial point (which was Weber's point): there must be judgment (Weber 1977:98–143). As a matter of logic, the process of justification could go on and on forever; there would simply be an infinite regress (Brown 1990). Yet judgments are made every day in a multitude of different contexts. Lawyers are not caught in the mental cramp of regress, and they are not frozen in place. That must tell one the following: legal judgment does not rest on a cognitive operation in which every possible authoritative premise is potentially put into dispute (Tully 1989). At some point, someone in a position of authority must decide the matter. This person must render judgment in a rich particular context and must utilize communally produced linguistic conventions to justify that judgment. That is why we call such persons judges.

My point about legal practices is not that any argument can be used or that anything at all might work (Patterson 1989). There are communally acceptable practices of argumentation, and there are unacceptable ones. It is unacceptable to lie to a judge; it is acceptable to ignore "authorities" from different sovereign entities because they are not binding in a particular jurisdiction. It is acceptable to pursue the facts of the situation by the use of elaborate fact-finding mechanisms— judicial, administrative, or legislative. It is not acceptable to grind opponents into the ground by burying them in meaningless paper. There is a world of difference between claiming that there is necessarily judgment in law and asserting that one can do anything at all. Indeed, any argument that decision makers can do what they please ignores the constraints of communal practices; that argument lapses into senseless solipsism. Practical judgment is indeed necessary to separate the acceptable from the unacceptable, but the necessity of practical judgment is just part of legal life (Patterson 1990, 1991).

In summary, to understand legal practice, one should think of law not as a structured body of rules existing in some texts that embody authority but as an interconnected flowing field in which legal components constantly interact (Teubner 1989). These components are lawyers' arguments and judgments, and in this interaction, the components continuously change each other. Lawyers' arguments shape judgments, which shape what can be argued, which in turn reflects back upon judgments, which shape arguments, and so forth (Ashmore 1989; Lawson 1985). Thus, both the internal pathways within the field and its external boundaries are constantly in flux. This dynamic is driven by the crucial component of legal life: practical judgment must be rendered in each rich, particular context, and judgment must be justified by recourse to communal practices of justification.

The Question of Professional Power: An Assessment

Given these practices, Freidson's and others' turn toward law asks both too much and too little of it. Power, authority, legitimacy, and similar concepts are universal in their potential use. When one asks, as we do in this book, "Does the medical profession in the 1990s in Australia, France, Greece, and other nations have power?'' we have narrowed the scope of our concepts. Yet plainly we are still discussing the medical profession by use of concepts. We can narrow the range of concepts still further by inquiring after power in the state, then the canton, the village, the hospital, and so on, all the while being sure to analyze within concrete, historical time. Nonetheless, the discussion can never escape the use of concepts, for our language must use concepts. Thus, the turn toward law to answer questions regarding medicine's power and legitimacy can be viewed in two ways. First, if law's aid is sought to help us get out of these concepts, then too much is being asked, for law can no more escape the use of concepts than can—as Freidson points out—sociology, political science, or economics (Freidson 1986a:20–35). If, in contrast, law is being asked to confirm or disconfirm empirically concepts of power and legitimation (Hafferty 1988; Light and Levine 1988; Mechanic 1991; McKinlay and Stoeckle 1988; Roemer 1986; Wolinsky 1988a) or to support the phenomenological description of the process by which these concepts are constructed (Abbott 1988:59–69; Freidson 1986a:35–36), then too little is being requested. Answers may be constructed, as they have been, by pointing to the texts of particular cases, statutes, and administrative decisions (Freidson 1983a, 1984, 1985, 1986a)—by pointing to the ''objective evidence'' that there are ''formal mechanisms'' to define ''the rules of the game'' (Freidson 1985:17, 26). Yet these answers are built around cognitive formal rules completely robbed of context—exactly the disembodied formal knowledge that alone cannot tell us very much about power, as Freidson has taught us so well (Freidson 1986a, 1989c:169–70). Such formalism teaches little because it cannot replicate what is ''realized in the concrete operation of the organization,'' a process ''that is critical'' (Freidson 1989b:69). Moreover, such answers necessarily group these judgments around categories. These categories necessarily rely on concepts. And it is here that we arrive full circle back at our initial question: Is the medical profession powerful, and is that power legitimate? In constructing this circle, the crucial step within legal practices—practical judgment—has been omitted, and it is that omission that does violence to law. Now so little is being asked of law that law simply evaporates. The theory of proletarianization and phenomenological description simply impose their questions, their categories, and their answers while eliminating the distinctiveness of law. They thereby trample law's perspective.

Power as Our Discourse about Power

Law cannot support a theory of proletarianization or a phenomenological description. Can it support some kind of debate concerning the power of the medical profession? Yes, but the concept of power must be formulated much differently than it has been in either McKinlay's theory of proletarianization or Freidson's phenomenological description. The law consists of linguistic practices; law is the use of words to persuade and to justify. A description of power in law cannot even begin to connect with law if it starts with the supposition that power is some mental and material resource, outside of language, that is available for manipulation to suit the wills or purposes of individuals, associations, or the state (e.g., Wrong

1988). Mental and material things are meaningless to us apart from our practices that give meaning, or, in other words, apart from our language (Weber 1977:102–15; Wittgenstein 1958). Therefore, a debate concerning medicine's power in law must begin with legal discourse, and it must claim that this discourse has both been persuasive and persuaded in a particular way (Foucault 1972, 1977). In legal discourse, the power of the medical profession is debated, as medicine comes to law with its own language of justification and its own brand of persuasion and as medical categories and legal categories interact (Foucault 1975). In economic discourse and in the recent boom industry of law and economics, a similar interaction is occurring in its own particular language (Frankford 1992). Legal opinions—and very important ones at that—reach out to the social sciences for evidence and concepts to justify their results (U.S. Supreme Court 1982, 1986, 1990). Thus, the chapters in this book, and prior work on professional dominance, proletarianization, and deprofessionalization, are and have been part of the legal discussion, for the sociological debates cross many disciplines and figure prominently in legal discourse (Capron 1985–86; Frankford 1989; Furrow 1989; Havighurst 1985; Law 1974; Mehlman 1990; Northwestern University Law Review 1988; Rosenblatt 1981). One must understand that, with regard to Freidson in particular, much of this legal literature has simply written a version of "Freidson" back to Freidson (Hall 1988; Havighurst 1978, 1985; Havighurst and King 1983; Kissam 1983a, 1983b); and Freidson, until very recently (Freidson 1989a, 1989b, 1989c, 1989d, 1990), has often cited this work without discussing whether his thought has been correctly characterized by these legal scholars when they have relied on it (Freidson 1983a, 1984, 1985, 1986a, 1986b).

Given this interplay, any debate of the medical profession's power in law must take itself into account; it must be reflexive. In our texts, we create or deflate claims of justified power; we shape the phenomena that our theories purport only to describe (Bové 1986). There is no historic dynamic at work in which some underlying forces grant and take power (e.g., Light 1991a:500). There are no ambiguous movements that mysteriously give rise to a phenomenon, such as "an emphasis on competition" (e.g., Freidson 1986b). Power is generated within our own work, by the traces of significance that our words impart, and there is no power apart from that work to be confirmed, disconfirmed, or described in a body of law. We can attempt to avoid the implications of *our* power by continually respecifying the nature of *their* power—administrative, economic, technical, cognitive, political, and so on (e.g., Freidson 1984, 1985). Our texts can abruptly lapse into the passive voice when describing a legal process by which formalized standards and rules are enforced by one carrier of knowledge against other such agents (e.g., Freidson 1989b:72–75). Yet it is our texts that make the agents disappear when we purport to describe any such "logic of operation" (Freidson 1989b:73). If we continue to write theories about a power that somehow effaces agency, our theories can go on and on and on (Hafferty 1988). Human action is distinctive in its agency, and we cannot eliminate this distinctiveness in a theory or phenomenological description of power.

Alternatively, we can face our power and use it explicitly by making suggestions regarding what should be done, what practices there ought to be. Do we, for example, urge that law encourage patients and doctors to square off in arms'-length relationships? Do we argue that law should instead encourage them to trust one another? Do we urge that this relationship of trust be couched within the bureaucratic authority of private association, or should it be bound primarily by public governance? As Freidson quite laudably seems now to recognize (Freidson 1989d:257–58), when we make such explicit use of our power to persuade, we are, as we should be, responsible for the law we create. The 1988 issue of the *Milbank Quarterly* that inspired this book is a witness to our power, for our writing has coalesced around the danger that McKinlay and Freidson in particular have excelled in identifying. There are very strong and numerous voices attempting to move the health care world toward a commitment to and standard of technical efficiency. Within the 1988 issue, Field's article summarizes the ironic and troubling possibility that we see: the massive bureaucratic apparatus of the former Soviet Union gave individual professionals tremendous discretion (Field 1988:188–94). Of course, our discussion of this possibility must be qualified to take into account the very different circumstances of different societies. Yet, as Field puts it, "One begins to wonder whether the Soviet situation is, to some qualified extent, a portent of things to come in the West as medical care becomes increasingly bureaucratized and corporatized" (p. 198).

It is our work that can show that there are other possibilities—that the human world is not reducible to the equations of neoclassical economics, quality assurance, or technology assessment. We must gather our voices together and sustain a chorus against these formulas. Many scholars, including both Freidson and McKinlay, from multiple disciplines have already embarked upon this course (Barer and Evans 1986; Barer, Evans, and Labelle 1988; Clark, Potter, and McKinlay 1991; Evans 1986; Field 1987, 1988, 1990; Freidson 1989a, 1989b, 1989c, 1989d, 1990; Glaser 1970, 1978, 1987; Kovner and Sigmond 1988; Potter et al. 1990; Rodwin 1982; Saltman and Otter 1987, 1989a, 1989b; Seay and Sigmond 1983; Stoeckle 1988). That direction, it seems to me, is the task at hand with regard to professions and the law.

4

How Dominant Are the Professions?

Eliot Freidson

This book is a welcome addition to the growing body of historical and comparative studies of the professions. It is only by such comparative study that we can refine and extend our understanding of the role of professions in the cultural, social, political, and economic affairs of advanced industrial societies. If comparative studies are to be fruitful, however, they must all provide comparable information; each writer cannot be seeking answers to different questions. It is true that a great many studies have explored the same general area—the relationship between professional status and power—but in the past they have been led to diametrically opposed conclusions.

Contradictory Visions of Professional Power

Consider the large literature that in one way or another claims that "experts" or "the professions" exercise enormous power over both state policy and the personal affairs of individuals. Some concentrate on the monopolization of particular kinds of work, like doctoring, by licensing, registration, and other exclusionary devices; others emphasize the power to create artificial dependence on professionals by determining state policy and controlling the way people perceive their problems and decide how to cope with them. Havighurst and King (1983:189–97, 267–68, 276–85, 288–89) link the two by claiming that licensing has created an "ideological monopoly," allowing the American medical profession to dominate both policy and lay perception of health problems and their solution. This view of professional dominance finds at least loose fellowship in Gramsci's conception of intellectuals and their "hegemony," in Foucault's work, and in some works on the professional "class" (e.g., Derber, Schwartz, and Magrass 1990).

The opposite view is that the professions are the passive instruments of capital, the state, or their individual clients and that they exercise little or no influence of their own over the substance and direction of institutional policy and everyday affairs. At most they merely administer those affairs, captive to the requirements of their masters, though to the extent that their members interact with lay clients of lesser status, some interpersonal power may remain in their hands. Akin to this position is one postulating trends toward powerlessness—a steady decline of professional power that is described as deprofessionalization, proletarianization, rationalization, bureaucratization, or corporatization. Some claim that the professions are losing their cultural authority due to increasing public skepticism, consumer activism and sophistication, and decreasing public respect. Others emphasize the professions' loss of exclusive jurisdictions to competitors, the increasing intervention of the state into the financing and administration of professional practice, and the increasing dependence of the professions on concentrated corporate and state economic power.

Heuristic Measuring Rods

The picture of professional powerlessness is a virtual mirror image of the picture of professional powerfulness. Which picture is true? I believe that question is unanswerable, in part because some are saying, "The cup is half empty" and the others, "The cup is half full." More important, most talk past each other because they are not attending to the same data. The problem stems from the most important consideration of all: the absence of common criteria by which to select systematically and analyze the data bearing on professional status and power. This lack has seriously confused past discussions of professions within individual nations and historic periods, and if it continues to be the case, it will prevent comparative studies from realizing their full potential.

If the participants in discussions about the status and power of professions employ the same internally consistent and systematic standard to guide their collection of data and use it to organize their analysis of the position held by different professions in different political economies, there would be some hope that we could arrive at greater consensus and more sophisticated understanding than is now the case. Such a standard should not, of course, be created out of one nation's historic experience, which, after all, is unique and time bound. It must be sufficiently abstract to be applicable to a variety of national and historical circumstances, and it must include a systematically related set of criteria surrounding a central issue. In short, it must be a logical, ideal, typical model. I suggest that the central issue of professional power lies in control of the work by the professional workers themselves rather than control by consumers in an open market or by the functionaries of a centrally planned and administered firm or state.

The character of such a model can be more easily visualized by first thinking of its opposite: the classic Marxist conception of the industrial proletariat composed of absolutely powerless workers. The industrial proletariat possess neither land nor capital but only their labor, so they have no choice but to work for those with capital in return for the wages by which they can gain a living. Their employers create, organize, supervise, and evaluate the work they must do, purposefully reducing it to simple tasks that any ordinary person can perform without special training so that the cost of labor is kept as low as possible. Thus, the proletariat possess only labor power, with no distinctive skill or body of specialized knowledge of their own and no control over the work they do. Furthermore, since their work is so fragmented by virtue of its simplification, they have little sense of its relationship to the productive whole or any sense of connection to their fellow workers or to society at large. Individually in the workplace and collectively in the marketplace and the political economy, they are totally without organization and power.

By contrast, professions with total power to control their own work are organized by associations that are independent of both the state and capital and that organize and administer the practice of an unambiguously demarcated body of knowledge and skill or jurisdiction, which their members monopolize. Those associations determine the qualifications and number of those to be trained for practice, the substance of that training, the requirements for satisfactory completion of training and admission to practice, and the terms, conditions, and goals of practice itself. They also determine the ethical and technical criteria by which their members' practices are evaluated and have the exclusive right to exercise discipline over their members. Within the limits of the rules and standards laid down by their authoritative associations, individual members are autonomous in their workplaces. And the professions serve as the ultimate authorities on those personal, social, economic, cultural, and political affairs that their body of knowledge and skill addresses. Their modes of formulating and interpreting events permeate both popular consciousness and official policy.

Scope and Method of Analysis

Both of these models are "ideal" in the sense that they are logically consistent extremes rather than faithful descriptions of any actual institution. Furthermore, they specify a number of different phenomena to examine, as well as the criteria for analyzing them. A truly comprehensive and authoritative appraisal of the power of any particular profession in time or place requires examining all the elements of the model rather than just one or two. In the case of the medical profession, for example, only part of its strength or weakness can be revealed by analyzing the formal administrative devices by which its services are organized and financed or by which its professional associations are linked with the state. As we shall see, without attention to the status of its specialized body of knowledge and skill and the character of its internal organization, one is unlikely to gain a complete and undistorted view of its powers, characterizing the whole by only a few of many equally significant but ignored parts.

Furthermore, it is essential that analysis not stop with gross, formal arrangements but examine both the full range of institutions that lie behind such global concepts as "the state" and "corporate capital," the characteristics of their personnel, and the concrete ways they formulate and implement policy. When an observer looks behind the facade of formal institutions to the way they are realized in practice, her or she gains a considerably more complex and precise view of the exercise of power or influence than is provided by official charters, tables of organization, and legislation.

Finally, a methodological point is important. In undertaking analysis, it is essential to avoid the use of a misleading kind of rhetoric that is common in the literature that analyzes contemporary professional power as historic process—a rhetoric that masquerades anticipation of the future as description of the present.

In historic studies of the process by which a profession developed over some period in the past, analysis is of events that have actually occurred. However, in studies of present-day professions that adopt a processual approach, the rhetorical emphasis of far too many is on events that have not yet occurred. For example, significance is read into newly instituted financial policies and administrative mechanisms designed to exercise more control over professional work largely on the assumption that they will continue and grow in the future. Yet the corridors of history are littered with policies that have been greatly modified, or even reversed, in the face of political challenge after their initiation, and others that have been subverted and turned to the advantage of those they were intended to control.

Furthermore, the significance of new and truly important recent events bearing on professional power is seriously exaggerated by the use of a rhetoric that implies their continuous growth into the future. In the case of health affairs in the United States, those who stress the significance of the activity of consumers in changing the balance of power in the consulting room use a rhetoric that does not describe the existing strength of the consumer movement but instead declares it to be "growing." Such relatively new institutional forms as for-profit, lay-investor-owned health care enterprises are described as "increasing rapidly." Although they are now proportionally few, they are discussed as if they will become the dominant form in the future. Yet we know from history that change is heavily contingent on unpredictable natural, political, and economic circumstances. Many institutions that were developed with high hope (or contemplated with despair) in the past have failed to become the norm—some disappearing entirely and others persisting only as a minor, specialized form. The assumption of steady, linear growth of any institution into the future is often unjustified.

We also know that some critically important circumstances affecting the position of professions occur cyclically rather than grow continuously or persist indefinitely. To take an obvious example, capitalist economies characteristically follow a cycle of boom, bust, and then, eventually, boom again. Thus, it is probably as mistaken to project the economic difficulties of the 1990s into the indefinite future as it was to project the boom (and social movements) of the 1960s into the present. Similarly, it is treacherous to assume that an "oversupply" of practitioners today will continue into the future and permanently affect the market position of professionals. The history of many professions in many nations shows that perceived oversupply stimulates efforts to restrict future supply and that demand itself can expand to create relative scarcity.

In sum, it is essential for fruitful discussion that analyses of the contemporary position of professions make a clear distinction between describing and appraising what actually exists today and prophesying the direction of change in the future. In describing the present, the most informative analysis is one guided by a systematic model, eschewing reliance on global concepts while emphasizing concrete institutions and the processes that underlie them. In the case of prophesying, or projecting trends into the future, due caution requires being aware of the danger of mistaking short-term, ephemeral trends for long-term trends and cyclical change for linear, progressive change.

The Complexity of Professions

The model of professionalism that I sketched contains a number of interrelated and sometimes interdependent parameters, but the literature analyzing the status and power of professions rarely goes beyond discussing the income, prestige, and working conditions of rank-and-file practitioners or the political and economic activities of corporate professional bodies. Those topics are certainly important, but there is much more to a profession. Its members do not constitute a homogeneous aggregate; rather, they are differentiated by substantive specialties and segments, by varying circumstances of practice, by their roles as rank-and-file practitioner, teacher, researcher, and manager, and by their relative preeminence as cultural, political, and intellectual leaders within the profession and in the lay world. These differences are often mirrored in separate associations, or sections within an association, including both associations devoted to the political and economic interests of their members and those devoted primarily to the advancement and communication of scientific or scholarly knowledge and procedures. In addition, some associations may be formally allied with particular political parties.

It is only when we conceive of the composition and organization of a profession in such broad terms that we can visualize the kind of influence claimed by those who invoke "technocracy" and the power of "technique" in shaping public policy (e.g., Ellul 1964), as well as those asserting professional "hegemony" and "monopoly of discourse" in shaping public consciousness (e.g., Illich 1980). The sole generic resource of professions is, like all labor, their capacity to perform particular kinds of work. They distinguish themselves from other occupations by the particular tasks they claim and by the special character of the knowledge and skill required to perform them. The authority of knowledge is central to professionalism and is expressed and conveyed by a variety of agents and institutions; it is not solely contingent on practitioner-client relationships or on the official activities of associations.

Furthermore, professions are differentiated by intellectual orientation and substantive emphasis, as well as by substantive specialty, work setting, and role. It must be assumed that any profession will contain more than one orientation toward its body of knowledge and skill, with contending theories and practices advanced by different formal specialties and informal segments or schools. Thus, different members of the same profession can advance markedly different ideas and still remain bona-fide members, even if of a minority school of thought that is ignored by the official representatives of the profession and deprecated by the majority. They may also have a separate association of their own that speaks independently of the one taken to represent the profession as a whole. One should not rule minority views within a profession out of bounds, or "unprofessional," because schools of thought and accepted practices shift in prominence and change over time. If minority views are ruled out, the capacity is lost to trace the many informal and unofficial ways by which segments of professional knowledge influence human affairs and professions themselves change. This is nowhere more apparent than in the relation of the professions to the state, for those in power may find a minority school of professional thought more compatible with their political ideology than the majority and initiate a considerable shift in the fortunes of the members of each.

The Activities of the State and Its Agencies

Comparativists have rightly noted that nations differ greatly in the degree to which the state and its agencies exercise centralized control over social and economic institutions. At one extreme is "high stateness" (Heidenheimer 1989:530–31), exemplified by a nation like the former Soviet Union. It had a centrally planned (command) political economy, governed unilaterally by the Communist party in conjunction with state agencies, and it permitted the existence of few if any independent, "private" associations or enterprises. Somewhat less extreme is a nation like France, which has a strong central government that engages in centralized control and planning but allows considerable room for independent economic and political activities. Still less centralized is Germany, with a federal structure in which a national government lays down and enforces basic rules within which strong provincial or state (*Länd*) governments exercise control over the economic and social activities within their jurisdiction through their well-developed civil service but allow much organized, private activity. At the other extreme is "low stateness," exemplified by the United States, which has a comparatively passive national government that allows extensive autonomy to federated state governments and to private associations and economic enterprises. National and state governments organize and control few social or economic enterprises of their own, relying instead on private agents to do so and acting more as referees than as active players in the political economy.

The tendency in the literature is to assume that in high-stateness nations professions have little power because they cannot organize themselves as private, autonomous groups. Indeed, largely for that reason Field (1957:45) describes medicine as having lost its professional status under the Bolshevik regime in the Soviet Union, and Jarausch (1990) claims "deprofessionalization" during the Nazi period (though he sees it as a process that began during the Weimar period and declares "reprofessionalization" after World War II).

The implication is that under conditions of high stateness, when professions have no formal association that is independent of the state and state agencies are responsible for legitimizing and directing their affairs, they lack power to influence state policy toward the way their members are selected and trained, their position in the division of labor and the labor force, their income and prestige, their working conditions, and their relations with their clients in particular and the public in general. But such a conclusion can be sustained only by ignoring the way states must function in large, complex industrial societies. Even under circumstances of high stateness, at least some professions, medicine among them, can wield important powers.

If one avoids a holistic concept of the state and asks how it actually functions, one is likely to find many places where professional knowledge is a critical resource. Björkman (1989:29) suggests a number of major channels through which professionals influence state policy and action. I note just a few here. In order to exercise complete control over its political economy, "the state" requires concrete agencies—ministries of education, for example, or ministries of health. Furthermore, in order to function effectively, those agencies must be staffed with personnel who know enough about their domains to be able to formulate relevant directives and understand and evaluate the information received from the practicing institutions under their jurisdiction.

In appraising the status of professions in circumstances in which they have no autonomous associations and are ostensibly creatures of the state, it is therefore critical to examine the qualifications of those chosen to direct and staff the agencies that formulate and implement policy in their domains. If the staff is composed solely of laypeople without any professional qualifications, then we can say that the profession whose activities it directs is indeed powerless on that level. But except in truly revolutionary times, and even then usually only during a brief period, laypeople have not been appointed to positions involving the formulation and administration of concrete policies governing the organization and operation of such professional institutions as schools, hospitals, courts, factories, and research institutes. In the case of health policy in the Soviet Union of some twenty years ago, Navarro's analysis (1977:64–65) indicates domination by a medical elite of academic and clinical professionals. This hardly supports a characterization of deprofessionalization.

It is true that even in low-stateness nations like the United States, agency heads or ministers are often laypeople chosen for their political acceptability and reliability (Freidson 1986a:191–99) and that professional credentials must be accompanied by acceptable political credentials. But within those constraints, if they or at least the bulk of their managerial subordinates are qualified members of the profession, we must recognize that the profession exercises an important degree of influence on state affairs. The need for the additional credential of Communist or Nazi party membership, or of being a conservative Republican, does indeed qualify the power of purely professional credentials, but that does not mean that professional knowledge is actually replaced by lay ideas.

Often, changes in the direction of the state bring changes in policies connected with professional affairs—changes that can be quite drastic following a political revolution. Those changes need not be, however, and are usually not in fact, based on substituting lay ideas for professional expertise. Instead, they usually entail a shift in emphasis from one cognitive strand or school of thought within the legitimate body of professional ideas to another, as when a regime empowers professionals to advance policies oriented toward preventive care and public health while displacing those representing academic and clinical medicine. Such a shift cannot be said necessarily to weaken or deprofessionalize "a" profession so much as weaken one of its segments.

Similar considerations should lead to caution in evaluating the imposition by the state of political criteria for admission to the profession and the distribution of jobs, for even there, some members of the profession might consider qualification for practice to require more than purely cognitive skills. For example, when the state intervenes to establish affirmative action policies that give priority to the admission of women, blacks, the children of peasants, industrial workers, or other previously deprived members of the population to professional schools and practice positions, it overrules the segment of the profession that prefers other criteria (such as Shils 1982), but it advances the preferences of another.

It is also implausible to assume that even under a high-stateness regime, government ministers and their staffs are merely passive instruments of those who are ultimately in command. It is far more reasonable to assume that they have some significant commitment to advancing the fortunes of the domain for which they are responsible—that the minister of health, for example, will struggle for greater recognition and increased resources for health affairs. In general, even in an authoritarian and centralized state, where there is a state ministry for a professional domain, there is also someone with considerable influence seeking to advance some version of a profession's, or a segment of a profession's, interests.

Turning from the general formulation of state policy to its implementation, one must ask again what agents are involved. Some analysts have argued that in continental Europe, professions have markedly different status and power from those in English-speaking countries because the state and its civil servants, rather than private professional associations or their agents, set the standards for entrance to professional training, qualifying for practice, and obtaining positions in which to practice. But formal administrative authority does not tell us enough. In many such nations, state service is a major career option for professionals because state agencies concerned with professional domains need qualified people to do their work. And where does the state get its standards? Who creates the curricula of the state professional schools and the criteria by which competent practice is evaluated? Who creates entrance examinations for professional schools and qualifying examinations for practice, and who grades them? Such agencies routinely rely on the advice of "outside" professional authorities (often the faculty of professional schools) for setting standards in general and for formulating, approving, and grading examinations in particular.

Examinations represent only a small element of a much larger and more consequential issue: the setting of official standards in general. The affairs of an advanced industrial nation are extremely complex and can avoid chaos only by the institution of common guidelines that allow some predictability and reliability in the production of critical goods and services and in the procedures by which they are evaluated. In the United States, many such standards are set by private professional and industrial associations (Freidson 1986a:199–205), but as is even more the norm for state-centered nations, others are formulated by state agencies. If, as is likely to be true for even the most totalitarian states, authoritative professional expertise provides the substance of those standards, duly tempered everywhere by political and economic considerations, we find additional evidence of its influence. That official standards are implemented or enforced by lay rather than professional functionaries is, of course, important, but this does not reduce the importance of the professional source of the standards they are obliged to follow.

I hope it is clear by now that when we avoid addressing the state as a formal monolith, look beyond the facade into its internal organization and the characteristics of its personnel, and examine how policy is implemented and by whom, we can see how professionals can exercise important kinds of control over the position of their profession. And we can see more potential for influence by examining the activities of those who have the ears of the powerful. No study worth its salt can afford to assume that state policy is made solely by formal committees and agencies. A leader, elected or unelected, exercises influence out of proportion to being merely one individual, and below the head of state there are other more than ordinarily influential ministers. But none of them, however absolute, tyrannical, or even mad, can function without the advice of others; there are too many issues and too many details for one person to command. In matters connected with the domains of the professions, therefore, we must ask: Who, beyond official representatives of the profession, has the ears of leaders, who are the trusted advisers without portfolio or public recognition? In scientific affairs in the former Soviet Union, for example, D. H. Lysenko's role as influential adviser was notorious, as were the roles of a handful of physical scientists in the United States during the 1940s and 1950s. Quite apart from the formal advice advanced by professional organizations and their official representatives, individual professionals who are considered to be the source of especially authoritative knowledge must be counted among the sources of influence that contribute to the sum of professional power.

The Concentration, Organization, and Disposition of Capital

Professions have no intrinsic resources other than their command over a body of knowledge and skill that has not been appropriated by others. However, cultural or human capital has no intrinsic material resources, so professions are dependent on economic capital as well as political power for their very survival, let alone their level of material and social comfort. How economic capital is concentrated and organized, therefore, cannot fail to influence the power professions have as corporate organizations and the autonomy that individual practitioners have in their workplaces. Nonetheless, its particular body of specialized knowledge and skill also plays a role in shaping a profession's position in the political economy.

When a profession's body of knowledge and skill is such that it can characteristically provide a personal service to individual clients, its members have more leeway to find work than would otherwise be the case. Members of professions like medicine and law have the option of practicing independently of organizations, of being self-employed. But such professionals as engineers, professors, clergy, and scientists must work in and for organizations.

Some analysts have taken the formal status of self-employment to be a major index of the capacity of professions to dominate the terms, conditions, and goals of work, but in fact this cannot be the case except under very favorable circumstances (Freidson 1986a:123–30). When economic resources are profusely distributed among a large population of individuals eagerly seeking a professional service and when the number of practitioners is relatively small, self-employment provides considerable freedom for professionals to control the content, terms, conditions, and goals of their work. The growth of such a favorable marketplace for medicine in the nineteenth century shifted dependence on a few very wealthy patrons who did not hesitate to impose their prejudices on those they consulted to dependence on a multitude of individuals able to pay fees out of pocket and willing to accept professional authority. Jewson (1974) suggests that the change from patronage by the few to patronage by the many (Johnson 1972:41–47) also changed the very content of medicine itself.

The twentieth century has seen yet another major shift in the organization of the medical marketplace from patronage by many to mediation between practitioner and consumer by concentrations of state or private capital. This, too, is likely to change some of the content of medicine and the strategy of its practice. Yet throughout the two centuries during which these two major changes have occurred in medicine, its practitioners in most capitalist nations have been nominally self-employed. This suggests that self-employment is too crude a measure of the degree to which professions are free to control their own work.

Neither is the formal status of being employed a useful measure of professional power. Both the structure of the marketplace and the organization of firms or agencies vary in ways that can make an enormous difference in the power of professionals to determine the content, terms, conditions, and goals of their work. The fact that professional skills are both discretionary in character and transferable from one work setting to another rather than being firm-specific in itself reduces dependence on any single institution for employment, particularly when both credentialism and conscious efforts to limit the supply of qualified professionals sustain high demand and when resources are plentiful.

Furthermore, considerable variation in the concrete ways organizations are administered and staffed cannot fail to have differential impact on practitioners. Organizations in which professionals work may be owned by the state, by a for-profit or nonprofit organization, or by some, if not all, of the professional workers themselves. They may be free-standing, like an engineering, architectural, or law firm, or a subordinate unit of a larger enterprise, like a research and development, architectural design, or law department in a firm or agency. Direction may be by either a lay or a professionally credentialed executive officer who may be selected by and responsible to either lay outsiders who exercise ultimate political or economic control or the professional members of the organization itself. Such variations in the concrete arrangements of employment seem far more consequential than the gross fact of being employed.

In no case that I know of has genuine ''proletarianization'' or literal deskilling of professionals been documented. A significant measure of discretion seems to be an intrinsic social requirement for the work professionals claim. This zone of discretion may create, in turn, the capacity to resist efforts at control by others. Fortescue (1987) described how, in the former Soviet Union, where the attempt was made to extend political control down into the workplace through party cells or primary party organizations, shared professional norms in scientific institutes seemed to subvert the effort. Analyzing scientific research in the former Soviet Union, he rejected both totalitarian and vanguard party theories of control after documenting both the influence of prominent scientists on policymakers and the zones of autonomy carved out by the working staff and their supervisors in research institutes. Unfortunately, no analogous studies seem to exist for the other major professions in the former Soviet Union, but since countless empirical studies elsewhere have shown how those in concrete settings can transform, if not entirely subvert, formal rules established by higher, remote policymakers, it is essential for analysts to study not only how policies are established on the level of the corporate board or the state ministry but also how they are actually carried out in the workplace.

A final element of importance lies in the absolute amount of capital—the re-sources—available in an economy at large and in individual work settings in par-ticular. Both depend on the state of the economy itself, which is beyond the control of professions but which may seriously affect the position of their members in the marketplace. When the marketplace is relatively free, professions whose services are considered essential rather than a luxury are likely to suffer less from a depressed or weak economy than others. Furthermore, both the state and investment capital may choose to invest more resources in one sector of the economy than in another, as the former Soviet Union chose to invest more resources in industrial defense production than in health care.

Investment decisions, of course, change, so what they are at one time cannot predict what they will be at another. Nor are they made unilaterally, in a political and economic vacuum. Both influential individual professionals and professional associations are likely to participate in influencing decisions involving the allocation of resources to their domain. When an association is unified, well financed, and able to mobilize its membership for collective action, it is likely to have more influence on decisions allocating resources, as Wilsford (1991) argues in his com-parison of France with the United States. Within their own domain or sector of the economy, segments of professions struggle with each other over how the resources made available to them are to be divided up.

Knowledge, Culture, and the Public

My discussion thus far has been seriously incomplete in that it takes no account of three critical elements: the bodies of knowledge and skill claimed by professions, the public, and the institutions that convey to the public the information and ideas that shape its members' conceptions of themselves and their world. These three elements are essential for explaining some of the variation in allocation of resources to sectors of the economy and to different institutions within any single sector. They are also essential for understanding the demand for different professional services and the value assigned to them, the support the public may provide to efforts by the state or capital to enlarge, restrict, or control professional enterprises, and the prestige and authority of professions themselves.

The most pressing need confronting the study of professions is for an adequate method of conceptualizing knowledge. Although the literature does provide some useful distinctions (Halliday 1985; Abbott 1988: 33–58, 177–211; Larson 1990), modes of analysis are not well developed, and there has not been much examination of the different ways bodies of knowledge influence policymaking, culture, and consciousness. I have already mentioned the importance of the process by which official standards are developed to guide both the production of the material goods we consume and the staffing of the institutions we rely on for critical services. Underlying it is an even more important process: the role of professional knowledge in creating and explaining the officially accepted "facts" about the social and physical world that form our consciousness.

Those who produce and convey professional knowledge are in interaction with the institutions that distribute knowledge to the public. Much of what the average person "knows" stems from the approved texts used to socialize children in the elementary and secondary grades. Much of what *we* "know" stems from the texts used to provide "higher" education and "cultivation" to the children of the more privileged classes attending postsecondary technical schools and universities. One may presume that those texts draw heavily on professionally approved knowledge, although politics everywhere qualifies and sometimes circumvents professional influence to a greater or lesser degree. In addition to official texts, and perhaps even more important for shaping common knowledge and consciousness, are the mass media. Although they are sufficiently independent, in democratic nations at least, to be able to advance a considerable number of ideas that run against professionally approved knowledge, I would guess nonetheless that they rely on professionals as their authoritative sources of knowledge and interpretation.

How Dominant Are the Professions?

How dominant are the professions? Given the issues and the varied actors and institutions, it is clear that the question can only be answered arbitrarily and stereotypically. When the focus is on practitioners interacting with demanding consumers, the likely conclusion is markedly different than when the focus is on prominent professionals advising policymakers or being interviewed on television. Contradictory as they may seem, both are true, but both are equally partial. The larger reality of which both are but part is too complex to be reduced to such simple and sweeping characterizations as "dominant," "hegemonic," "proletarianized," "corporatized," "bureaucratized," "rationalized," or "deprofessionalized." Which segment of the profession is one referring to, at what level of analysis, and in what arenas? In no case in any industrial country today, including those with command political economies, can any one of those words accurately characterize all segments, at every level, and in every arena. They are too gross to characterize such a complex whole as a profession.

It is true that over the past forty years the rank-and-file practitioners of some professions have lost some of their privileges in many industrial nations, so one can rightly argue a relative decline in their position. On the other hand, when one looks at some of the other members of their professions in other arenas in those same nations, where both the state and capital depend on professional knowledge for formulating, directing, and legitimizing policy, one can argue for an increase in professional power over the same period.

But note my use of the word *argue*. It rightly implies rhetoric, the deliberate use of language to persuade. This, I believe, is at the bottom of the character of much of the discussion about the power of professions. We need a large, simple, but intrinsically vague idea to characterize a position in a striking manner. Such rhetoric is especially useful for teaching undergraduates, which cannot fail to affect how ideas are presented. It creates simple oppositions that provide convenient pigeon-holes into which students can sort varied data that otherwise can be overwhelming. And it is convenient for multiple-choice examinations. It is also a useful tool for scholarly activities, for scholars too need ways of labeling data in a simple and striking fashion and ways of attracting the attention of colleagues by presenting a stereotyped intellectual position against which to advance its opposite.

Simple opposites, however, are a poor guide for understanding. Because the value and integrity of knowledge depend on maintaining a comprehensive and sophisticated view of what is analyzed, we ought to avoid such simplification wherever we can. Before we even pretend to be able to determine whether professions are powerful or powerless, we must examine the entire range of professional institutions and their connections with the ultimate sources of power: the state and capital. Should we do that scrupulously, and examine the workings of the state and of corporate capital rather than merely their formal structure, and the actual professional labor process rather than the formal administrative procedures said to control it, we would avoid much of the sterile debate that has exercised us for so long and instead collect and exchange new, richer information that will be considerably more enlightening, even if not so striking or entertaining.

Acknowledgments

Dedicated to the memory of Dr. Magdelena Sokolowska, late of the Polish Academy of Sciences, who knew how to get good work done under state socialism. I am indebted to Helen Giambruni and Frederic Hafferty for helpful criticism of a draft of this chapter.

II

CROSS-NATIONAL
CASE STUDIES

5

Countervailing Power: The Changing Character of the Medical Profession in the United States

Donald W. Light

The medical profession appears to be losing its autonomy even as its sovereignty expands. With the more frequent use of physician profiling and other comparative measures of performance, together with the ability of sophisticated programmers to capture the decision-making trees of differential diagnosis on computers so well that they can check out and improve the performance of practitioners, theories of professionalism that rest on autonomy as their cornerstone need to be reconstructed from the ground up (Light 1988).

Although physicians play a central role in developing tools for scrutinizing the core of professional work, they work for purchasers who use them for the external measure of quality and cost-effectiveness. Thus, not only autonomy but also the monopoly over knowledge as the foundation of professionalism is thrown into question. The computerized analysis of practice patterns and decision making, together with the growth of active consumerism, constitute deprofessionalization as a trend (Haug 1973; Haug and Lavin 1983). Patients, governments, and corporate purchasers are taking back the cultural, economic, and even technical authority long granted to the medical profession.

The sovereignty of the profession nevertheless is growing. Evan Willis (1988) was the first to distinguish between autonomy over one's work and sovereignty over matters of illness. The sovereignty of medicine expands with advances in pharmacology, molecular biology, genetics, and diagnostic tools that uncover more and more pathology not known before. Although chronicity is the residue of cure and the growing proportion of insoluble problems is providing a new legitimacy to nonmedical forms of healing, care, and therapy, no other member of the illness trade has a knowledge and skill base that is expanding so rapidly as is the physician's.

This chapter describes the changes in the American medical profession over the past two decades and outlines the concept of countervailing power as a useful way to understand the profession's relations with the economy and the state.

Some Limitations of Current Concepts

In the special issue of the *Milbank Quarterly* out of which this book emerged, Sol Levine and I reviewed the concepts of professional dominance, deprofessionalization, proletarianization, and corporatization (Light and Levine 1988). Each has its truth and limitations. Each captures in its word one characteristic and trend, but this means that each mistakes the part for the whole and for the future. One set predicts the opposite of the other, yet neither can account for reversals. This is best illustrated by the oldest concept among them, professional dominance.

Professional dominance captured in rich complexity the clinical and institutional grip that the profession had over society in the 1960s, a formulation that supplanted Parson's benign and admiring theoretical reflections of the 1940s and 1950s (Freidson 1970*a*, 1970*b;* Light 1989). But the concept of professional dominance cannot account for decline; dominance over institutions and resources leads only to still more dominance. As the very fruits of dominance itself weakened the profession from within and prompted powerful changes from without, the concept has become less useful. In its defense, Freidson (1984, 1985, 1986*e*, 1989) has been forced to retreat from his original concept of dominance, by which he meant control over the cultural, organizational, economic, and political dimensions of health care, to a much reduced concept that means control over one's work and those involved in it. Even that diminution to the pre-Freidson concept of professionalism may not stand, given the fundamental challenges to autonomy.

Space precludes reiterating the limitations of the other concepts, but it is worth noting the danger of conflating many by-products of professional dominance after World War II (such as increasing complexity, bureaucratization, and rationalization) with recent efforts by investors to corporatize medicine and by institutional payers such as governments and employers to get more effective health care for less money. The concept of corporatization in particular includes five dimensions that characterize medical work today as segmented and directed by the administrators of for-profit organizations that control the facilities, the technology used, and the remuneration of the physician-workers (McKinlay 1988). As the empirical part of this chapter shows, this characterization is not typical and does not capture the complex relations between doctors and corporations.

The Concept of Countervailing Powers

Sociology needs a concept or framework that provides a way of thinking about the changing relations over time between the profession and the major institutions with which it interacts. The concept of countervailing powers builds on the work of Johnson (1972) and Larson (1977), who analyzed such relations with a dynamic subtlety not found elsewhere. Montesquieu (de Secondat Montesquieu 1748) first developed the idea in his treatise about the abuses of absolute power by the state and the need for counterbalancing centers of power. Sir James Steuart (1767) developed it further in his ironic observations of how the monarchy's promotion of commerce to enhance its domain and wealth produced a countervailing power that tempered the absolute power of the monarchy and produced a set of interdependent relationships. One might discern a certain analogy to the way in which the American medical profession encouraged the development of pharmaceutical and medical supply companies within the monopoly markets it created to protect its own autonomy. They enriched the profession and extended its power, but increasingly on their terms.

The concept of countervailing powers focuses attention on the interactions of a few powerful actors in a field in which they are inherently interdependent yet distinct. If one party is dominant, as the American medical profession has been, its dominance is contextual and likely to elicit countermoves eventually by other powerful actors in an effort not to destroy it but to redress an imbalance of power. "Power on one side of a market," wrote John Kenneth Galbraith (1956:113) in his original treatise on the dynamics of countervailing power in oligopolistic markets, "creates both the need for, and the prospect of reward to the exercise of countervailing power from the other side." In states where the government has played a central role in nurturing professions within the state structure but has allowed the professions to establish their own institutions and power base, the professions and the state go through phases of harmony and discord in which countervailing actions emerge. In states where the medical profession has been largely suppressed, we now see their rapid reconstitution once governmental oppression is lifted.

Countervailing moves are more difficult to accomplish and may take much longer when political and institutional powers are involved than in an economic market. Nevertheless, dominance tends to produce imbalances, excesses, and neglects that anger other countervailing (latent) powers and alienate the larger public. These imbalances include internal elaboration and expansion that weaken the dominant institution from within, a subsequent tendency to consume more and more of the nation's wealth, a self-regarding importance that ignores the concerns of its clients or subjects and institutional partners, and an expansion of control that exacerbates the impact of the other three. Other characteristics of a profession that affect its relations with countervailing powers are the degree and nature of competition with adjacent professions, about which Andrew Abbott (1988) has written with such richness, the changing technological base of its expertise, and the demographic composition of its membership.

As a sociological concept, countervailing powers is not confined to buyers and sellers; it includes a handful of major political, social, and other economic groups that contend with each other for legitimacy, prestige, and power, as well as for markets and money. Deborah Stone (1988) and Theodore Marmor with Jonathan Christianson (1982) have written insightfully about the ways in which countervailing powers attempt to portray benefits to themselves as benefits for everyone or to portray themselves as the unfair and damaged victims of other powers (particularly the state), or to keep issues out of public view. Here, the degree of power consists of the ability to override, suppress, or render as irrelevant the challenges by others, either behind closed doors or in public.

Because the sociological concept of countervailing powers recognizes several parties, not just buyers and sellers, it opens the door to alliances between two or more parties. These alliances, however, are often characterized by structural ambiguities, a term based on Merton and Barber's (1976) concept of sociological ambivalence that refers to the cross-cutting pressures and expectations experienced by an institution in its relations with other institutions (Light 1983:345–46). For example, a profession's relationships to the corporations that supply it with equipment, materials, and information technology both benefit the profession and make it dependent in uneasy ways. The corporations can even come to control professional practices in the name of quality. Alliances with dominant political parties (Krause 1988b; Jones 1991) or with governments are even more fraught with danger. The alliance of the German medical profession with the National Socialist party, for example, so important to establishing the party's legitimacy, led to a high degree of governmental control over work and even the professional knowledge base (Jarausch 1990; Light, Liebfried, and Tennstedt 1986).

Countervailing Powers in American Medicine

In the case of the American medical profession, concern over costs, unnecessary and expensive procedures, and overspecialization grew during the 1960s to the "crisis" announced by President Richard Nixon, Senator Edward Kennedy, and many other leaders in the early 1970s. President Nixon attempted to establish a national network of health maintenance organizations (HMOs) bent on efficiency and cost-effectiveness. He and the Congress created new agencies to regulate the spending of capital, the production of new doctors, and even the practice of medicine through institutionalized peer review. All of these were done gingerly at first, in a provider-friendly way. When, at the end of the 1970s, little seemed to have changed, the government and corporations launched a much more adversarial set of changes, depicted in Table 5.1. The large number of unnecessary procedures, the unexplained variations in practice patterns, the unclear answers to rudimentary questions about which treatments were most cost-effective, and the burgeoning bills despite calls for self-restraint had eroded the sacred trust enjoyed by the profession during the golden era of medicine after World War II. To some degree, the dominance of the medical profession had been allowed on the assumption that physicians knew what they were doing and acted in the best interests of society. Unlike the guilds of earlier times, however, the medical profession had failed to exercise controls over products, practices, and prices to ensure uniformly good products at fair prices.

The reassertion of the payers' latent countervailing powers called for a concentration of will and buying power that was only partially achieved. Larger corporations, some states, and particularly the federal government changed from passively paying bills submitted by providers to scrutinizing bills and organizing markets for competitive contracts that covered a range of services for a large pool of people. The health insurance industry, originally designed to reimburse hospitals and doctors, was forcefully notified that it must serve those who pay the premiums or lose business. Today, thousands of insurance sales representatives are now agents of institutional buyers, and insurance companies have developed a complex array of managed care products. Hundreds of utilization management companies and entire divisions of insurance companies devoted to designing these products have arisen (Gray and Field 1989:Ch. 3).

Table 5.1. Axes of change in the American health care system

Dimensions	Provider driven	Buyer driven
Ideological	Sacred trust in doctors	Distrust of doctors' values, decisions, even competence
Economic	Carte blanche to do what seems best; power to set fees; incentives to specialize, develop techniques	Fixed prepayment or contract with accountability for decisions and their efficacy
	Informal array of cross-subsidizations for teaching, research, charity care, community services	Elimination of "cost shifting"; pay only for services contracted
Political	Extensive legal and administrative power to define and carry out professional work without competition and to shape the organization and economics of medicine	Minimal legal and administrative power to do professional work but not shape the organization and economics of services
Clinical	Exclusive control of clinical decision making	Close monitoring of clinical decisions—their cost and their efficacy
	Emphasis on state-of-the-art specialized interventions; disinterest in prevention, primary care, and chronic care	Emphasis on prevention, primary care, and functioning; minimize high-tech and specialized interventions
Technical	Political and economic incentives to develop new technologies in protected markets	Political and economic disincentives to develop new technologies
Organizational	Cottage industry	Corporate industry
Potential disruptions and dislocations	Overtreatment; iatrogenesis; high cost; unnecessary treatment; fragmentation; depersonalization	Undertreatment; cuts in services; obstructed access; reduced quality; swamped in paperwork

These changes have produced analogous changes among providers: more large groups, vertically integrated clinics, preferred provider organizations (PPOs), health maintenance organizations (HMOs), and hospital-doctor joint ventures. When the federal government created and implemented a national schedule of prospective payments for hospital expenses, termed diagnosis related groups (DRGs), doctors and health care managers countered by doing so much more business outside the DRG system that they consumed nearly all the billions saved on inpatient care. Congress more than ever now regards doctors as the culprits, and it has countered by instituting a fee schedule based on costs. In response, the specialities affected have joined hands in a powerful political countermove designed to water down the sharp reductions in the fee schedule for surgeons and technology-based specialists (like radiologists).

Thus, although the buyers' revolt depicted in Table 5.1 spells the end of dominance, it by no means spells the end to professional power. Closely monitored contracts or payments, corporate amalgamation, and significant legal changes to foster competition are being met by responses that the advocates of markets, as the way to make medicine efficient, did not consider. Working together (or, as the other side terms it, collusion), appropriate referrals (known as cost shifting to somebody else's budget), market segmentation, market expansion, and service substitution are all easier and often more profitable than trying to become more efficient, particularly when the work is complex, contingent, and uncertain (Light 1990). Moreover, most inefficiencies in medicine are embedded in organizational structures, professional habits, and power relations so that competitive contracting is unlikely to get at them (Light 1991).

On the buyers' side, the majority of employers and many states have still not been able to take concerted action, much less combine their powers. The utilization management industry has produced a bewildering array of systems and criteria, which are adjusted to suit the preferences of each employer-client. The Institute of Medicine (IOM) study on the subject states that the Mayo Clinic deals with a thousand utilization review (UR) plans (Gray and Field 1989:59), and large hospitals deal with one hundred to two hundred of them. Who knows which are more "rational" or effective? Moreover, the countervailing efforts of institutional buyers rest on a marshland of data. "Studies continue to document," states the IOM report, "imprecise or inaccurate diagnosis and procedure coding, lack of diagnostic codes on most claim forms, only scattered documentation about entire episodes of treatment or illness, errors and ambiguities in preparation and processing of claims data, and limited information on patient and population characteristics" (Gray and Field 1989:48).

In spite of this morass, a profound restructuring of incentives, payments, and practice environments is beginning to take place, and more solid, coordinated data are rapidly being accumulated. The threat of denial, or of being dropped as a high-cost provider in a market, has probably reduced treatments but in the process increased diagnostic services and documentation, a major vehicle for the expansion of medical sovereignty. Accountability, then, may be the profession's ace card as governments and institutional buyers mobilize to make the profession accountable to their concerns.

Changing Practice Patterns

Cost and Income

If the first round in the struggle to control rising medical expenditures consisted of tepid and unsuccessful efforts to regulate capital and services in the 1970s, then providers again emerged as the winners of the second round in the 1980s. They expanded services, took market share away from hospitals, packaged services to the most attractive market niches, featured numerous products developed by the highly profitable companies specializing in new medical technology, and advertised vigorously. Eye centers, women's centers, occupational medicine clinics, ambulatory surgical centers, imaging centers, detoxification programs: these and other enterprises caused medical expenditures to rise from $250 billion in 1980 to about $650 billion in 1990. This equals 12 percent of the nation's entire gross national product

(GNP), one-third higher than the average for Western Europe. There seems to be no way to avoid health expenditures' rising to 16 percent of GNP by 1995.

At the level of personal income, many physicians tell anyone who will listen that one can no longer make "good money" in medicine, but the facts are otherwise. From 1970 to about 1986, their average income stayed flat after inflation, but since then it has been rising. The era of cost containment and dehospitalization has actually been an opportunity for market expansion. Although physicians' market share of national health expenditures declined from 20 to 17 percent as hospitals' share rose between 1965 and 1984, it has climbed back up to 19 percent since then (Roback, Randolph, and Seidman 1990:Table 105). The profession appears thoroughly commercialized (Potter, McKinlay, and D'Agostino 1991), doing more of what pays more and less of what pays less. Although the profession likes to think it was more altruistic in the golden era of medicine after World War II, this was a time when physicians' incomes rose most rapidly and when it controlled insurance payment committees.

In addition, the range of physicians' incomes has spread. For example, surgeons earned 40 percent more than general practitioners in 1965 but 57 percent more in 1985 (Statistical Abstract 1989). As of 1989, surgeons earned on average $200,500 after expenses but before taxes, while family or general practitioners earned $95,000. All specialties averaged a sixty-hour week. Beleaguered obstetricians, even after their immense malpractice premiums, are doing well. They netted $194,300, up $14,000 from 1988, which was up $17,500 from 1987.

Despite the success so far of the profession in generating more demand, services, and income, the tidal force of population growth is against them. The number of physicians increased from 334,000 in 1970 to 468,000 in 1980 to 601,000 in 1990. By the year 2000, there will be about 722,000 physicians (Roback, Randolph, and Seidman 1990:Table 88). Although about 8.5 percent are inactive or have unknown addresses, the number of physicians in America is growing rapidly nevertheless, as it is in many European countries. There is no slowdown in sight, given the number of doctors graduating from medical schools and the nation's ambivalence about reducing the influx of foreign-trained doctors, many of whom are American born. In fact, between 1970 and 1989, foreign-trained doctors increased 126 percent compared to a 72 percent increase in American-trained doctors, and they constituted 130,000 of the 601,000 doctors in 1990 (Roback, Randolph, and Seidman 1990). As a result, the number of persons per physician is steadily dropping, from around 714 people per doctor thirty years ago to about 417 today and 370 in the year 2000. Will 370 men, women, and children be enough to maintain the average doctor in the style to which he or she is accustomed—about five and a half times the average income—in the face of countervailing forces? And how will the gross imbalance between the number of specialists and the need for their services play itself out? Today we have what could be called the 80-20 inversion: 80 percent of the doctors are specialists, but only about 20 percent or fewer of the nation's patients have problems warranting the attention of a specialist. Nearly all growth depends on an increasing number of subspecialties in medicine and surgery, and there are now about two hundred speciality societies, many not officially recognized but vying for legitimacy and a market niche (Abbott 1988). Thus, the rapid growth of physicians and their specialty training has set the stage for sharp clashes between countervailing powers.

Trends in the Organization of Practice

The post-Freidson era, from 1970 to the late 1980s, saw a steady trend of dehospitalization and a long-term shift back to office-based care. Most doctors (82%) are involved in patient care, and despite all the talk today about physician-executives, the data show no notable uptrend in numbers (Roback, Randolph, and Seidman 1990:Table A-2). Office-based practice has been rising slowly since 1975 (from 55% to 58.5%), and full-time hospital staff has declined from 10.4 to 8.5 percent in the same period. Hospital-based practice still makes up 23.6 percent of all practice sites because of all the residents and fellows in training. These data underscore the immense role that medical education, practically an industry in itself, plays in staffing and supporting hospital-based practice. The total number of residents has grown since 1970 by 60 percent, and they are a major source of cheap labor. They grew in use during the golden age of reimbursement, and curtailment of the work-week from 100 hours to 80 or fewer is already raising costs.

An increasing number of the 58 percent of doctors practicing in offices (that is, not a hospital or institution) do so in groups. Since the mid-1960s, when private and public insurance became fully established and funded expansion with few restraints, more and more doctors have combined into groups and formed professional corporations. The motives appear largely to have been income and market share. There were 4,300 groups in 1965 (11% of all nonfederal physicians), 8,500 in 1975, and 16,600 in 1988 (30%, or 156,000) (Havlicek 1990:Ch. 8). Supporting this emphasis on economic rather than service motives, an increasing percentage have been single specialty groups, up from 54 percent in 1975 to 71 percent in 1988. They tend to be small, from an average of 5 in 1975 to 6.2 in 1988, and their purpose seems largely to share the financing of space, staff, and equipment and to position themselves for handling larger specialty contracts from institutional buyers.

The future of groups will be affected by demands of the buyers' market. For example, almost all fee-for-service care now is managed by having an array of monitoring activities and cost-containment programs. These complex and expensive controls favor larger groups, and Havlicek (1990:8–38) believes we will see more mergers than new groups in the 1990s. He also suspects there will be more cooperative efforts with hospitals, which have more capital and staff but are subject to more cost controls.

Capitalist Professionals

An important, perhaps even integral, part of the rapid expansion of groups since the mid-1970s has involved doctors' investing in their own clinical laboratories (28% of all groups), radiology laboratories (32%), electrocardiological laboratories (28%), and audiology laboratories (16%). (Additionally, 40 percent of all office-based physicians have their own laboratories.) The larger the group is, the more likely it owns one or more of these facilities. For example, 23 percent of three-person groups own clinical laboratories and 78 percent of all groups with seventy-six to ninety-nine doctors. Large groups also own their own surgical suites: from 15 percent of groups with sixteen to twenty-five people to 41 percent of groups ranging from seventy-six to ninety-nine physicians. The hourly charges are very attractive (Havlicek 1990).

Growth of HMOs, PPOs, and Managed Care

The countervailing power of institutional buyers has forced practitioners to reorganize into larger units of health care that can manage the costs and quality of the services rendered. Health maintenance organizations, first developed in the 1920s, became the centerpiece of President Nixon's 1971 reforms to make American health care efficient and affordable. Medical lobbies fought the reform; when they saw it would pass, they weighed it down with requirements and restrictions. By 1976, there were 175 HMOs with 6 million members, half of them in just six HMOs that had built a solid reputation for good, coordinated care (Gruber, Shadle, and Polich 1988). Among them, PruCare and U.S. Health Care represented the new wave of expansion: national systems of HMOs run by insurers as a key "product" to sell to employers for cost containment or run by investors for the same purpose. Moreover, most of the new HMOs consisted of networks of private practitioners linked by part-time contracts rather than a core dedicated staff.

By December 1987, there were 650 HMOs with about 29 million members. Both Medicare and Medicaid revised terms to favor these groups as a way to moderate costs, as did many revised benefit plans by corporations. HMOs keep annual visits per person down to 3.8 and hospital inpatient bed-days down to 438 per thousand enrollees, well below the figures for autonomous, traditional care (Hodges, Camerlo, and Gold 1990). There were now forty-two national firms, and they enrolled half the total. The proportion of these firms that use networks of independent practitioners rose from 40 percent in 1980 to 62 percent in 1987. To increase their attractiveness, new hybrid HMOs were beginning to form that allowed members to get services outside the HMO's list of physicians if they paid a portion of the bill.

Preferred provider organizations come in many varieties, but all essentially consist of groups of providers who agree to give services at a discount. Employers then structure benefits to encourage employers to use them. For example, they offer to pay all of the fees for PPO providers but only 80 percent of fees from other doctors.

PPOs became significant by the mid-1980s, and by 1988 they had 20 million enrollees (Rice, Gabel, and Mick 1989). This figure is only approximate because patterns of enrollment are constantly changing. Perhaps more reliable are data from employers, who say that 13 to 15 percent of all employees and half their dependents are covered by PPOs (Sullivan and Rice 1991). Increasingly insurers are using PPOs as a managed care product, and they are forming very large PPOs—in the range of 200,000 enrollees each with 100 to 200 hospitals and 5,000 to 15,000 physicians involved in their systems. From the other side, physician group practices derive from 13 to 30 percent of their income from PPOs as group size increases. Besides volume discounts on fees, half to three-quarters of the PPOs use physician profiling (to compare the cost-effectiveness of different doctors), utilization review, and preselection of cost-effective providers.

In response to the "buyers' revolt" and the growth of HMOs and PPOs, a growing number of traditional, autonomous, fee-for-service practices have taken on the same techniques of managed care: preadmission review, daily concurrent review to see if inpatients need to stay another day, retrospective review of hospitalized cases, physician profiling to identify high users of costly services, and case management of costly, complex cases. By 1990, the most thorough study of all small, medium, and large employers, including state and local governments, found that only 5 percent of all employees and their families now have traditional fee-for-service physicians without utilization management (Sullivan and Rice 1991).

Conclusion

The countervailing power of institutional buyers certainly ends the kind of dominance the medical profession had in 1970, but by no means does it turn doctors into mere corporatized workers. The medical profession's relations with capital are now quite complex. Physicians are investing heavily in their own buildings and equipment, spurred by a refocus of the medical technology industry on office or clinic-based equipment that will either reduce costs or generate more income. Employers and their agents (insurance companies, management companies) are using their oligopolistic market power to restructure medical practice into managed care systems, but physicians have many ways to make those systems work for them. Hospitals are using their considerable capital to build facilities and buy equipment that will attract patients and their physicians, whom they woo intensively.

The state is by far the largest buyer and has shown the greatest resolve to bring costs under control. The federal government has pushed through fundamental changes to limit how much it pays hospitals and doctors. Each year brings more stringent or extensive measures. At the same time, the state faces a societal duty to broaden benefits to those not insured and to deepen them to cover new technologies or areas of treatment. And the state is itself a troubled provider through its Veterans Administration health care system and its services to special populations.

Both buyers and providers constantly attempt to use the legal powers of the state to advance their interests. Thus, regulation is best analyzed from this perspective as a weapon in the competition between countervailing powers rather than as an alternative to it. At the same time, competition itself is a powerful form of regulation (Leone 1986). However, Galbraith warned that the self-regulating counterbalance of contending power-blocs works poorly if demand is not limited, because it undermines the bargaining power of the buyers or their agents. This is another basic reason why institutional buyers are, so far, losing.

In response, buyers and the state are using other means besides price and contracts to strengthen their hand. Even as providers keep frustrating the efforts of institutional buyers through "visit enrichment," more bills, and higher incomes, a fundamental change has taken place. The game they are winning (at least so far) has ceased to be their game. Most of the terms are being set by the buyers.

The paradox of declining autonomy and growing sovereignty indicates a larger, more fundamental set of countervailing powers at work than simply the profession and its purchasers. As the dynamic unfolds, capitalism comes face to face with itself, for driving the growing sovereignty or domain of medicine is the medical-industrial complex, perhaps the most successful and largest sector of the entire economy. It is Baxter-Travenol or Humana versus General Motors or Allied Signal, with each side trying to harness the profession to its purposes. Different parts of the profession participate in larger institutional complexes to legitimate their respective goals of "the best medicine for every sick patient" and "a healthy, productive work force at the least cost." The final configuration is unclear, but the concept of professionalism as a countervailing power seems most clearly to frame the interactions.

6

Continuity in Change: Medical Dominance in the United Kingdom

Gerald V. Larkin

The preeminent position of the medical profession as a major factor in an understanding of the evolution of systems of health care now characterizes an international literature in the social sciences. In addition to this assumed centrality in the organization of health care, the profession has drawn the attention of sociologists interested in tracing the broader links of knowledge, work, and processes of social control in modern societies. In contrast to other occupations, medicine apparently has increased its autonomy, controlled its own knowledge base, and elevated its broader social status so as to exemplify one of the most developed forms of professionalism. As influentially analyzed by Freidson (1970a, 1970b) and Johnson (1972), among others, the profession has also gained a substantial degree of influence over its clients and control of an extensive range of variously allied subordinate occupations. Through all of these features, it has, until now, significantly escaped the managerial and bureaucratic organization that characterizes most other forms of paid work. These other occupations, by contrast, typically are exemplified by higher degrees of surveillance and control in both their immediate tasks and the context of their execution.

Although Freidson and others emphasized the importance of national variations in this picture, the professional ascendancy of medicine in both Britain and United States has been widely linked to doctors' convincing the modern state to grant them substantial autonomy. Against this background of a delegated trust, significant discord on medical autonomy has developed between the medical profession and government policies in Great Britain. Through the 1980s the U.K. government pursued a number of linked and accumulating themes emphasizing managerial effectiveness, cost containment through competition, and "value for money" in health care (Davies 1987). The outcome has been a closer surveillance of medical consultants' contracts, patterns of work organization, and clinical behavior. Under a declared intention to make the National Health Service more consumer responsive, lay managers, under centrally controlled performance contracts, have been promoted from formerly residual zones of administration to confront any opposition to these developments. In response, major medical associations and groups of eminent medical practitioners have openly and expensively advertised their opposition, most recently to the implementation of the government's preferred "internal market" in health care (Department of Health 1989), which makes hospitals, previously directly managed by health authorities financed by central government, compete for business from those authorities and general practitioners. Hospital managers, now charged with ensuring profitability for their unit, are thus encouraged to review medical activities. Changes in the boundaries between lay and professional control and the relative influence of varying medical specialties are underway.

In the United States, more government intervention in health care may appear on political agenda, but in Britain, the government is supposedly trying to reduce its previous centralized control by an advocacy of market principles. In reality, beneath these apparently contradictory policy rhetorics lie similar processes of intensifying governmental regulation of health care. Both are linked to common fears of escalating costs, ineffective uses of resources, and the range of ever-growing unmet needs in both countries. It is thus timely to ask whether a fundamental change in the nature of medical professional power is occurring in the United Kingdom, as may be developing elsewhere. However, given a possible convergence in state concerns and problems in modern societies, it is also important to acknowledge the significance of historical differences among them. These national variations will inform answers to such questions as to whether there are limits to any convergent trends, whether the medical profession is changing, whether the state is altering with consequences for medicine, or in fact that both are involved in an interactive process of mutual reconstruction variously involving harmony and discord. In answering these questions in the British case, a dearth of analytic studies of the recent rapid waves of policy changes can be noted, so appraisal of any possible long-term diminution in medical authority must be tempered with caution. As Hunter (1991) comments, the full interactive combination of professional responses to changes over the past decade and the accumulation of intended but also perverse policy effects has yet to be determined.

The variants of the professional disestablishment thesis, whether termed "deprofessionalization" (Haug 1988) or "proletarianization linked to corporatization" (McKinlay and Stoeckle 1988), together with their empirical foci, are discussed elsewhere in this book. As Elston (1991) points out after reviewing British evidence, neither of the two major alternative accounts amounts to a satisfactorily developed theory amenable to rigorous testing. Nevertheless, they are valuable perspectives and partly illuminate significant developments, and they may prod British sociologists to augment the paucity of analytic studies of recent changes in the major institutions of medicine in the United Kingdom.

Advocates of both the continuity of professional dominance (Freidson 1985) and its diminution (McKinlay and Arches 1985) may in part share a common misconception, as well as disagreements with each other, because of a common tendency to view medical professional dominance as strong in the past, whatever their assessments of recent qualitative changes in its character and context. In the British case at least, this assumption is questionable, insofar as medical authority over the past century has been both state sponsored and state circumscribed through a complex relationship of developing autonomy and control.

Asserting a change in or a continuity of medical dominance requires not only a sensitivity to historically different national experiences but also a clarity as to the base points and periods of change that are employed for comparative purposes. Theoretical positions drawing principally on American experiences in many ways are applicable but also require extensive qualification when applied to the British context, even if applied to the same time periods. Contrary to both "waxing" and "waning" accounts, both of which see professional dominance and state intervention as antithetical, state and professional power have developed together in the United Kingdom. Rather than assuming an inverse relationship, as Johnson (1982) points out, the professions are emergent as a condition of state formation, and state formation is a major requirement for professional autonomy. Within Johnson's perspective of an interdependence in mutual evolution, contemporary developments that constrain medical authority may seem to be less novel than similar occurrences elsewhere. They may be viewed at least as reemergent tensions rather than radically different features of the profession-state relationship.

The past one hundred years in the United Kingdom have seen both the evolution of a complex health care division of labor and the intensifying development of the modern state. The two are almost inextricably connected, and as such characteristically and inevitably fuel both the expansion (Freidson 1970*a*) and the enclosure of medical dominance (McKinlay and Arches 1985). Demonstrating this thesis is a major historical task in all the dimensions of change specified by either deprofessionalization or corporatization theses. Standing in contrast to accounts of professional authority in the nineteenth century, there is a shortage of empirical studies of the twentieth century. The former period was more characterized by Johnson's (1972) categories of oligarchic and collegiate modes of organization and the less-studied later epoch by state mediation, which both inflates and constrains professional power. By accepting Freidson's (1985) account, which narrows his earlier account of professional dominance more specifically to control over subordinate health workers and the powers of licensure as applicable within this century, it is possible to trace at least these facets through a linked and in other ways complex period of state mediation and medical power.

Medical dominance, Freidson confirms, primarily refers "to the relation of the medical profession to most other health care occupations in the division of labor." To establish and preserve such a dominance, the profession has to incorporate and subordinate actual or potential producers of health care. In Freidson's depiction, allied or cognate occupations were subjected in everyday medical practice to very close supervision and normally acted, in effect, under instruction. If allowed some autonomy, this in turn was constrained within a few degrees of carefully specified occupational freedom. Both immediate or everyday subordination and tolerated minor forms of autonomy in perhaps medically marginal activities were contained within an overarching national licensing system, which expressed and integrated medical professional control. In this argument the medical profession "stays ahead," by allowing only developments in the licensing system and patterns of interoccupational behavior that express those changes necessary for its own continuity. A continuing political agency is required, which in turn presupposes "the cohesion of the medical profession during its twentieth-century prime." This adaptive cohesion, as Freidson points out, is not inevitably preserved in current and future conditions of health care and its broader social context. There are dangers of professional fragmentation associated with ever-increasing specialization, diminishing market shares, and a failure to control rivals. Despite these perils, Freidson argues, the overwhelming evidence is for an adaptive persistence of medical dominance.

There is much in this account that illuminates the different British case, particularly regarding professional dominance over other occupations. Nonetheless, a closer examination of some key features of the past also may reveal some differences. A continuous struggle is evident through the entire modern history of medical professional ascendancy. In Britain, the medical profession sought, but did not historically win, any enduring direct control of other occupations within the broader health care field. The British Medical Association, for example, cannot match the role of the American Medical Association in licensing educational programs for allied health professions. Professional dominance in the United Kingdom was achieved through and with the state rather than expressed in a separate zone of autonomous activity. Its particular form of authority was state sustained, and although very influential in the drawing up of particular interprofessional boundaries, did not amount to a direct control over the broader development of the division of labor (Larkin 1983). With this distinction in mind between direct and indirect forms of professional dominance, the extensive historical role of the medical profession and some limits within its formative development may be traced.

A Profession-State Partnership

During the nineteenth century, with the exception of a limited number of urban voluntary hospitals, most formal medical care in Great Britain was provided through solo or very small practices. By the early 1900s doctors were facing the linked challenges of meeting a rising demand for health care and of establishing a new organizational framework that could control and deliver more effective forms of medical treatment. Against a framework of substantial scientific and social changes, hospitals and clinics were expanding with state support. These offered increased possibilities of treatment and standards of care, but in turn they required an elaborate work force to sustain their activities. At this point, neither the medical profession, seeking to stay ahead in the market, nor the state, in wishing increasingly to sponsor health care, possessed a formula for managing its growing work force. Instead, given their joint interests and within these particular historical circumstances, together they had to construct an organizational mode for an expansion of numerous occupations allied to medicine.

The partnership that developed between medicine and the state has several identifiable stages, reflecting the changing balance of interdependency between both parties. By the second half of the nineteenth century, the relatively organized character of the medical profession effectively limited any state choice of another agent of control over the growing health care division of labor. It was the first recognizably modern health care occupation to acquire state registration or licensing through the 1858 Medical Act. This placed within one framework of education, qualification, and regulation the increasingly convergent ancient "castes" of apothecary, surgeon, and physician. The unitary, if not entirely unified, profession was thus able to standardize its training and coordinate its activities, particularly as the accumulating scientific discoveries of previous and subsequent decades began to alter the character of medicine (Waddington 1990). The discovery of the principles of asepsis, of anesthetic and other more refined drugs and their uses, of further insights into the microprocesses of human biology, of aspects of x-ray and laboratory technology, placed the leading allopathic sect in nineteenth-century medicine in an advantageous position to respond to broader changes.

The 1858 Medical Act, which preceded many of those developments, had invested substantial self-regulatory authority in the emergent profession. This form of licensing nonetheless should not be confused with a full form of occupational sovereignty. The Act, while devolving the monitoring of standards of education and practice to a practitioner-dominated General Medical Council, also firmly tied the profession to the administrative responsibilities of the state. The standardization of agreed qualifications, for example, consolidated a bureaucratically identified class of registered medical practitioners, authorized as agents of the state to record the official existence of birth, sickness, and death. Professional emergence and state surveillance were linked in relation to the broader citizenry, and subsequently this link gathered force in the extension of medical services. The growing involvement of the state itself in the provision of these services in part was fed by the accumulating and increasingly recorded evidence of the social inadequacies of laissez-faire policies. An alleged physical deterioration of the population, as progressively becoming statistically evident through the latter part of the century, became central to policy concerns (Thane 1982). Ironically, although the British Medical Association officially opposed an associated tendency toward state intervention in health care, in reality doctors were in an oversupply for the private sector by the 1900s. Thus, they joined the expanding local authority hospitals, clinics, and government-backed insurance schemes that accumulated up to the inception of the Emergency Medical Service of 1939, prefacing the National Health Service a decade later.

The establishment of the Ministry of Health in 1918 led to a number of developments in the alliance of mutual interests between the medical profession and state. The expansion of hospital services and the development of new treatments requiring an elaborate supporting labor force brought a need to regulate potentially competitive occupational groups in the enlarging medico-bureaucratic order. Cooperating with the state in this task was a necessary part of market control for the medical profession, given a central vulnerability in its position in the preceding years. Despite the recognition secured by the 1858 Medical Act, its statutory protection through this measure was only one of title, a weak form of market closure. Through the Act, the medical profession had not achieved a government-backed monopoly of all medical services. It had no conferred legal authority to proscribe or in any way limit new and rival occupations implementing new medical technologies or perhaps older unorthodox types of practice and associated theories of healing judged incompatible with allopathic medicine. The profession thus had to capitalize upon its limited rights under law to realize their value. It opposed similar forms of legal recognition, however weak, for other occupations while it transformed its own titular monopoly into a criterion of state employment. Thus, whatever value was gained by holding a protected title of registered medical practitioner in a free market, its worth grew as that market diminished in relation to an expansion of government-sponsored services.

The credentialist requirements of a state-sponsored system provided an opportunity to upgrade a limited nineteenth-century market advantage into a twentieth-century monopoly of practice in the public sector. At the same time, this successful escalation of advantage pointed up the modernizing medical profession's dependency on state patronage. The greater value given to state registration within this beneficial dependency had to be protected against other groups such as herbalists and osteopaths seeking its extension to themselves (Larkin 1992). Medical dominance under state patronage was also evident in the structuring of relationships with orthodox but subordinate allied practitioners. Following the state registration of nurses in 1919 and dentists in 1921, many other emergent skill groups sought similar forms of legal status. The dentists in particular were an attractive example in their achieving not only a protection of the title "registered dental practitioner" but also a prohibition of all unqualified dental services. These advantages appealed to other groups in the marketing of services, such as ophthalmic opticians (optometrists) and chiropodists (podiatrists) who floated ensuing bills of their own. For a while, particularly through the 1920s, the new Ministry of Health supported the adamant opposition of medical interests to a further fragmentation and proliferation of professions. By the 1930s, however, these arguments came to be seen as somewhat atavistic and self-serving. For example, the medical profession's counterclaim for a monopoly over ophthalmic refraction tests was obviously untenable. There were simply too few doctors competent in its administration, and thus their claims impeded the effective delivery of optical benefit under the expanding provisions of insurance schemes. To regularize matters, a ministry-recognized official register of ophthalmic opticians was established in 1936. At this stage, the official recognition fell short of a statutory form of state registration, although both measures were vehemently opposed by the medical profession. The former limited development, however, emphasized some official reservations over medical monopolistic tactics that too clearly conflicted with state interests.

The conditional character of state support for medical dominance also became increasingly apparent in the hospital sector in the interwar period. By the late 1920s interoccupational tensions between doctors and what were then termed "medical auxiliaries" were subject to open debate within the British Medical Association. As argued by its council chairman, doctors required subordinates, and thus they should be active in shaping their emergent roles rather than simply rejecting their ambitions and aspirations (*British Medical Journal* 1928). This position stimulated a further series of debates over eight years culminating in the British Medical Association's founding the Board of Registration for Medical Auxiliaries in 1936. The establishment of the board was encouraged by the Ministry of Health, but as a mechanism for interoccupational control it was fundamentally flawed, by both continuing internal medical divisions on its necessity and the conditional character of governmental support afforded to its development. In the former respect, the profession remained divided between those who opposed any recognition for allied occupations and those who feared that such reactionary attitudes were likely to lose an opportunity to channel inevitable change through licensure in a direction favorable to medicine. To balance these internal tensions, the constitution of the board stipulated that it had complete control of all policy matters and that all registrants had a duty to work exclusively under medical direction. In reality, affiliating and aspiring medical auxiliary organizations were offered professional approval in return for a form of interoccupational fealty.

The terms of entry to medical approval so subordinated applicants that many would not join the new board. In other cases, paramedical associations were divided by the issue of affiliation. Additionally, the compensatory value of medical legitimacy in exchange for occupational obeisance depended on the scarcity value of that legitimacy, which would be diluted by the board's expansion. The main weakness of the British Medical Association's board, however, and the principal obstacle to its success was the voluntary character of participation. Although the Ministry of Health encouraged allied professions to join, it did not require them to register or make it a condition of employment in the expanding state-sponsored health care sector. Up to the inception of the National Health Service in 1949, the British Medical Association thus lobbied for a grant of statutory powers for its own regulation of all nonregistered health occupations. In response, this ambition, as in the case of medical control of ophthalmic services, again was judged to be unrealistic as the ministry's direct role in managing health services intensified. Ministry officials, some of whom were doctors, shared the medical profession's aversion to a plethora of state registration acts, with numerous associated supervisory councils for rival occupational jurisdictions. On the other hand, much as in earlier years, government officials were not prepared to support any total medical control of the private market; they were now unable to diminish the state's own managerial position by intensifying medical control over occupations increasingly in direct government employment (Larkin 1983).

By the late 1940s the British Medical Association's policy of dominance over the many emergent professions in health care was in disarray, insofar as its coverage was limited and any correcting extension conflicted with state interests. The recommendations of the Cope Enquiry (1951), established by the Ministry of Health but heavily influenced by the British Medical Association's pressure for strengthened control over allied occupations, were quietly dropped by the government, anxious to avoid antagonizing the latter in the new national health service, which began in 1948. Through the 1950s, with decreasing credibility, the premier profession unsuccessfully tried to oppose the state registration of opticians in 1958 and a further eight professions supplementary to medicine two years later. Medical dominance up to 1960 thus did not extend to either prohibiting developments in or totally controlling the emergence of other occupations. Nonetheless, it remained influential in their terms and pace of development. The medical profession was allowed a substantial but not determining minority presence on the final registration boards of other groups. No provision existed of the reverse kind through, for example, representation on the General Medical Council from other health professions. In addition, newly emergent licensed professions were limited from any encroachment on doctors' carefully guarded responsibilities of diagnosis and prescription, through codes of conduct enforced by the registration boards.

The state thus regulated medical dominance, in some important ways preserving medicine's premier position without endorsing medicine's preferred policies, to consolidate the extended occupational structure required for modern health care. This evolving policy of modifying medical authority to sustain its reformed continuity also received some support from within the medical profession. For example, the *Lancet,* through its editor (Fox 1956), welcomed a policy based on an ordered commonwealth of health professions in a partnership of senior and junior equals rather than a rejection of other groups' claims in line with majority medical opinion. In reality, the profession had no power to reject an extension of state registration to other occupations, and its opposition to such measures was decreasingly influential. Thus, in this sense, medical hegemony was modified in the postwar period (Armstrong 1976) but in continuity with some previous limits to professional dominance. The state had both constrained and promoted medicine's development through this century. Within this tension, the state's interest lay in the medical profession's role as a proxy manager for a division of labor increasingly subject to government supervision. A bureaucratized medical order thus developed, based on modified and dispersed forms of professional dominance linked to a hierarchy of internally autonomous but externally circumscribed occupations.

Developments in the 1980s and 1990s

From its position as a profession with a sizable proletariat of insecure and impecunious practitioners prior to the 1911 Insurance Act, doctors became collectively wealthier and established with each step in the evolution of Britain's state system (Klein 1990). With these benefits came a gradually attenuated tutelage over other occupations in the associated division of labor. Despite the existence of some earlier historical limits to medical dominance, nonetheless it can be argued that there is an accelerating rather than novel erosion of medicine's position in recent years. Evidence in support points to the new intrusions of nonclinical managers in organizing medical work, the resurgence of popular forms of alternative medicine, the growing range of vocal consumer and self-help groups, and problems of professional cohesion posed by ever-growing specialization (Elston 1991). These may amount to a threat of deprofessionalization, particularly if the premier profession is willing to respond in only terms that invoke past halcyon days of professional dominance over patients, administrators, and allied health professions (Armstrong 1990). However, professional responses to these developments are not complete, particularly with regard to doctors' now-encouraged involvement in budgetary management (Department of Health 1989), which may afford some medical groups further influence. Thus, their effectiveness in preserving the medical profession's position through change cannot yet be fully assessed. The establishment of the National Health Service in 1948 and the 1911 Insurance Act, although presented by medical leaders as damaging professional authority at the time, in retrospect can be seen to have strengthened it. After the apparent conflicts and reforms of the 1980s, the terms of a new concordat between both parties may yet emerge, representing a further mutation in, rather than sudden deflation of, professional dominance.

Whatever the contemporary character of the doctor-state relationship, interoccupational relationships may continue to change. The professions allied to medicine increasingly have set their sights on higher education and graduate rather than simply licensed status for their membership. This process is continuing, and these educational ambitions and the increasingly sophisticated nature of paramedical skills together could suggest new challenges within the medical division of labor. However, the base point for these developments should be noted, such that in the mid-1980s only 1.7 percent of nonmedical or dental health professionals qualified through university equivalent programs in England (Department of Health 1985). The overwhelming majority of health professionals are still trained in apprentice-type programs attached to National Health Service schools. However, it is also unclear whether further upgradings of training as such will result in major changes to the social organization of medicine rather than a generating of further strata in its division of labor. Within each profession, a minority group of graduates may take leadership roles, while initial entry standards and qualifications are lowered. Thus, "reskilling" and "deskilling" may be linked by policies aimed at increasing both graduate requirements and a much greater number of lesser-paid and -trained aides.

A combination of professional aspirations and government interests in restraining wage costs may extend the occupational hierarchy rather than dislodge doctors from the apex of the medical division of labor. However, changes in the local financial management of health services being implemented (Department of Health 1989) may create further pressures for forms of professional dilution. Since 1948, health service administrators have mostly accepted spending priorities as determined by professional interests (Harrison 1988). Up to the present, there have been no local financial benefits or other inducements—for example, retaining the benefits of reduced wage costs—that might challenge the structure of occupational monopolies in the workplace. Much professional activity, it could be argued, does not require such extensive training, which rather mystifies, and justifies as natural, an expensive range of restrictive practices. Nurses, for example, could take over aspects of medical work, possibly at a cheaper cost. The same case could be made across the range of professions and to some degree would receive some support from the winners in such a process. After all, moving into another group's occupational territory is a normal form of professional advancement. Technological changes fuel this process, as new areas of responsibility are created and older, jealously guarded occupational boundaries are abandoned.

Role boundaries, skill mixes, and professional monopolies as developed over decades have been funded from a national budget, but these may now locally be viewed differently. Following an accumulation of policy changes through the 1980s, amounting to a "celebration of managerialism" (Hunter 1991), the recent establishment of hospital trusts, permitted to opt out of national agreements on wages and conditions, may be particularly significant (Department of Health 1989). These units manage their own budgets within central constraints as trading entities within the National Health Service. Whatever their future, linked as they will be to the political fortunes of their promoters, it is intended that pay will be locally determined. This, however, will lead to plant bargaining if implemented, which is not necessarily tantamount to any form of deprofessionalization. Furthermore, any cost-driven attempts to break professional barriers in employment practices face constraints. These rest on the complex nature of many health care tasks, the continuing presence of professional mystification, and the legal liabilities of hospitals for the quality of treatment. In addition, the national government has not yet attempted any statutory overhaul of the web of existing national legislation that would be required for local agencies to take advantage of a deregulation of occupational monopolies.

The brief and controversial history of hospital trusts and allied policies leaves much unclear; however, it is difficult to anticipate any reversal of Britain's recent tradition of assertive managerialism, given the international ascendancy of the corporate rationalizers in systems of health care (Alford 1975). Similar pressures, linking cost containment to medical practice while meeting rising public expectations, face superficially varying political parties in the United Kingdom. Whether their electoral appeals are based on advancing or excoriating any extension of market principles to health care, all parties in the election year of 1992 emphasized effective management rather than a reemphasis of professional control as their way forward. Some caution, nonetheless, is still required before asserting an associated fundamental erosion of medical authority. Managements cannot deliver treatments, and, more basically, medical authority in a strong perception was an effect, not a cause, of an earlier period of partly mythical expanding budgets. Any forceful impression of medical professional influence in Great Britain in part was a product of an immediate separation of treatment choice and ensuing costs as carried into a national budget. Correspondingly, the recent and increasingly localized management of clinical budgets may indeed be perceived by practitioners as a diminution of their professional freedom. It is, however, a mutation in, and not necessarily an advance of, state control, and in part it represents a return to a pre–National Health Service era, when doctors faced many constraints on the cost of their practices. The national and local balance in containing medical authority and its effects on treatment costs has varied across time as state policies have responded to a host of factors outside health care.

In a number of ways, closer bureaucratic control may also endorse rather than dislodge the premier position of doctors in the medical division of labor. Although particular instances may be cited of medical activity's being placed under greater scrutiny, as, for example, in the monitoring of clinical outputs and their effectiveness, bureaucratic surveillance affects all professions. Those forces that reduce medical freedoms are more likely to have an even greater impact on originally less powerful or less established professions. For example, nurses in many National Health Service areas appear to have lost some powers of both intraprofessional management and their wider, albeit tenuous, involvement in overall health care planning through the 1980s (Strong and Robinson 1990). They appear also to have less effective professional defenses against continuous productivity pressures and associated staff cuts. The continuity or disestablishment of medical professional authority must also thus be related to a broader occupational context and an evaluation of the differential impact of any changes across a number of cases. There are difficulties, however, in assessing these because nonmedical health occupations, forming the majority of the National Health Service work force, have been notably less subjected to sociological scrutiny than the medical profession, while being perhaps most affected by the new managerialism.

State scrutiny, through a centrally monitored but invigorated local management of all health care activity, is intensifying through the National Health Service in Britain. On the other hand, state involvement has continuously both constrained and consolidated medical authority in ways that distinguish Britain from other countries. Coburn's view (Coburn and Biggs 1986) that a process of decline in the power of the medical profession is linked to state involvement may clearly apply when its power was deployed and indeed developed in a "free market" only latterly subject to governmental regulation. However, if at earlier stages the state supervised the emergence of a nationally coordinated service, in particular historical circumstances it may actually but conditionally promote medical hegemony. The medical profession is then employed in a managerial role within an expanding but also subordinated relationship, subject to neither a complete empowerment nor any opposite process of complete disestablishment. Thus, in Britain, all three concepts of professional dominance, deprofessionalization, and proletarianization need theoretical elaboration and empirical review to capture the full range of trends in state-profession relationships. Certainly all three perspectives require careful grounding in and qualification by varying historical contexts before major changes may be confirmed.

7

Professional Powers in Decline: Medicine in a Changing Canada

David Coburn

The changing nature of Canadian medicine cannot be understood simply through a historical analysis of events internal to the medical profession. The development of medicine in Canada is part of changing provincial, national, and international contexts.

Canadian medicine is functioning in an era of the triumph of capitalism on a world scale along with the hegemony of the United States as the leading capitalist nation. The international mobility of capital has brought reduced power for peripheral nation-states and for national working-class movements, and Canada has reflected these international trends. Neoconservative governments gained power federally and in a number of the provinces. Most recently, reformist social democratic (New Democratic party) governments have been elected in British Columbia, Ontario, and Saskatchewan and now govern provinces and territories containing more than half of Canada's population. Furthermore, the current (1992) Progressive Conservative federal government is the most unpopular that Canada has ever had, favored by only 12–16 percent in national polls. However, the more general neoconservative trend, economic recessions, the threatened secession of Quebec, and the effects of the recent free trade agreement with the United States (and potentially also with Mexico) colors all developments in Canada. The future of the Canadian polity and Canadian society, and medicine within it, is uncertain.

A major event influencing medicine was the implementation of government-sponsored health care insurance in Canada, itself a product of class struggle (see Coburn, Torrance, and Kaufert 1983). National health insurance has produced substantial change in the health care power structure. The medical profession is threatened both by government involvement (in Canada) and by market forces (in the United States).

Medicare (referring to national, universal, free, health care insurance, financed partly by the federal government out of general tax revenues but administered by the provinces) is not embedded in stone. In a time of fiscal crises, a conservative federal government is reducing the funds it pays to the provinces in support of medicare (and regarding higher education and social welfare). Decreased federal financing leads to declining federal leverage in ensuring that the provinces, which are constitutionally responsible for health matters, actually adhere to national medicare policies. This increase in provincial powers (and consequent possible national fragmentation in health policies) is being aided by those who argue that the only way to "preserve" Canada is to hand over to Quebec (and, some would argue, to all the provinces) powers formerly reserved to the federal government. The situation is fluid.

Social theorists in various countries disagree regarding the changing social position of medicine. Is medicine declining in dominance, deprofessionalizing, or being proletarianized? In fact, these concepts are not congruent, and medicine shows national variations. Here I use medical dominance as an orienting concept with which to analyze change in Canada.

Freidson (1970*a*) has described dominance (implicitly) as consisting of control over the content of care, clients, other health occupations, and the context of care. But Freidson's early contention that medicine is dominant in the health field failed to explain adequately the reasons for that dominance and to situate medical dominance within a broader theory capable of explaining changes in the role of medicine. Freidson's later (1985, 1986*a*) claims that medical power (in the United States) is not in decline are fatally weakened by his slide from a defense of the notion of medical dominance (control over others) to a defense of the more restricted idea of medical autonomy (freedom from control by others), partly due to a confounding of these concepts in his earlier work. Freidson's recent writings reveal an implicit admission of medical decline, one with which, in respect to Canada, I agree.

This chapter focuses on the possible decline of medical dominance since there seems agreement that Canadian medicine did rise, or professionalize, in the nineteenth century and did consolidate its power in the twentieth (Coburn, Torrance, and Kaufert 1983).

In this century, depression and war had important consequences for health care in Canada and for the medical profession. In the postwar era of general social reforms, universal access to health care became a prominent political issue. But the period before and shortly after World War II was characterized by close connections of medicine, state bureaucracies, and governments. Medicine was a "private government" (Taylor 1960) administering government-funded systems, opposing direct government intervention in care or in payment, and spreading its own physician-controlled (nonprofit) health insurance plans. Medicine was dominant within health care, although this dominance was contingent on the support of external forces such as business interests and the state.

Health care was to change. Change was signaled by the doctors' strike in Saskatchewan in 1962 in protest against the introduction of a (provincial) government-sponsored medical insurance plan (after the earlier implementation of hospital insurance, first in Saskatchewan in 1947 and then nationally in 1958). The strike failed in its major aims, although it forced some government compromises. A system of universal government-administered health insurance was in place. This successful provincial plan was to be "like Banquo's ghost" (Taylor 1978:353) at every subsequent national discussion of health care.

In crucial public battles after 1962, medicine could not halt or drastically modify the implementation of medicare on the national level. Once medicare was in place, the profession failed to prevent the banning of user fees (direct charges by physicians or hospitals to patients) and extra billing (billing patients for amounts above what the health insurance plan would pay). Given the financing of health insurance through general taxes and increasing costs, state involvement in health care broadened steadily, from an initial focus on costs and physicians' fees to a later emphasis on the restructuring of health care.

Medicine faced challenges not only from the state but also from emergent health occupations, the feminist movement, and patients. These external challenges, along with a more fragmented medical profession, brought the decline in the power of organized medicine that I examine here.

Medicine after Saskatchewan

In attempting to counter the spread of Saskatchewan-style medicare, medicine advanced its own doctor-sponsored voluntary plans. It also pressed the provincial governments that were ideologically opposed to national health insurance (among them, British Columbia, Alberta, and Ontario) to implement provincial programs that conformed to the profession's vision. Medicine wanted the use of existing voluntary plans, the freedom of doctors to opt out and to extra-bill, unilateral fee setting by the profession, and a predominant medical voice in administration.

The major event of the 1960s, however, was initiated by the Royal Commission on Health Services (Hall 1964). Health care professions were well represented on the commission, and the medical profession did everything in its power to influence the commission. Hence, the RCHS's recommendations for a universal, free, government-sponsored and -administered plan, hit the profession like a bombshell. It was to be seven years later, in 1971, and only after determined opposition by medicine, before health insurance was fully implemented on a national level (Taylor 1978). Despite the fact that health was constitutionally a provincial responsibility, one after another the provinces enrolled in a national plan. The provinces could hardly resist 50 percent federal funding for health care (in return for which they promised to fulfill the requirements of universality of access, government administration, and others).

Enacted at the beginning of a period of economic problems for Canada, health insurance was to be the last major social reform of the postwar era. Planned action on such matters as a guaranteed annual income were submerged in the surging tide of business power. Later, previously universal social programs such as family allowances and old age pensions were to be tied to income; that is, higher income families (as defined by the government) were to have their family allowances and pensions reduced or eliminated entirely.

Health insurance was, in essence, a financing matter. But costs, now publicly visible rather than hidden in the market, led to an increased rationalization of health care. The drive for efficiency directly influenced medicine's position as controller of health care.

The Industrialization of Health Care

Medical insurance was not the only impetus to change. World War II brought the beginnings of the "industrialization" of health care. These changes would have influenced Canadian medicine (though in exactly what ways is open to speculation) even in the absence of government-financed health insurance.

Costs rose, from 5.5 percent of gross national product (GNP) in 1960 to 8.7 percent of GNP in 1983 (declining to 8.5 percent in 1985). Hospitals become larger and more bureaucratic "health factories" (Torrance 1987). Between 1947 and the early 1980s, the average size of hospitals doubled. By 1981, Canadian hospitals employed more people than did automobile manufacturing, iron and steel mills, and pulp and paper mills combined.

Research monies increased dramatically with the formation of huge teaching research complexes. In Ontario alone nearly $150 million was spent on biomedical research in 1984–1985. Of this amount, 92 percent was channeled through faculties of medicine, leaving nursing less than one-seventh of the total devoted to veterinary medicine. Medical dominance partly rested on control of the research endeavor.

The pharmaceutical industry and the medical supply industry were massive undertakings. The major medical journals, and hence their sponsor, the Canadian Medical Association (CMA), were heavily dependent on drug advertisements. Over the years the CMA has strongly supported drug industry initiatives.

Health care was being transformed from a cottage industry to a big business ranging from medical school–teaching hospital complexes to medical equipment and supply industries serving a universal market. The entire industry was dependent, directly or indirectly, on the state funds administered by the "corporate rationalizers" of the provincial departments of health. In this transformation, medicine, once controlling most of the levers in a simpler system, became less central.

Medical Insurance: Its Immediate Effects

The onset of medicare prompted a huge number of provincial and federal studies, including the Castonguay-Nepveu Commission in Quebec (1966–1971), the Ontario Committee on the Healing Arts (1970), and the Task Force on the Costs of Health Services (1969). Almost universally the reports noted the ineffectiveness or inefficiency of the health care system and suggested that better health care could come about only with a reduction of the overwhelming control of medicine.

Medicine had the power to ensure that the actual reforms that followed these reports were much less radical than the recommendations made (for Quebec, see Renaud 1987). However, a surprising number of these recommendations, such as the regionalization of care and the use of community health centers, did not die completely but lay dormant, to be revived during the 1980s. Faced with fiscal crises, governments in the 1980s were now more determined to reduce health care costs, and they faced a more malleable, and more fragmented, medical profession. In their search for efficiency, governments were drawn, step by step, ever deeper into the restructuring of health care.

Extra Billing and User Fees

By the mid-1970s, two issues came to dominate medicine's external relationships, extra billing and user fees. The battle over these issues became symbolic of an underlying struggle for control over the health care system between the state (largely supported by public opinion) and the medical profession, one that, in the long run, the profession could hardly win. This conflict took place within a changing Canadian political economy.

In 1982 the Canadian GNP plunged to −4.8 percent, the worst showing since 1933. In the same year unemployment and inflation soared to approximately 11 percent. Economic policies after the mid-1970s signaled the end of Keynesian attempts to manage the Canadian economy (Wolfe 1984). Postwar efforts to balance the interests of capital and labor were "replaced by a one-sided preoccupation with the concerns of business" (Wolfe 1984:75). Health care restructuring formed only one aspect of attempts by a government-business coalition to cut all social expenditures.

Governments faced contradictory pressures. On the one hand, they sought to reduce expenditures; on the other, they faced strident calls from health care providers for increased health care funding. The result was a commission to reexamine health insurance (the Hall Commission, 1980). The profession strongly argued to this commission that the quality of medical care had declined because of underfunding. Its position, however, was publicly contradicted by both the Canadian Hospital Association and the Canadian Nurses Association (CNA). The Canadian Medical Association was particularly troubled by the CNA brief, which, in addition to denying the system was underfunded, called for the abolition of extra billing, greater use of nurses as first-contact health care providers, and for all health care practitioners to be put on salary.

After political battles pitting medicine and conservative provincial governments against a heterogeneous collection of social movements under the rubric of the "Health Coalition," the Canada Health Act, which followed the Hall Commission report, was passed in March 1984. The Act financially penalized provinces that permitted extra billing, and a year later, only Ontario and Alberta still allowed this practice. In 1985, the Ontario Conservative party, which ideologically supported medicine's fight to preserve extra billing, was replaced by a minority Liberal government supported by a social democratic party, the latter completely opposed to extra billing.

The bill to ban extra billing in Ontario, introduced into the Ontario legislature in late 1985, provoked the most virulent and public reaction from medicine since the Saskatchewan doctors' strike nearly twenty-five years earlier. The outcome was little different. A twenty-five-day strike, observed at most by 60 percent of Ontario's doctors and overwhelmingly opposed by the public, collapsed in disarray.

In spite of this defeat, the strike paradoxically indicated that medicine was far from powerless. The government did make concessions, which the profession, in the heat of the strike, unwisely declined. Nonetheless, the failure of the strike publicly confirmed a decline in the authority and influence of organized medicine.

It set the stage for discussion not only on fees but also on physician numbers, payment methods, geographical distribution, and even total physician costs.

Physician Fees, Incomes, and Costs

Given national health insurance, the provincial medical associations became the bargaining agents for their members. The medical associations became separate from those organizations, the provincial colleges (controlled by elected members of the profession) embodying the self-governing aspects of medicine. The colleges, in those provinces in which they had existed, represented the profession's control over educational standards, registration of practitioners, and the disciplining of its members. The associations came to be viewed as physicians' unions, while the provincial colleges began to assume the facade, if not the reality, of quasi-public bodies. Over time the colleges increasingly were constrained by government regulations or standards. Lay representation on college governing councils increased, as did lay membership on various college committees, including in some provinces on committees hearing patients' complaints against physicians. Governments defined new limits to professional authority.

Although in the two decades prior to 1971, when medicare came into force nationally, physicians' fees had risen 26.6 percent, between 1971 and 1985, relative to the consumer price index, "physicians' fees *fell* by 15.9 percent." In comparison, during the same time period, fees of doctors in the United States rose 15.6 percent (Barer, Evans, and Labelle 1988:19). (There were large interprovincial differences; physicians in British Columbia showed increases, and doctors in Quebec had the greatest declines [Barer and Evans 1986].) Incomes also shrank in the immediate postmedicare period, though not as much as fees, for physicians increased their utilization and mix of services to compensate for the lower fee increases (Barer, Evans and Labelle 1988). Yet fees are highly visible, and so confrontation between the medical associations and their provincial government paymasters became common.

The involvement of the state in health insurance brought vast increases in government health care bureaucracies. The physicians in government service were soon swamped by the new tide of corporate rationalizers: lay planners, accountants, and managers. Medicine, which had never completely controlled politicians but had greatly influenced health care bureaucracies, lost its previous close association with public officials. Conflicts over fees and the decline of physician influence on the bureaucracy produced ever-cooler state-profession relationships.

The concerns of state health planners moved from fees, to income ceilings, to distribution and staffing, and then to total physician costs. When control over fee levels failed to control costs, governments turned to individual income ceilings for physicians. When this measure too proved ineffective, physician fees began to be adjusted in response to physician income growth. Eventually provincial policies (especially in Quebec and Ontario) focused on placing a global cap on the amount that physicians in the province as a whole could bill (Barer, Evans, and Labelle, 1988). Barer, Evans, and Labelle (1988:46) conclude their study of physician fees and incomes across Canada by noting that "attempts to control fees lead progressively into more extensive management of medical care—controls *do* beget further controls."

Further limits to medical dominance emerged in hospitals, whose budgets were strictly controlled by provincial treasuries. Hospitals in Canada were never publicly owned, and yet they have never been profit-making enterprises. Doctors, once in de facto control but not legal owners of hospitals, soon experienced the limits and penalties of nonownership. Their control of hospitals was challenged directly by provincial concerns about hospital budgets, the regionalization and government allocation of technology and resources, new strata of planners and administrators at the provincial and hospital levels, and hospital-based occupations seeking increased autonomy. Physicians were also being co-opted into the administrative hierarchy of hospitals through the appointment of full-time heads of service. Physician-administrators had different interests from practitioners.

The Health Care Division of Labor

Medicine faced challenges from other directions too. Once-subordinate health occupations were struggling for independence. Nursing, traditionally controlled by medicine, began to seek "separate but equal" status. It attempted to develop an independent theory of nursing care (as opposed to cure), raised its own educational requirements, and emphasized nursing research. Nurses not only gained self-governing powers and control over their own organizations (in which doctors had previously had representation) but publicly challenged medical dominance over health care.

Similarly, other healers, such as chiropractors, have been gaining in public and official acceptance despite medical opposition (Baer 1984; Coburn and Biggs 1986). In Ontario and other provinces, chiropractic has secured official recognition as a self-governing health occupation (though at the expense of a narrowing of scope of practice). Even occupations always part of the formal health care system, such as physiotherapy and pharmacy, are seeking autonomy (e.g., to have physiotherapists rather than physicians as head of physiotherapy departments) or expanded roles (clinical pharmacy).

These occupational challenges were reflected in changing professional regulations. Quebec was only the first of a number of provinces to grant a whole series of health occupations self-governing powers on a par with medicine, although this new self-regulation was much less than that medicine had previously enjoyed.

In 1991, legislation passed in Ontario mandates a new system of twenty-four self-regulating colleges to cover twenty-four health occupations, from medicine to midwifery to massage therapy (Ontario, 1991). The legislation defines new scopes of practice that "will, to a significant degree, shift away from the governing bodies of a small number of licensed professions . . . the authority to draw lines of demarcation between professions' scopes of practice" (Health Professions Legislation Review 1988:16). That is, individual professions have the exclusive mandate to perform only a series of specifically mentioned licensed acts—thirteen in all. These licensed acts are much narrower than the scopes of practice that the health professions had previously claimed. Any "nonlicensed act" can be carried out by any of the health occupations. The boundaries between the health professions have been loosened.

The Ontario legislation also includes a much widened public scrutiny of the self-governing professions. For example, there will be almost as many laypersons as physicians on the Governing Council of the College of Physicians and Surgeons. All meetings of college councils and disciplinary hearings are opened to the public, an entirely lay board to hear appeals from decisions of the colleges' complaints committees (which hears complaints by patients or by practitioners denied registration) is continued, and an entirely lay board is established to advise the minister of health on professional matters. The legislation also gives the minister the power to require the college to carry out activities that the minister (now almost invariably a nonphysician) believes are in the public interest.

These developments strike at the heart of what it means to be self-governing. The organizations that defined professional autonomy have been infiltrated by public authority. Whatever Freidson's claims that, in the United States, medicine as an organized profession is completely autonomous, such is clearly not the case in some of Canada's largest provinces. (There is a good deal of interprovincial variation.)

Still, medicine remains the most inclusive health profession; it can perform more licensed acts than can any other profession. Thus, although professional power was diminished and medicine's control over even the content of work was touched, much power remains with the profession.

Patients

Pressure on medicine came not only from the state and other health occupations. The efficacy of medicine and its curative rather than preventive emphasis are being questioned by the general public. Patients seek to recover birth (alternative birthing centers and home births) and death (the living will, euthanasia) from medical control. The women's movement in particular has supported both more self-care by patients and more assertiveness by the largely female health professions.

Psychiatric patients have successfully challenged medical legal prerogatives regarding compulsory hospitalization or treatment. In Ontario, patient advocacy systems were proposed and in some instances instituted (in the Ontario mental health system), and new methods to enforce informed consent were proposed (in Ontario). Patient representatives came to be common in general hospitals.

Legal reforms followed these trends. The Supreme Court of Canada in the 1980s changed the criteria to be applied in judging whether adequate consent to medical treatment had been given from the information a "reasonable doctor" would give to the information a "reasonable patient" would want. These changes have not yet had much substantive effect, but they are potentially important and have a significant symbolic effect.

Legal actions and formal complaints against doctors reflect the general trends. In 1956 there were only 10 writs (a document indicating an intention to begin a legal case) issued against physicians. These numbers rose rapidly to 80 in 1970, reaching a peak of 915 in 1987. In the entire period from 1932 (when damages first began to be paid) to 1970, the total damages awarded all patients in Canada amounted to less than $2 million. Damages increased rapidly, to over $5 million in 1979 and over $25 million in 1988, according to the Canadian Medical Protective Association. The public, in groups or as individuals, is much less likely now to accord the medical profession, or individual doctors, a privileged social position.

Health Policy Innovations

The National Health Service in Britain had been introduced on the assumption that health care costs would decline as the population became healthier (due to better medical care). Neither health status nor costs have conformed to these predictions. Faced with ever-increasing utilization and with restricted revenues, governments in Canada reacted by revising their health policies. It was no longer assumed that more money for health care meant a healthier population. The 1980s brought a torrent of reports pointing to the social and life-style determinants of health status; *health promotion* and *healthy public policy* became the bywords (Pederson et al. 1988:8).

Organized medicine was faced with powerful pressures from within health care to rationalize and reorganize; from without, it faced public and official skepticism about the efficacy of orthodox medical treatments. There was increasing pressure to emphasize prevention. The official direction of health policy, although not necessarily the reality of day-to-day care, had slipped from the hands of practitioners to academic physicians and to the new corporate rationalizers.

Changes within Organized Medicine

Medicine itself is fragmenting. More physicians are being recruited for administrative posts. Many physicians now work in community health or public health and in the medical education complex (though the vast majority of physicians remain in private practice), groups with quite different goals from practitioners (Freidson 1986a).

There is an incipient split between general practitioners (50% of all doctors in Canada) and specialists regarding hospital privileges, relative fees, and professional–state issues such as extra-billing or the proposed induction of midwifery. Like other national groups, medicine also shows a deep split between medical organizations in Quebec and those in the rest of the country.

Medicine is changing in gender composition. In 1987, about 42 percent of Canadian medical graduates were women, and in that year women formed 47 percent of the entering class at Canadian medical schools. This continued a trend toward the feminization of medicine that had begun in the 1960s. The work patterns of female physicians suggest they are open to more routinized forms of medical practice, perhaps because of their double burden of work outside and work (and reproduction) inside the home. Medicine is being segmented and stratified by gender.

Medicine's Changing Context

Broader sociopolitical events also had their influence. In 1984, a newly elected Conservative prime minister, pro-business and pro-American, boasted to Prime

Minister Margaret Thatcher of Great Britain that Canada had business governments from coast to coast. This did not last long—both Ontario and Quebec turned Liberal—but this new liberalism was more conservative than the old. Throughout this period there were continuing tensions between Quebec and the rest of Canada. The separation of Quebec medical organizations from those in English Canada reflected the reality of this dualism.

The international mobility of capital (in Canada largely continentalism), paradoxically accompanied by an increasing Canadianization of Canadian labor organizations, led to more or less open class conflict over the Conservative party's proposed free trade agreement with the United States. Health care formed a major focus for the 1988 election campaign on free trade, an election in which the Conservatives, with massive help from their business allies, won a majority of seats (but not a majority of votes) from a fragmented opposition. The free trade agreement weakens those forces (such as the labor movement) that have traditionally supported national health insurance and strengthens the sovereignty of market forces. The power of capital was strengthened by threats to "disinvest" in Canada.

In the 1980s business began to make openly reactionary declarations that social measures destroyed initiative. The claim was no longer that welfare measures ameliorated the inequalities brought about by capitalism; rather, it was now said that government taxes and expenditures were crippling the private market. Inequality was held up as a "necessary" part of a capitalist market system. The class struggle became a more open fight, but big business now bestrode international boundaries whereas labor did not. The strength of neoconservative forces encouraged a greater interest in the privatization of health care, though much of big business still viewed national health insurance in a positive light (since it "socialized" health care costs rather than devolving these onto individual corporations).

Although the business view of reality was predominant, it was not unopposed. Efforts to reduce the labor movement to passivity in Canada were not successful; the percentage of the labor force unionized remained nearly 40 percent (well above that in the United States). White-collar and state-employed workers (particularly nurses) unionized and became more militant in the face of government financial restraint.

Medicine in Canada had fought any government involvement in health and health care. In the 1980s it sought, largely unsuccessfully, to follow the general neoconservative trend in attempts to roll back what it saw as intrusive and unnecessary government involvement. But opposition forces were powerful enough to make even conservative governments agree that medicare, and a health care system in which government and the public played an increasing role, were part of their sacred trust.

Conclusions

In the postwar era organized medicine focused much of its attention on health insurance. A major consequence of health insurance was medicine's loss of unilateral control over the context, the terms, and the conditions of medical practice. But control over context cannot be separated from other aspects of medical dominance. The industrialization and rationalization of health care produced decreased medical control over other health occupations, declining control over clients, and even challenges to exclusive medical determination of the content of care (through computer protocols for treatment, control by planners over the use of new equipment, and more restricted definitions of scope of practice). Medical organizations central to self-regulation and professional autonomy, such as the provincial colleges, came under greater state influence.

Never monolithic, medicine itself showed more visible cracks and strains. Different group interests were increasingly manifest as physicians carried out varied medical work in many different kinds of work contexts. Viewed in both interest group and class terms, medicine grew more heterogeneous.

I have emphasized those developments that indicate a decline in medical dominance, yet there have been contrary indications. Medicalization could be viewed as a countertrend. Similarly, many current reforms in health care, such as regionalization and reforms of professional self-regulation, are not yet fully worked out or are specific to some of the larger provinces. The trend, nevertheless, is clearly away from medicine.

Although there are general declines in medical power, there are suggestions that organized medicine might regain elements of its former glory. Some within medicine view greater professional control as synonymous with greater privatization. The effects of the free trade agreement, the support of conservative provincial governments, and pressure from some more affluent Canadians may facilitate efforts to privatize the health care system. But even if these efforts are successful, which is unlikely, medicine will not return to its previous position at the pinnacle of health care.

Dominance can be viewed as part of a continuum of control, with dominance at one end, subordination at the other end, and autonomy in the middle. Freidson asserts that medicine will still be dominant provided that it controls other occupations and no other occupation controls it or that it still has organized autonomy. This is an unnecessarily narrow focus, but, even given these arguments, medicine has certainly moved closer to a situation of autonomy rather than one of dominance regarding interoccupational rivalries. In parts of Canada at least, medicine has lost substantial elements of its previously almost untrammeled self-governing powers.

Does this decline signal the proletarianization of medicine? If proletarianization refers to the beginnings of a process of loss of control, yes; if it implies a slippery slope, with an ever-increasing loss of control as more or less inevitable, no. Medicine is part of a process involving numerous other professional occupations. These are increasingly wage labor and less petit bourgeois, yet they retain or fight for relative autonomy in the labor process. The individual outcomes of these struggles are not predetermined. While many health occupations are struggling up to medicine's level, medicine is striving to prevent a further downward slide. We are witness to the general class structuration of white-collar workers in which one segment has been reasonably successful in professionalizing while the lower levels are more subject to rationalization and resulting unionate forms. In this process the attempt to professionalize by some produces or enhances the proletarianization of others. Interoccupational struggles are part of the process of proletarianization itself.

Medicine currently is isolated both occupationally and regarding class forces.

It has no occupational allies in health care (apart from, perhaps, dentistry). It has no contacts with the organized working class or with unions, nor are these groups allies. This situation contrasts sharply with that of teachers and nurses, whose militant unions are now at the forefront of labor struggles. The medical profession has little to expect from big business and only ideological support from small business. Medicine's principal interest links seem to be with other professions, which may, but I think not, as yet form a new class (Derber, Schwartz, and Magrass 1990).

This examination of the profession of medicine points to areas that have been previously underemphasized. The importance of occupational organizations as the sites for struggles for control over the occupation from groups within and from without is noteworthy. More links need to be made with welfare state theories. The role of medicine as an international discipline and occupation requires further exploration. For example, are there limits to national variations brought about by the internationalization of scientific knowledge and of medical organizations? Although national case studies are laudable, we need more international comparisons. Those authors in Part III commenting on the case studies presented in this book will point the way.

Acknowledgments

This chapter was developed from a larger study, "The Rise and Fall of Medicine in Canada," funded by the Social Science and Humanities Research Council Grant Number 410-85-0539. I owe much to discussions with C. Lesley Biggs and to her archival skills and to George Torrance and Joseph Kaufert for their collaboration on an earlier paper on the topic. I extend thanks also to Elaine Gort and Rick Edwards for their aid in this research.

8

The Medical Profession in Australia

Evan Willis

This chapter addresses the question of how best to make sociological sense of the changing social character and position of the medical profession (henceforth referred to as doctors) in Australia. The conceptual debate broadly has three related positions: deprofessionalization, proletarianization, and the maintenance of professional dominance. That the medical profession is undergoing major changes is not under dispute. What is disputed is what these changes mean in general and in the specific context of particular nation-states. What is happening to Australian doctors in relation to this debate?

The Debate

In order to situate the Australian evidence to make this argument, it is necessary first to review and take a position in relation to the conceptual debate. In considering the changing social position of the medical profession in Australia or any other country, it is necessary to locate them in the political economy of that society; for most, that means advanced capitalist societies. It is necessary to consider the four levels of analysis McKinlay (1988:4–5) outlined: financial and industrial capital (together with the class that controls it), the state, medicine itself, and the public. Each of these levels has an impact on the medical profession as each shapes the nature and character of the health sector in advanced industrial societies. Furthermore, to use McKinlay's game analogy, control over the center field, which the medical profession has, does not imply control of the game itself and necessitates considering the other levels of analysis in addition.

Deprofessionalization

The conceptual confusion with the terminology has been considerable. Since the mid-1970s there has been fairly general agreement that professionalization is part of the development and maintenance of the class structure; it is a process aimed at collective upward social mobility through social closure and monopolization. For Larson (1977), in addition, the process has an ideological component. What professions have in common is an occupational ideology staking a claim to autonomy (the "sacred cow" for Freidson) in the performance of their work and in regulating their affairs. Such autonomy, as Johnson (1977:229) argues, is based on the historical process whereby occupationally generated definitions of professional service ("health") become official, state-patronized ones. The process of professionalization as a mode of occupational control (for Johnson, the institutionalization of colleague control in medicine) "took place in the nineteenth century when social conditions associated with the rise of 'private' capitalism were conducive to 'professionalism' and occupational definitions of client need" (p. 229). Professionalism is therefore both a material practice and a set of ideas that justify that practice—in short, an ideology ("it is right and proper that . . ."). Professionalism reproduces what Habermas (1970) calls the "ideology of expertise." This ideology emphasizes technological rationality, effectiveness, and individualism, which result in a claim that "knowledge is beneficent power" yet legitimate inequality and elitism, as Larson (1977:241–43) has shown.

From this point of view, then, deprofessionalization would be represented as a historical process in which state patronage of professionalism resulted in a decline in both autonomy and the expression of professionalism as an ideology. Contrary to this, I would argue that, in Australia at least, the ideology of professionalism has been more stridently expressed, particularly by general practitioners, whose status and income are being most adversely affected. It takes the form of an ideological rearguard action to preserve the position of the medical profession in the face of challenges to its position.

Proletarianization

This has been taken to mean that with the development of capitalism, the petit-bourgeois class location of doctors is increasingly threatened. This argument, however, makes most sense within an orthodox Marxist position, which does not adequately account for the continued existence and flourishing of an intermediate class location in advanced capitalist societies. Within this class grouping, a distinction is needed between the old or traditional middle class (small business persons, family farmers, etc.) and the new middle class comprising major professional groups. Proletarianization, the consequence of the concentration and centralization of capital, has occurred mainly to the former group. In the latter group, as Freidson (1977:28; 1986a) has argued, self-employment or employment status per se is less important as an analytical issue than the process by which control over work is established and maintained. Doctors, as important members of the new middle class, have not been proletarianized because of their involvement in the maintenance of ideological hegemony. Doctors must be seen as organic intellectuals who, along with other professional occupations, have emerged in association with a new dominant class in advanced capitalism. These professions exercise "the subaltern functions of social hegemony and political government" (Gramsci 1971:12). They are what Merrington (1968:154) calls "experts on legitimation." They rationalize and provide a justification for the nature of that society, thus acting "as the mediators of the realities of capitalism into values" (Davidson 1968:45). In the specific case of doctors, the basis for state patronage lies in the role of doctors in the reproduction of labor power, mediating relations between individuals and their bodies, on one hand, and the state, on the other. This is, after all, how medicine acts as an institution of social control.

Professional Dominance

This position in the debate, as developed in Freidson's (1970a) seminal work, accords doctors a position of dominance in the health sector, which is based on esoteric knowledge and state patronage. As I have argued elsewhere, however (Willis 1989a), the problem with the original formulation of this position is that it is inadequately located in a theory of class relations, which is central to an analysis of autonomy and professionalism. In McKinlay's terms, the level of financial and industrial capital is underrepresented in his analysis. For those reasons, although acknowledging the importance of Freidson's account, I have referred to the phenomenon as medical dominance in order to differentiate it. With this expansion to the broader politico-economic context, my interpretation of the evidence on the changing social position of doctors in Australia is that it still is best analyzed sociologically within the professional dominance tradition.

What I have called medical dominance is sustained at three levels. The first is autonomy; at the level of control over their own work, doctors are not subject to direction and evaluation by other health occupations. The second level is authority over the work of other health occupations, exercised either directly by supervising and directing the work of others or indirectly by medical representation on registration boards or denial of legitimacy. The third level, medical sovereignty, involves the sustenance of medical dominance in the wider society. Doctors are institutionalized experts on all matters relating to health. For a decline in medical dominance to have occurred, a discernible diminution in the control of doctors at each of these levels should be apparent.

The Historical Process

The specific historical circumstance of the different societies considered must be analyzed to provide the backdrop against which changes in the social character of the medical profession in various countries can be elucidated. A brief historical background to the provision of health services in Australia is relevant. Medical dominance is, after all, the end point of a long historical process of the establishment of control. (Because of the federal structure of Australia, there are state differences in particular historical detail; I have chosen examples from the state of Victoria.)

Since the arrival of white settlers just over two centuries ago, health services in Australia have been provided on the basis of a mixture of public (state funded) and private suppliers. In the nineteenth century, the English tripartite medical system of apothecaries, surgeons, and (a few) physicians was transplanted to Australia. Consolidation into a recognizable medical profession occurred in 1862 in the state of Victoria, for instance, with the passing of a registration act modeled on the 1858 English act. Until early in the twentieth century, however, state patronage for doctors was relatively limited. Internal divisions within medicine promoted disunity. A general lack of effectiveness in treatment meant that early doctors had difficulty distinguishing themselves in other than status terms from homoeopaths, their main competitors. In addition, an ideology of laissez-faire individualism prevailed consistent with the economic times, rendering unsuccessful several attempts to ban unqualified medical practice in the late nineteenth century.

From the early twentieth century, however, consistent with a general trend in many Western capitalist countries toward the beginnings of a transition from laissez-faire to monopoly capitalism, the state began to adopt a more interventionist role in regulating the affairs of Australian society. A significant step in the state of Victoria, for instance, was 1908 legislation effectively regulating the size of the medical work force with controls placed on the number of foreign doctors joining the medical register. The medical board established in the 1862 act was given partial autonomy, able to act as an internal regulatory body in certain cases.

A position of dominance in the health division of labor having been achieved by 1908, the next decades were ones of consolidation as the state became increasingly interventionist. The second decade of the century saw a major struggle to control the terms and conditions of practice. To do this, doctors had to gain control over the demand for medical services in the marketplace and achieve professionalism as a form of control over work. Friendly societies or lodges, based on the English model, were the major alternative entrepreneur of medical care, employing doctors on a salaried rather than on an individualized fee-for-service basis. In lodges, doctors experienced a mediated form of work control, thus limiting their autonomy. Industrial action in the form of withdrawal of labor followed, organized through local branches of the British Medical Association. A royal commission followed at which the friendly societies capitulated, thus ending salaried practice. (See Pensabene 1980; Green and Cromwell 1984.)

By the 1930s the professionalization process reached the stage of achieving professionalism as the form of control over work. In 1933 in the state of Victoria, legislation granted full autonomy for internal regulation to the profession through the medical board with the passing of an infamous conduct clause. By such a sanction containing the threat of being struck off the register, doctors were able to supervise the professional behavior of members without recourse to outside authority.

Since World War II, the tendency toward state intervention in health care has increased, particularly under social democratic–type Labour governments. An attempt in the late 1940s to introduce a national health service broadly along British lines was prevented only by a high court ruling that such a scheme would involve civil conscription of doctors, something the Australian Constitution proscribes. The long period of conservative government in the 1950s and 1960s saw health care funded through private health insurance companies, a development initiated by the doctors themselves in conjunction with the government to preserve their autonomy. This period arguably represents the heyday of medical dominance. At this time, an important medical pressure group emerged comprising conservative refugee doctors from the United Kingdom who had fled the establishment of the British National Health Service to settle in Australia and were determined not to see a similar health service established.

In the mid-1970s, however, the reformist Whitlam Labour government, in the teeth of medical opposition, introduced a national health insurance scheme, Medibank. It reimbursed a substantial proportion of medical fees but did not interfere with autonomy or fee-for-service payment for medical services. This scheme was wound down with a return to private health insurance under the Fraser Liberal-National party coalition in the late 1970s and early 1980s but reintroduced in a slightly modified form by the Hawke Labour government on its election in 1983. Now called Medicare, the scheme either refunds part of the fee paid by patients to doctors, or directly pays the doctor at a slightly lower rate. This latter practice, known as bulk billing, cannot be said to affect the autonomy of doctors.

The evidence available supports the contention that medical dominance is being maintained, although its form and mode of operation is changing. A consideration of each of the four levels of analysis, examined in terms of the impact of changes in autonomy, authority, and sovereignty, will illuminate the effect on medical dominance.

Levels of Analysis

The Public

Traditionally, the medical profession has enjoyed substantial autonomy in the performance of its work from a largely acquiescent public. The normative expectations of the traditional doctor-patient relationship enshrined medical care as something that doctors did to patients, who were expected to accept unquestioningly that the doctor knew best and was acting in their best interests. The change in these normative expectations has been in the direction of casting the relationship as more of a partnership: the doctor and patient together bringing about the required end of improved health. These changes have occurred in considerable part through the growth of the consumer movement, particularly the women's health movement, which has been important in questioning the unbridled autonomy that doctors have historically enjoyed. Consumer representatives have been appointed to state bodies affecting doctors, including research fund allocation committees as well as ethics committees, exerting some influence over the direction and conduct of medical research in the sense of restraining the previously unfettered right of medical researchers to be answerable only to their medical colleagues for the direction and conduct of their research. Consumer representatives have also been incorporated within state health authorities themselves, often serving alongside medical officers. One substantial consequence has been a decline in the impact of the ideology of professionalism, particularly as it involves the "doctors know best" ideology of expertise. The political experience of organized medicine's strident opposition to the introduction of the Medibank and Medicare health insurance schemes has been to implant firmly in the public mind the notion that the organization of health services was essentially a political rather than a technical problem in which doctors did not necessarily know what was best for the rest of the populace.

Public regard for the status of the medical profession, as measured by public opinion polls, nonetheless remains high. While other occupations have regularly received a higher or lower ranking of public esteem over time, doctors have maintained their position at the top of the list. In a recent assessment of public opinion carried out by the Gallup method in 1986, 74 percent of Australians placed doctors at the top of the list when asked to nominate the five occupations they held in highest regard. In a previous poll, conducted in 1984, doctors topped the list for 63 percent of Australians (Australian Public Opinion Polls 1986). In occupational status hierarchy rankings, the medical profession retains its traditional position at or near the top of the hierarchy, being surpassed in the most recent ranking only by judges (Najman and Bampton 1991).

Medicine

The autonomy of doctors has also been affected by intraoccupational changes within the profession itself. There appears to be a concentration of power in the hands of academically oriented specialists and away from general practitioners and even private specialists. This trend has been apparent for a long time but appears to have accelerated more recently. Very few general practitioners do any surgery other than in fairly remote rural areas. As in other countries, general practitioners increasingly are becoming a screening mechanism for referral to specialists for the management of most health conditions. In the speciality fields, the social relations of the increasingly sophisticated medical technologies, such as randomized control trials, is concentrating power in the hands of academic, salaried specialists backed up by technicians of one sort or another (including biostatisticians) and away from specialists engaged in private practice who rely on the academically oriented specialists and technicians to interpret the meaning of the studies.

At the level of authority in relation to other health occupations, changes are also evident. The idea of a team approach to patient care, for long mainly ideological rhetoric, appears to be more common, although the doctor remains very much the captain of the team and there is considerable variation between rural and urban areas. In this respect, I agree with Freidson's (1977:28) contention that "interdependence does not necessarily corrode dominance." There has been a marked growth in militancy among paramedical groups, particularly nurses, who are largely abandoning professionalism as the strategy for occupational advancement in preference for trade unionism. The consequences of such a change were reflected in the state of Victoria in a seven-week nursing strike at the end of 1986. Part of the settlement of that industrial action, in addition to significant increases in remuneration, was the establishment of a Professional Issues Inquiry to consider workplace issues not amenable to settlement by industrial action. For example, one of the nurses' grievances was that they were not consulted about which technology is introduced or how it is used, yet they are often required to operate it and deal with patient discomfort and other ramifications. The inquiry reported in 1988, and many of its recommendations are being gradually implemented, such as creating and increasing nurse representation on many decision-making bodies, including the senior executive of the state health bureaucracy. Certainly it appears that the traditional role of nurses as handmaidens to doctors has been eroded, and to that extent the doctors' authority has diminished. Authority changes in relations with other health occupations are also apparent, though perhaps to a lesser extent than with nurses. A small, concrete result of some decline in authority and growth of inter-dependence of doctors with others (lamented by many doctors) is the loss of priv-ileged parking access for medical staff at some city hospitals, meaning that doctors have to take their chances with the rest of the health work force.

The other health occupation sometimes considered a threat to medical dominance involves health administrators who are not also medically qualified. Certainly there has been a something of a trend toward employing chief executives of hospitals, both public and private, who are nonmedically qualified administrators. There also has been a trend toward corporatization of private hospitals identified elsewhere, with the entry of several American multinational hospital companies into Australia. The question is whether such changes of ownership and direction have led to a decline in medical dominance. My argument is that the form of dominance has changed from overt to (relatively) subtle. Medical committees within hospitals remain very powerful. Administrators may be able to implement budget cuts of one sort or another, but the medical committees have a powerful voice in how this occurs. The size of the budgetary cake to be divided up might be smaller as a whole, but that does not mean a redistribution in the relative size of the slices.

The other area in which it could reasonably be said that medical authority has declined is with patients regarding alternative or complementary medicine. Utili-zation of complementary practitioners (such as chiropractors, osteopaths, natural therapists, and practitioners of traditional Chinese medicine) has been growing rapidly (Willis 1989*b*) even in spite of, or even perhaps because of, medical op-position. Chiropractic is a good example; it now has statutory registration in every part of Australia and within the state-funded tertiary education system. The legit-imation of chiropractic, both legally and clinically, has long been opposed by organized medicine, although it is clear that individual referral relationships have existed for a long time. Medical opposition to the statutory registration of chiro-practic was ineffective, largely because of the gradual process of the separation of medicine and the state. Whereas traditionally legitimation was dependent on medical approval, complementary modalities have increasingly looked directly to the state for legitimation.

Yet this decline in medical authority should not be overstated. Practitioners of complementary health care modalities so far have been unsuccessful in gaining access to the hospital system, public or private. Furthermore, a number of rec-ommendations by government inquiries for research monies to be made available to investigate properly the efficacy of these complementary modalities have fallen on the deaf ears of medically dominated research funding bodies (Willis 1989*b*).

The State

In the development of the Australian health care system, the relationship between the medical profession (represented by its organization, the Australian Medical Association) and the state has been a fickle one. It was closest when conservative political parties occupied the legislative arm of the state, as it did through most of the 1950s and all of the 1960s. Since the 1970s, the relationship has been more problematic, coinciding with relatively long periods of less conservative governments' being elected. State patronage as the underlying basis for medical dominance has never been threatened, however. What has occurred is that the relationship between the profession and the legislative and bureaucratic arms of the state has become a less cosy and more wary one. Furthermore, the government at times has shown itself willing to act against the advice of organized medicine, as seen in the statutory registration of chiropractors, the reduction in medical dominance of health administration, and the reform of the financial basis to health care provision through the introduction of Medibank and Medicare. Part of the opposition by doctors to their introduction was a perceived threat to their autonomy with a third party intervening in the relationship between doctor and patient. Effective record keeping, it was believed, would make doctors vulnerable to charges of overservicing patients. Experience has shown, however, that although there have been some prosecutions for blatant overservicing, the autonomy of doctors has not been affected.

This last point raises the issue of the third level of medical dominance, sovereignty at the level of the state. As in most other Western capitalist economies, the fiscal crisis of the state has led to attempts, under pressure from dominant classes at the level of financial and industrial capital, to reduce government expenditure in such areas as health and welfare. An example is a recent attempt to remove cosmetic surgery items from the schedule for which medicare benefits are payable. In the past, the close identification of doctors with the state has been based on class affinities, the compatibility of medical knowledge, and sympathetic governments occupying the legislative arm of the State, all of which provided the basis for medical dominance having reached its peak in the 1960s. Since that time, however, the state increasingly has become a terrain on which struggles over social expenditure have taken place. As doctors try to maintain their position, the possibility has emerged of coalitions between doctors and patient groups to preserve social expenditure in the face of dominant class pressure to reduce it.

The pressure for restraint on spending is also having some impact on the autonomy of doctors, particularly in hospital settings. Decisions about what surgical procedures should be performed on whom have to be taken with an eye to the cost allocation. Many hospital-based doctors, particularly the more junior ones, are now required to "clock on and off" and to restrict as much as possible the overtime they work.

For now, however, at the level of the state, medical sovereignty largely continues. Medicine retains its role as an institution of social control. Nonmedical representation on state health bodies remains largely token, and medical certificates from doctors are required to legitimate all sorts of state benefits in the health arena. Only in the area of legitimation of absence from work for illness has there been some erosion, with some employers accepting certificates from practitioners other than doctors.

Financial and Industrial Capital

In 1988 McKinlay and Stoeckle identified the process of corporatization of the medical profession as it became more consolidated into capitalist production relations. In the past decade in Australia, and the past few years in particular, this trend has become more obvious. In the hospital sector, the sale of private for-profit hospitals by doctor-investors has become common. This has occurred first to local capital and more recently to international capital, particularly American private hospital companies.

In the primary health care sector, the trend is even more pronounced. From about 1985, chains of investor-owned primary health care clinics have been established in the major metropolitan centers and have rapidly spread to most suburbs of larger cities. Despite some early controversy over ownership and the best-known original doctor-entrepreneur (known for his flamboyance) eventually being jailed and struck off the medical register, these clinics have become a part of the primary health care scene. They are likely to remain so despite an ongoing hostile campaign over their very existence by the more traditional general practitioner section of organized medicine. The exact ownership structure of these clinics is difficult to ascertain, but some have only token medical representation in their management structure. In one chain, the capital is provided by property development interests. The process of establishing new clinics involves paying careful attention to location to maximize passing trade; the clinics are open extended hours (often never closing), advertise extensively, routinely bulk bill all patients, and have a wide range of services available under one roof ("one-stop medical care"), usually including pharmacy, pathology, radiology, and weight control and often including physiotherapy, optometry, and other services. If pathology services are not available on site, kickback arrangements with local pathology companies are common, according to journalistic accounts. The doctors work shifts within the center, for either an hourly wage or a percentage of the Medicare fee, or some combination of the two. Many of the doctors are recent graduates, but others are well-established older general practitioners who work a shift or two each week, more or less as semiretirement.

Historically, this development represents the beginning of the end of the petty commodity, cottage industry basis on which general practice in Australia has operated throughout its history. Australia is following a trend toward the penetration of capitalist production relations into the human services field, which is much more developed in other countries, including the United States. State patronage, together with the ideology of professionalism, has allowed particularly the general practitioner segment of the Australian medical profession to resist successfully the concentration and centralization of capital that has steadily occurred in most other areas of society. As a result, as much as a third of all general practitioners in the state of Victoria are still engaged in solo practice (Medical Board of Victoria 1988). General practitioners are and feel particularly threatened by the emergence of the entrepreneurial chains in their neighborhoods. Their responses so far have been varied. Some are bemoaning what is in effect the passing of the more English style of professionalism, which has characterized Australian professional life, and its replacement with a more aggressively commercial American style. In this case, the ideology of professionalism is even more stridently expressed as a rearguard action. This group has had little success in persuading either the Australian Medical Association or the state to take action against such chains. Other general practitioners have responded competitively by joining together, offering more services and longer opening hours, moving to bulk billing all patients, and instituting a greater division of labor with the employment of specialized record keepers and accountants to take advantage of the benefits of more centralized management of their practices. Others have quietly shut up shop and gone to work in the chain clinics. In one instance, a local doctor took his receptionist and worked one day a week in the local chain clinic to supplement his income.

The crucial conceptual question of this development is the implication of this trend toward corporatization for the maintenance of medical dominance and in particular for the autonomy, authority, and sovereignty upon which such dominance rests. Although evidence is difficult to obtain, two aspects appear particularly relevant insofar as they are likely to affect the autonomy of individual doctors to practice as they see fit when confronted by demands or encouragement from the center management to practice in a manner that will maximize profitability: the potential for management demand to increase productivity by speeding the through-put of patients and the potential for doctors to be directed or encouraged to practice in a manner other than solely on their professional judgment.

Clearly an extensive study of these issues would be valuable, but enough evidence is available to conclude that these are real possibilities for affecting the autonomy of doctors. On the first point, in a journalistic account of the operation of one such center, the receptionist reported being required to take out of the center computer before leaving work for the day a printout of the number of patients each doctor saw that day. Overnight, the management examined this daily production schedule; doctors who had reached the daily target of one hundred patients for the day had a happy face drawn next to their names and those who had "failed" a sad face. On the second point, there is pressure in many of these centers, according to journalistic accounts, to maximize the number of pathology tests ordered, thus maximizing profitability. This practice, combined with the pressure on throughput of patients, may affect the application of doctors' skills away from clinical judgment on the basis of careful history taking, which their textbooks taught them, using pathology tests only where considered necessary and likely to be a useful adjunct to clinical diagnosis, toward the routine ordering of pathology tests to make a more technological diagnosis. The consequences of this trend are apparent in the large number of complaints that are made by dissatisfied consumers to state health authorities complaining of peremptory treatment, inadequate diagnosis, rudeness, and poor communication. A large proportion of those complaining did not even know the name of the doctor who treated them (personal communication).

Corporatization may also have implications for authority relations with other health practitioners, since all are responsible to the center management. How much this affects medical dominance is not known, although it seems likely that the doctors will still be very much the captain of the team. At the level of financial and industrial capital, changes in the social character of the medical profession appear increasingly likely, though the extent to which these actually mean a decline in medical dominance is less certain. Nevertheless, the vast bulk of primary medical services are provided by self-employed general practitioners working in a partnership of other doctors or alone.

Conclusion

Considering the changing social position of the medical profession requires analyzing developments not only within the field of medicine itself but also at the three other levels of the public, the state, and financial and industrial capital. Furthermore, the levels are arranged in a broad order of determination over the health sector. Although all levels affect what occurs within the health sector and are interrelated, structural changes at the level of the state and capital are likely to be of greater importance than those at the level of medicine or the public.

Yet despite the structural changes identified in the character of the medical profession, particularly the trend toward corporatization, the most useful way to make sociological sense of the changing social position of doctors continues to be the professional dominance tradition of explanation, referred to here as medical dominance. Such medical dominance, the end point of a historical process of the creation and maintenance of medical control, probably peaked in the 1960s in Australia and has been waning since. At the same time, the decline in medical dominance has not been sufficient to suggest that either deprofessionalization or proletarianization is a preferable means of making sociological sense of what is occurring to doctors in Australia. Both of these conceptual tools indeed have substantial limitations, as outlined. Instead, medical dominance has changed its form and become more subtle and indirect. At the level of autonomy, for instance, although some changes are evident, the level of personal autonomy that individual doctors experience does not seem to be greatly affected. Changes in the form of medical dominance do not mean changes in its applicability as a whole.

In the light of the structural changes, it is necessary to go beyond the conceptual debate thus far to analyze how the position of doctors is being maintained or undermined as the nature of health care changes in the final years of the century. It is necessary to consider the implications of changes at the various levels for the labor process of doctoring: how relations of domination and subordination are created and maintained, how the nature of the employment relationship will influence the autonomy experienced by doctors, as well as the implications of production relationships for the maintenance of the traditional skills of doctors and the role of technology in affecting those. In this way the detail can be painted in of what it means to be a medical practitioner in late-twentieth-century Australia.

9

Struggling for Control: The State and the Medical Profession in New Zealand

Geoff Fougere

How do doctors come to exert or lose control over their own work and the work of others involved in the funding, production, and consumption of health services in different national contexts? And how does the form and extent of this control change over time? In this chapter I draw on the New Zealand experience of the past fifty years to illuminate aspects of these questions.

The New Zealand health system, like those of most other developed countries, is the target of major reform (Scott, Fougere, and Marwick 1986). In New Zealand, these reforms are part of a general response to a deep economic, political, and ideological crisis that has resulted in a fundamental and continuous restructuring of relations within society and between state and society since 1984 (Bollard and Buckle 1987; Holland and Boston 1990; Easton 1989). The current government seeks to shift the health system from a combination of direct state provision of hospital care (organized largely on a command basis, although there is also a small private hospital sector) and subsidized primary care (organized largely on a market basis) toward a new inclusive system organized in terms of managed competition among public and private funders and providers of health care (Upton 1991).

The major pressures for this reform come from the general crisis outside the health system but also intersect with and are refracted in specific ways by pressures within the health field itself. This moment of reform is an opportunity to explore how forms of professional autonomy and control become embedded in health systems, how their exercise shapes the ways in which health services are provided, how these consequences become implicated in pressures for reform, and how in turn particular reforms reshape patterns of autonomy and control.

The account presented here weaves together two themes, one analytic and the other historical. The analytic theme shows how the kinds of autonomy and control that doctors have over their work is an outcome of particular configurations of relationships between doctors and other core actors comprising a health field. In New Zealand, these core relations include those with state actors, private funders,

managers, other medical workers, and clients. The historical theme traces how these
relations change over time and the consequences of their change for professional
autonomy and control. The major focus is on the changing relations between doctors
and the state between 1938 and the present.

Installing the Current Health System Regime

The legislative and institutional framework of the current New Zealand health system
was created between 1938 and 1941 (Fougere 1984). Its particulars were less the
result of design than the outcome of a protracted and often bitter conflict between
a reforming Labour government and a resistant medical profession.

By the 1930s, doctors dominated the provision of health care and the making
of health policy in New Zealand, a situation well described by historian Michael
Belgrave:

> Work in the health sector was . . . stratified and institutionalised. At the top were the
> doctors. . . . The doctors dominated the country's major health institutions—the hos-
> pitals and the Department of Health. Then there were commercial entrepreneurs—
> the chemists and the opticians. Nurses, physiotherapists and midwives aspired to
> professional status and had gained recognition of their professional skills and even
> some control over their registration, but they remained in the semi professions because
> of their largely salaried and female status. . . . Alternative therapies and independent
> practitioners had been pushed to the outside, where they continued to survive but
> did not flourish. . . . Despite the creation of new bureaucracies, doctors continued to
> practice largely as independent fee collecting practitioners. . . . [They] were able to
> dominate the health system and ensure that most other health workers either worked
> under their direction or were in some way subordinated to them. Because of their
> training, their professional status and their commitment to science, doctors saw
> themselves as having the authority to direct and control all others within the health
> economy. (Belgrave 1991)

In 1935, the first Labour government was elected in the midst of world depression. It remained continuously in office until 1949. Crucial to this electoral success
was a series of wide-ranging and interlocking social and economic reforms of which
the reform of health care formed a small but, for doctors and electors alike, significant part.

Labour sought to institute a tax-financed health system that provided all citizens
access to free health care on the basis of need. Doctors, clearly necessary to the
policy's implementation, organized to oppose the legislation. They correctly saw
state funding of health care as threatening to undermine their direct, fee-for-service-
based relationships with their clients and, by bringing the state much more directly
into the health care system, giving state actors a long-term stake in the oversight
and control of their work.

The result was a three-year struggle ended by partial compromise. All citizens
would have access to public hospital care financed from taxation, while tax-financed
subsidies would be made available to those choosing to use private hospitals.
Primary care would not be directly funded by the state. Instead, a variety of patient
subsidies would be paid covering all or most of the cost of a consultation, fully

subsidizing prescribed pharmaceuticals, and gradually extending to subsidize in full or part a range of other diagnostic and therapeutic services. This compromise largely preserved Labour's universalistic approach but drove an enduring wedge in forms of funding, organization, and careers between primary and secondary care (Hanson 1980; Fougere 1984).

How the Regime Has Worked

The first effect of the new regime was greatly to increase access to existing medical services while laying the financial basis to underwrite later increases in the intensity of servicing. Tax funding freed the health system from its dependence on direct payments to providers for specific services and instead linked its expansion to the growth in wealth of the society as a whole. As absolute gross domestic product (GDP) expanded, so did the share of it devoted to health expenditure. Currently health expenditure amounts to about 7 percent of GDP and tax funding to almost 80 percent of all health expenditure (Muthumala and McKendry 1991). The result, as in other developed countries, has been an enormous quantitative and qualitative expansion of the health sector.

The second effect of the new health sector regime was to entrench those forms of professional autonomy and control that doctors had already secured. This entrenchment was most obvious in primary care. General practitioners continued to enjoy the right to practice where they chose, as they chose, for the prices they chose, while being able to draw on extensive state subsidy of their fees and of the resources, especially pharmaceuticals, that they used in their practice of medicine. Such market advantages were enjoyed by none of their actual or potential competitors, such as osteopaths, chiropractors, or nurse practitioners. In addition, the position of general practitioners was strengthened within the medical division of labor by the elaboration of their role as gatekeepers, providing state-subsidized access to the services of other health care providers, such as physiotherapists. Ironically, general practitioners, who had initially been most opposed to the Labour government's reforms, gained through them an apparently open-ended commitment to protect them from competitors and to underpin financially whatever form of service they thought appropriate to provide.

In the hospital sector, the entrenchment of medical autonomy and control was less obvious but no less pervasive. Specialists have been largely free to combine salaried public hospital and fee-for-service private hospital employment, switching their time and attention to the better-paying private sector according to the amount of demand for their services (Fougere 1978, 1984). As in primary care, unquestioning acceptance of the doctrine of clinical freedom has left specialists free to make decisions about how resources are allocated among patients. The absence of effective information systems or even of effective forms of peer review has meant that such decisions are essentially unmonitored (Coney 1988). Similarly, specialists enjoyed a virtual monopoly in defining new forms of medical need and the new services and technologies required to meet these. Decisions about the kinds and form of development of hospital services consequently were seen as matters for specialists to decide, although lay representatives and government officials might have some voice in the timing and extent of new service provision (McKinlay 1980). As hospital-based services expanded, so did the authority of the profession within the increasingly extensive medical division of labor of the hospital and in society as a whole.

The third effect of the 1938 regime, the reconstitution of the role of the state in the health system, was partly a direct result of the legislation and partly a result of the consequences of the first two effects: the widening and deepening of access to health services and the entrenchment of professional autonomy and control. If the new regime constituted state actors as the guarantors of the free access of citizens to an extensive and expanding range of professionally defined and provided health services, it also simultaneously constituted them as the principal, potential source of resistance to such expansion (Fougere 1984).

The basis of this resistance can be simply stated if not simply analyzed. State actors are enmeshed not only within the set of relationships defining the health system but also within the wider sets of economic and political relations that structure the relationship between state and society. These define the capacity of the state's taxing and borrowing power, as well as articulating the various demands (including those of the health sector) made on state revenues. As a result, health budgets are only marginally flexible in the short term. State actors find themselves up against budget constraints, which within the current health regime largely define the rate of health system expansion.

But if state actors face a budget constraint on one side, they face on the other an apparently open-ended guarantee to provide citizens with access to adequate health care on the basis of need, and they do so in a context in which the embedding of high levels of professional control and autonomy within the health system means that they have few levers to control directly what health services are produced or how these services are delivered. The resulting tension has proved by turns a source of debilitating pressure and a spur to institutional creativity.

This creativity has evolved around three strategies. The first, dependent on both the growth of the economy and the growth of taxing power, has been to devise new ways to expand the health budget. The second has been to seek to rationalize the health care system itself, so that it can deliver more for the same input of resources. The third strategy has been to shift the cost of expanding the health system budget on to others' shoulders. Although all three strategies have coexisted since the birth of the 1938 health system regime, different strategies have had a greater or lesser emphasis at different times. In particular, the growing economic crisis in New Zealand, manifest from the mid-1970s, has turned attention from budget expansionary to cost shifting and rationalization strategies. In turn, the pursuit of these different strategies and their varying mix has differentially affected patterns of professional control and autonomy.

In primary care, state actors, having lost the initial battle to rationalize and control provision through contracting directly with general practitioners, found themselves drawn into the provision of patient subsidies as a means of guaranteeing access. Consequently, the demands on their budgets depended less on their own decisions than on those made by practitioners. In the case of payment for phar-maceuticals, the effect was quite straightforward. Doctors prescribed as they thought clinically appropriate, and the state paid the cost of the drugs. Weak efforts have been made at state monitoring of prescribing and, of late, to encourage doctors to provide peer review of each other. Attempts to influence directly doctors' choices between higher- and lower-priced drug equivalents have so far been successfully resisted (Davis 1992).

The subsidy of doctors' fees, the other major component of primary care expenditure, has traced a somewhat different path. High inflation in the 1970s and 1980s allowed the subsidy to lag behind fee increases, shifting the burden of payment to patients. This shift, in turn, encouraged the rapid growth of a market for private gap insurance, and now almost 50 percent of New Zealanders have such coverage. But those who were most disadvantaged by the increasing out-of-pocket cost of seeing the doctor, particularly the poor and the chronically ill, were also those who had the most difficulty in getting access to gap insurance. Consequently, success in cost shifting by state actors exposed them to new political pressures to increase and to target subsidies in the name of social justice. Each new round of subsidy increase quickly bled out as it provided a new floor under doctors' fees. Consequently, there has been renewed interest in incorporating general practitioners within contractual obligations so that increased state subsidy of fees is accompanied by some state control over the rate of fee increases and over the obligations that doctors have to patients. Again, steps in this direction have so far been successfully resisted by general practitioners.

The playing out of and the interactions among these strategies generate ambivalent and contradictory responses from state actors and general practitioners alike. Cost shifting by state actors, and especially the growth of a gap insurance industry, which increases its refunds to policy holders in line with increases in doctors' costs, leaves doctors free to charge what they like and practice as they wish. But it also leaves them with a substantial pool of patients who have great difficulty in paying and who, if the doctor is not to deny them medical care, must be treated for a reduced or no fee. Doctors therefore generally favor state subsidies but want them to be free of restriction. State actors, on the other hand, meet their budget targets by cost shifting but then find themselves held responsible for the inadequate access to medical care of the poor and the chronically ill. Being pressured to raise the subsidies for care directs their attention to ways of gaining some overall control of the system, at both the level of doctors' charges and obligations and, in a more muted way, at the level of their clinical practices. In turn, this situation brings them into conflict with doctors. Meanwhile, the terms and conditions of access for patients reflect the playing out of this conflict, as first one side and then the other implicitly holds patients as hostages to gain compliance from its bargaining partner.

In secondary care, state actors have consistently pursued a cost shifting strategy but with only limited success. Through a series of subsidies and tax breaks, attempts were made from the 1950s into the 1980s to encourage first the rebirth of a private hospital sector (the numbers of private hospitals had steeply declined after 1938) and then the development of private gap insurance so as to widen private sector access. For specialists, particularly surgeons, the substitution in whole or part of private sector work for their public sector employment offered them greatly increased income and much more control over their immediate work environment. But despite the encouragement of the state and the willing participation of doctors, private hospital care still amounts to less than 4 percent of all hospital expenditure in New Zealand (Muthumala and McKendry 1991). Moreover, this cost shifting strategy is not without its contradictions. The private sector developed as a complement to, rather than a substitute for, the services offered in public hospitals. Private hospitals emphasize routine, nonacute surgery for which there is demand simply because such surgery is given low priority by public hospitals and consequently generates long waiting lists. The result has been that while the cost shifting strategy moved some low-cost procedures off the state budget, it has also made state actors the exclusive target of demands for the most capital intensive and costly of hospital procedures (Fougere 1984).

The limitations of cost shifting strategies in the public hospital sector increasingly focused attention on how to rationalize and control its functioning. The gradual implementation through the 1980s of a population-based funding formula that distributed funds for hospital care among regions on the basis of their population (adjusted for crude measures of health status and other factors) turned out to provide an effective means of capping global budgets for hospital care. Its implementation, however, revealed new weaknesses. State actors could control overall levels of spending but not how funds were spent. Holding the line on budgets was intended to stimulate increased productivity, but to the public it seemed more often to result in the cutting of services. At the same time, shifts in the pattern of economic management that emphasized rapid reduction of the fiscal deficit meant new pressure to reduce rather than just hold the line on health spending by the state.

Consequently state actors were faced with increasing pressures to develop more direct managerial control over health service delivery and organization. These pressures coincided with a general rethinking of issues of management and control within the state sector as a whole. Since 1988, a new administrative framework, bundling together responsibility for public health and hospital services within a network of regionally based area health boards, has been created, together with the introduction of general management along the lines of the British National Health Service. At least as important, comprehensive management information systems based on new information technology are being developed and implemented within boards. National health goals were promulgated, along with steps toward much more extensive monitoring by central government of the performance of its providers in the regions (Walsh and Fougere 1989).

These different strategies and their mix within the hospital sector have had ambivalent and contradictory effects for professional autonomy and control. The expansion of private sector hospital care as a partial consequence of cost shifting opened up an arena of almost total professional control for doctors in terms of their charges and forms of practice. But the limits on the kinds of services provided in the private sector meant that their opportunities for high technology or state-of-the-art clinical work largely lay in public rather than private sector work. Similarly, the attempts by state actors to control global budgets undercut the resources available to doctors for providing services to their patients in the public sector but simultaneously increased the demand for their services in the private sector. And the attempts to rationalize and control services more directly within the hospital through an emphasis on developing management hierarchy and the implementation of management information systems has, paradoxically, emphasized the reliance of managers on the cooperation of doctors for meeting their targets. Even the new information technology, with its ability to document precisely the cost of individual doctors' work practices, is as likely to be useful to doctors seeking to demonstrate management's wastefulness as it is to managers seeking to demonstrate the need for control of clinicians' decisions. And it is likely to serve both in making claims for more resources from central government, undermining the basis of global budget controls.

The latest moves to gain greater control over the budgetary risks posed by the health care system were announced by a newly elected government in July 1991 (Upton 1991). The proposed policies have appeared to many as quite revolutionary in approach, and indeed their proponents do seek to break decisively with the 1938 welfare state regime for health care provision. From a slightly different perspective, however, the proposals can also be seen as new twists to state actors' old strategies of seeking to rationalize health sector provision and to shift responsibility for its costs to others' shoulders.

Among the key measures, the government proposes creating regional health authorities whose appointed members will be responsible for using their health sector, management, and financial skills to purchase most hospital and primary care services for all citizens in their regions. These services will be provided by a mix of for-profit and not-for-profit providers (including what were previously public hospitals, now reorganized as crown health enterprises). All providers will be dependent on winning contracts for the provision of specific services from regional or other funders to keep them in business. The resulting competition is expected to squeeze inefficiencies from the system, lead to innovation in delivery, particularly at the boundary between primary and secondary care, and generally increase the power of purchasers over providers in the system.

Competition in funding is also envisaged. Citizens will be able to opt out of regional health authority coverage, taking a risk-adjusted voucher from the regional health authority to a rival private insurer (a health care plan) that offers alternative cover. Competition among insurers is intended to make their managers vigilant in demanding value for money from health system providers and innovative in how they bundle the services they offer to clients. Equally crucial, the development of rival plans opens the way for state actors to opt out of funding or providing health care altogether. In this case citizens' taxes would no longer be used to fund health care plans or regional health authorities. Instead, citizens would pay premiums directly to the insurer of their choice. Although the state would retain regulatory authority, its only funding responsibility would be to ensure that poor people had sufficient income support to allow them to buy insurance coverage.

The government's proposals are intended to diminish the control of doctors and other providers within the health system and increase that of collective purchasers and health service users. But they are as likely to lead to a much less favored outcome. The competition envisaged between funders may make them more responsive to users but also much weaker in bargaining with doctors and other providers who can play one funder off against another. Funders' difficulties in getting leverage over professional providers and (because they are many rather than one) their lack of responsibility for overall health system outcomes also encourage them to compete with each other by shedding bad risks and shifting their costs to others rather than by wringing efficiencies from providers. This outcome is made more likely by the fact that the public regional health authorities but not the private health care plans are required to act as insurers of last resort. If the new regime does develop in this way, it will result in an increase, rather than a decrease, in the ability of doctors individually and collectively to maintain autonomy and exert control within the system (Evans 1984; Scott, Fougere, and Marwick 1986). It is also likely to lead to rapid cost inflation and a markedly two-tier system of health care based on the line between those able to gain coverage from private health care plans and those dependent on public regional health authorities.

Conclusion

The introduction, fifty years ago, of a welfare state–based health care regime in New Zealand embedded existing forms of medical autonomy and control within a new configuration of relationships among doctors, state actors, and users of health services. It also created an ongoing struggle between state actors and doctors over how control would be exercised and how the financial and other risks generated by the new system would be distributed. The results of these struggles have shaped and reshaped the organization of health service provision, as well as augmenting and undermining, often simultaneously, patterns of professional control.

The current drive by state actors to break out of the structure of the 1938 regime and to move toward a new system of managed competition reflects wider ideological changes and a new design for economic management. But it is also recognizably a response to some of the consequences and forms of professional autonomy and control characterizing the current health system. (In the current New Right lexicon fashionable in New Zealand, the phenomenon is called ''provider capture'' and is understood, mistakenly, as pertaining to state-organized but not market-organized health systems.)

In the analysis offered here, professional autonomy and control of work has appeared less as something that doctors win or lose than as a constantly challenged outcome of relationships between core actors within the health system. In one view of the New Zealand case, this construction of professional autonomy and control is always fragile and contingent, differing from one segment of the health system to another and changing over time as the strategies of actors intersect to produce intended, unintended, and often contradictory outcomes. From another point of view, little changes over long periods of time. Professional autonomy appears deeply embedded in relatively enduring institutional arrangements. These define actors' interests and resources and shape their strategies but leave little room for major change, except in periods involving the major restructuring of the whole society. The current period in New Zealand, like the last such period in the 1930s, may be such a time.

Acknowledgments

My thanks to Kevin White and particularly to Terry Austrin, Peter Davis, and Else Oyen for helpful comments on an earlier draft of this chapter.

10

The State and the Medical
Profession in France

David Wilsford

Health care policy in France is emphatically state led and has been so from the earliest moments in modern medicine's history. This state-led pattern has been reinforced in the postwar period as France has established and expanded comprehensive schemes of national health insurance. Although the 1920s and 1930s constitute, to a degree, the golden parenthesis of liberal medicine in France, powerful forces have moved in the postwar period to close that parenthesis.

Abetting the state's dominance in making health care policy in France is the historical weakness of organized medicine. It has been weak since the earliest days of the nineteenth century because medicine has, except for the occasional moment, been deeply fragmented organizationally and poorly mobilized politically. These organizational variables cut across the generic imperatives embedded within the professions, such as technical expertise, which establishes the doctor as a key figure in the hierarchy of service providers. Organizational variables are particularly important when professionals must mobilize politically, and especially in the face of strong, focused opposition. In the French case, fragmentation and poor mobilization have weakened the influence of organized medicine, and by extension the profession as a whole, in the health policy universe.

High State Autonomy in Health Care

Although any national health service or insurance system must be more state led than a free enterprise or mixed system counterpart, the French case is distinguished by a particularly high degree of state autonomy in making health care policy. The state's agencies and institutions (state structures, in the political science vocabulary) that are charged with a given policy domain are relatively homogeneous and operate according to clearly defined agendas. There is a clear and consensual conception of the state's mandate in the policy arena, and the state's structures benefit from clear, effective policy instruments that give them a certain number of tactical advantages against actors from society, especially the physicians in this instance. There are other conditions as well for state autonomy: a functional mandate for the state agencies involved rather than a clientele mandate, state agencies' activities centered around the execution of long-standing, clearly defined laws and regulations that are not subject to constant negotiation with societal groups, and an in-house capacity to generate, use, and evaluate technical and scientific information independent of the societal associations (Wilsford 1988, 1989; Atkinson and Coleman 1989:52).

In France, the organization of the national health insurance system has been largely in place since the years immediately following World War II. During this period, the French engaged in a significant remaking of their social and welfare system. One primary focus of this social security engineering was health care. Yet this national health insurance system was not cut from whole cloth. Its contours were influenced by earlier, more skeletal forms of collectivized health care from the interwar period.

The French think of their medical system as a treasured mix of socialized access to health care, which fulfills the important goals of social solidarity, combined with the private practice of medicine, which preserves the freedom and independence of the patient and of the physician. This latter aspect is known as *la médecine libérale* ("liberal medicine"). *La médecine libérale* is composed of the four sacred principles of French medicine first set forth in the 1927 manifesto known as the Medical Charter, or *Charte médicale:* (1) freedom of physician choice by the patient, (2) freedom of prescription by the physician, (3) fee-for-service payment, and (4) direct payment by the patient to the physician for services rendered. These principles have governed health care delivery by private practitioners, both generalists and specialists, since that time. Private practitioners constitute roughly 57 percent of French physicians. They are private not because their incomes are financed privately—except in rare cases they are not—but because they work on the fee-for-service basis in their own offices and are paid directly for their services by their patients, who are then reimbursed by the sickness funds. Nonprivate practitioners—mainly the hospital doctors and public health service personnel—are salaried functionaries of the state.

In France, a large proportion of medicine is practiced in hospitals, in addition to the private practices. Hospital physicians constitute roughly 35 percent of the practicing medical corps. Eighty percent of French hospitals are public; their administration falls under the purview of the national health ministry and is highly centralized. In general, once a private practitioner admits a patient, the salaried hospital staff takes over the case. Public hospitals range from small, provincial establishments in rural areas to the most prestigious and very large research hospitals in the large university cities, such as Paris. The remainder, 20 percent, are private hospitals, or *cliniques,* owned and operated for profit. Patients in them are covered by the national health insurance but at a markedly lesser rate. *Cliniques* may charge whatever they want.

Currently, the main sickness fund, the *Caisse nationale de l'assurance maladie des travailleurs salariés* (CNAMTS), covers the health care expenditures of 80 percent of the French population. The remainder are divided between the agricultural regime and other specialized regimes. At the national level, the CNAMTS governs a system of 16 *caisses régionales* and 129 *caisses locales.* The regional sickness

Table 10.1. Average level of reimbursement fixed by the CNAMTS, 1985

	Reimbursement level	Patient copayment
Physician fees	75%	25%
Other personnel expenditures	65	35
(e.g., nurses, physical therapists)		
Hospitalization	80	20
Prescription drugs	70	30
Special medications	100	None
Eyeglasses, prostheses	70	30
Laboratory analyses	65	35

Source: CNAMTS.

funds coordinate preventive health measures and the development of hospital facilities and public health clinics, although decisions about infrastructure and capital
investment are made in the national Ministry of Health. The jurisdiction of the local
sickness funds usually corresponds to the French departments (the main administrative unit of France, somewhat like states or provinces, though a good bit smaller).
They oversee the enrollment of those covered by the system and the collection of
the employee-employer contributions. They also are charged with the reimbursement
of all claims. The national sickness fund fixes all general fiscal policy, often at the
direction of the government, regarding levels of contribution, levels of reimbursement, and levels of charges and fees. It also generally oversees the administration
of the system. This system is vast. In 1985, there were over 100,000 administrators,
agents, clerks, and physician-inspectors employed by the CNAMTS. Of these,
76,000 worked in the local funds. In 1984, 393 million payment operations were
executed. The average levels of reimbursement are displayed in Table 10.1. In
1984, the CNAMTS administered 267 billion francs in payments.

For their patients to be reimbursed for their services, physicians in private
practice in France must adhere to the *convention,* the standard fee schedule for all
procedures and consultations, which is periodically negotiated between the sickness
funds and organized medicine. Physicians are paid directly by their patients, except
for most surgical procedures and hospital consultations. If the physician is *con-
ventionné,* and virtually all French doctors are, the patient is then reimbursed the
specified percentage of the scheduled fee by the sickness fund.

As of December 12, 1984, 69,094 physicians, or 79.7 percent of private practitioners, had signed the 1984 fee agreement. Another 7,186 physicians (8.3%)
benefited from a sanctioned right to exceed the fee schedule without the loss of
their patient's right to reimbursement (the *droit de dépassement*). These are usually
physicians who are either very celebrated in their specialty or practice a specialty
in exceedingly great demand. The *droit de dépassement,* however, is no longer
granted. Another 9,740 physicians (11.2%) had opted for Sector II, a parallel fee
system created in 1980 that permits physicians who choose it to exceed the negotiated
fee schedule "with tact and reasonableness." In return, they must pay their own
social insurance premiums. In practice, Sector II physicians generally exceed Sector
I fees by about 35 percent. They tend to be physicians from specialties in demand
or those who enjoy a stable surplus of patients, much like the physicians who were

formerly granted the *droit de dépassement*. Sector II replaces the *droit de dépassement* as a safety valve, or exit option, for physicians in high demand to get around the restrictions of the national health insurance system. The state and the sickness funds assumed that with a large and growing supply of physicians, fees in Sector II would be kept more or less in check. Further, the financing of the higher fees of Sector II would fall on the consumer, who would be reimbursed by the sickness fund at the Sector I rate (CNAMTS 1985). These figures do not count hospital or other salaried physicians.

Although this portrait of the national health insurance system seems to indicate that the French state has built a certain degree of decentralization into the system— in particular, a system of *caisses* administers the system, and at the national level day-to-day decision-making power resides with the sickness fund rather than with the government—in fact, the state authorities have always been very careful to reserve final decision-making powers to themselves. By law, the Social Security Code, which governs the national health insurance system, assigns to the government the general responsibility for the fiscal integrity of the system and the specific responsibility to ensure that employer and employee contribution levels are sufficient to cover expenditures. Therefore, state officials are always shadowy but important figures in the ongoing operation of the CNAMTS and other sickness funds, and they play an indirect but exceedingly important role in all fee negotiations with providers.

A number of agencies and ministries are involved in the execution of the health care mandate. The *directions,* or line agencies, divide policy jurisdictions functionally. The Direction de la pharmacie et du médicament, the Direction générale de la santé, and the Direction des hôpitaux fall under the general rubric of the Health Ministry, sometimes included in a larger functional ministry called Social Affairs. Political appointees go down as far as the heads of these line agencies, but although these officials are politically appointed, they are usually career civil servants.

Other government agencies have a deep interest in health policy as well. The most important is the Ministry of Finance. The escalating cost of health care (Figure 10.1) has led the Ministry of Finance to play a leading role in pressuring other government agencies to limit spending. In containing health care costs, France has done comparatively well when contrasted with the United States but not nearly as well as Japan or Britain.

In the French political universe, the Ministry of Finance is generally regarded as the most powerful ministry. The sickness funds govern the private practitioners and, under the government's direction, set employer and employee contribution levels to the funds. They also negotiate fee schedules (the *convention*) with the private practitioners. Finally, although hospital funding is the responsibility of the sickness funds, hospital budgets and personnel are controlled through the Direction des hôpitaux, medical education is controlled through the Ministry of Education, and enrollment quotas are set by mutual agreement between Education and the Ministry of Health. All of these organizational features of the French health care system highlight its centralization and rationalization when compared to its American counterpart. Policy in almost all health domains is leveraged from the top.

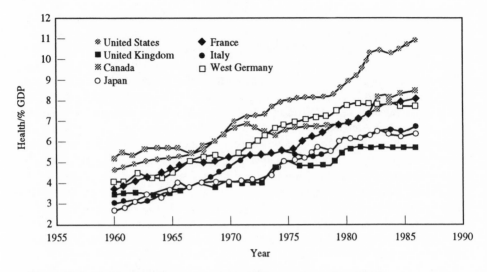

Figure 10.1. Health expenditures as percentage of gross domestic product

Organized medicine thus assumes a distinctly reactive posture, one that is compounded by many deep and lasting divisions within the medical corps.

Poor Interest Mobilization of the Medical Profession

In the face of high state autonomy in health care policy, the providers of health care—in this instance, the medical doctors—are organizationally weak. The chief indicators of this weakness are the divisions within the profession and the manifest divisiveness characterizing the profession's organized political structures and activities. Both division and divisiveness are deeply rooted in the history of the medical profession in France.

I refer to these two dimensions together under the rubric of interest mobilization. To what extent are the interests in the sector under study characterized by unitary organization, high rate of membership, sufficient resources for collecting and analyzing political and technical information, and the ability of the organization to speak authoritatively with the government on behalf of its members? This last characteristic means that the association can, in effect, negotiate effectively with the government because it can ensure the cooperation of members in implementing any accord that it reaches with the state authorities.

Along these dimensions, the fragmentation of the French medical profession and its organizational weakness are striking. The first form this fragmentation takes is a splintering of organized medicine into competing medical *unions,* as well as into functional divisions. There are today three major medical unions that compete with each other to represent private practitioners—both generalists and specialists. A number of minor unions exist as well. In addition, there are a number of other unions representing the hospital and salaried sectors, often in competition with each other.

The oldest and largest medical association representing private practitioners in France is the Confédération des syndicats médicaux français (CSMF). It was founded in 1928 and had momentarily consolidated a tenuous preeminence by 1930. One of the most persistent problems facing the CSMF is how to handle the competing pressures, both internally and externally, of union forces within the medical profession that compete against it. By the 1980s, the CSMF had managed to consolidate a truce of sorts with its main rival, the Fédération des médecins de France (FMF), enabling it to cooperate, or at least coordinate its activities, with the rival group. Yet by the end of the 1980s, an antagonistic sentiment among general practitioners within the CSMF had grown so strong that a new rival union split off and regrouped under the label MG France (Médecins généralistes de France). This group began in a small number of provincial departments and within two or three years had gathered strength and was represented in most departments nationally. In the universe of medical profession forces, MG France was considerably strengthened when the minister of social affairs designated it as a representative union, granting it official status for the 1989, and subsequent, fee negotiations.

Additional dimensions of fragmentation characterize the medical corps as well. The first is common to all advanced health systems: the segmentation of the medical corps into general practitioners, the various and diverse medical specialities, hospital staff, and the biomedical research community. This functional segmentation is one centrifugal force damaging to the unity of the medical corps. In some countries—Germany, Japan, and the United States, among others—the profession's political structures have done a better job of containing these centrifugal forces. In France, they have not.

The second additional dimension of fragmentation is also functional but in a different way. Ethical responsibilities and accountability have been reserved to an organization entirely separate from organized medicine, the Ordre des médecins. Insofar as ethics and ethical questions could potentially serve as a powerful unifying force to the profession, its organizational isolation from the profession's political structures deprives the profession of an important source of unity and cohesion.

Moreover, the French medical profession is fragmented demographically in the face of a very high supply of physicians. Generational fragmentation—young versus old—pits older, more established doctors against young, struggling doctors in a resource environment characterized by extreme scarcity. Young doctors in France face great difficulties establishing a practice. Further, all doctors, young and old, compete with each other for patients, who are perfectly willing to shop around. The shopping takes the form of seeking the physician who will provide the desired treatment—the right prescription drugs, the authorized medical leave from work, the better bedside manner, and so on. French physicians also operate within a fee-for-service structure characterized by very low fees. Comparative income data show that French physicians make notably less than their American counterparts—about one-half using purchasing price parities to wash out exchange rate differentials (Wilsford 1991:25).

One important variable that has led to the oversupply of physicians, and thus to generational and other divisions within the profession, is the way in which the state has not hesitated to manipulate the supply of physicians through medical school enrollments. Through the 1960s and early 1970s, the state intentionally increased the quotas of medical students permitted to pass from first-year medical studies to second year. Medical school enrollments constitute an important area of health care policy, of special concern to practitioners in the labor market, over which organized medicine in France and the medical profession in general play almost no role.

A final source of fragmentation of the French medical profession is the increasing feminization and increasing salaried basis of the medical corps. The French profession is not unique in the Western world in this regard. Yet the feminization and "salaryization" of the medical corps has served to introduce entire new sets of needs, incentives, and perspectives into the French profession, increasing its heterogeneity and diluting the cohesion of the various medical unions even further.

Early History of State-led Health Care in France

The history of the French medical profession and its relations with state authorities underscores the two distinguishing characteristics of the French case: state autonomy in health policy and interest mobilization of the medical profession. This history illustrates how deeply rooted these characteristics of state-profession relations are and puts forth the evidence to substantiate the two general claims of this chapter, that of high state autonomy and poor interest mobilization of the medical profession in France.

The character of the French health care system is heavily public. In fact, state intervention in health care has a long history in France. Henri IV issued an edict dated May 16, 1604, establishing salary deductions from miners' wages so that a surgeon could be employed and medicines bought to care for those injured in mining accidents. According to the edict, "The injured poor could [thereby] be freely cared for, and by this example of charity, others shall be the more encouraged to work." In 1673, Colbert issued similar ordinances concerning sailors of the merchant marine.

With the rise of industrialization in France—in the mines, steel, shipbuilding, heavy construction, textiles—coupled with advances in medicine and science, a collective protection of the health risk gradually supplanted individual and familial protection. Emile Zola, in works such as *Nana* and *Le Ventre de Paris,* gives compelling accounts of the dangerous conditions surrounding the industrial workplace in France during the latter nineteenth century and of how workers suffered. But there was a more utilitarian concern as well: injured workers are not productive. The law of April 9, 1898, instituted workers' compensation and required industrial employers to subscribe to private insurance for industrial accidents.

The first *syndicat médical,* or medical union, in France was formed in the Vendée, a provincial region in 1881. This union was illegal; French associational law at the time was based on the June 1791 Le Chapelier law forbidding any political association. In August 1792 the formal privileges of the professional guilds were suspended. The practice of medicine was thus no longer protected, regulated, or restricted, and total free enterprise ruled. In 1884, almost a hundred years later, workers' unions were finally legalized, but the liberal professions were excluded.

The creation of the first Vendée medical union exhibits key characteristics common to the organization of the medical profession to the present day. In the face of a strong and unyielding state, the syndical movement sprang up from the grass roots and took the form of contestation, or an extrasystem challenge to the state authorities. Between March and December 1881, eleven (illegal) departmental unions had been formed; there were no formal ties between them. In 1884 there were approximately 150 departmental unions with a total of 3,500 physician members. In November 1884, 40 of these departmental unions joined together to form the Union des syndicats médicaux de France (USMF). But in a judgment rendered by the circuit court of appeals (*cour de cassation*) on June 27, 1885, confirming two lower court decisions, the USMF was declared illegal under the terms of the Chapelier law.

While medical unions continued to exist and to form, it was not until the comprehensive law of November 30, 1892, that they were declared legal by specifically applying the previous occupational unions law to physicians. The 1892 law also established conditions of practice and penalties for malpractice, but this law also contained restrictions. Groups were required to register with the state by filling their bylaws and other organizational information with the city hall. And although physicians could now unite in syndical organizations in defense of their interests, they were not permitted to exercise this right against the state, its departments, or its communes.

Medical unions formed in this period to combat two principal problems. First, physicians typically worked during the latter nineteenth century as salaried employees of private mutual aid societies, which had been established for different occupations to collectivize certain risks, such as health care expenses. There were mutual aid societies for hairdressers, shopkeepers, metalworkers, weavers, carpenters, and many others. In the department of the Loire-Inférieure (now the Loire-Atlantique), for example, mutual aid societies numbered in the several hundred. One of the chief demands of the medical unions was for doctors to be paid for their work for the mutual aid societies on a fee-for-service basis. Because competition among orthodox physicians was very stiff, physicians often had to bid quite low to get mutual aid society work, and their incomes consequently were low. Second, competition to orthodox physicians came from healers, witches, and other unorthodox health care practitioners. The early medical unions in France took a more and more active role in pressing legal complaints against these charlatans. From the very beginning, however, centrifugal tendencies plagued the medical unions. In a typical story, one of the first associations of local unions, in the Loire-Inférieure, organized in April 1884. By July, the union from Saint-Nazaire had already left to form an independent group.

From 1884, the USMF attempted to represent collectively the rapidly developing regional associations; however, organizational fragmentation affected the USMF in two ways. First, from the beginning, syndical organizers wished to see another structure created within the profession, independent of the USMF, to license and police the practice of medicine. Eventually this came to pass with the creation by Vichy in 1940 of the Ordre des médecins, which still today, though reformed in 1945, enforces the ethical code and administers licensing. Thus, the French medical profession never combined the powerful disciplining and licensing prerogatives with union activities and representation, as did the American Medical Association. Perhaps more important, it never wanted to. Second, these unions grew up from the grass roots in provincial areas, and their associations were both loose and fragile. Subsequently, great schisms periodically rocked organized medicine at local, regional, and national levels, further diminishing its effectiveness.

Opening the Liberal Parenthesis

The first, but not last, serious schism in French medical syndicalism afflicted the USMF between 1915 and 1928. During this lengthy period of social policymaking in health care, two sides formed. On the one hand, USMF loyalists argued—in agreement with successive governments—that the adaptation of Alsace and Lorraine's comprehensive health care system to the rest of France should include such Bismarckian features as collective contracts between physicians and local sickness funds and third-party payment by the funds directly to physicians for patients' treatment. The dissidents based their opposition upon the four sacred principles of the "Medical Charter," which I have already outlined. In 1926, in the midst of this debate, the dissidents established a rival organization to the USMF, the Fédération des syndicats médicaux de France (FSMF). After fifteen years of controversy, the 1930 social insurance law was enacted, and it included the four principles of the Medical Charter. This national health insurance was essentially a legislative support for the numerous previously private sick funds. Employees covered were required to enroll in a fund, and the state paid the premiums out of taxes levied on wages and employers. At this juncture, the two organizations reunited, taking a name first used in 1928, the Confédération des syndicats médicaux français.

Based on this consolidation, the 1930s opened for French physicians the golden parenthesis of liberal medicine. Limited national health insurance was not passed in the interwar period until organized medicine agreed to its terms. However, there persisted forces of division and contestation characterizing relations both within the medical profession and between the profession and the state authorities. These recurrent strains meant that the French profession was ill suited to consolidate gains when achieved and incapable of effectively defending the liberal parenthesis as it came under attack by the state authorities.

Closing the Liberal Parenthesis

With the Nazi occupation, the Vichy government dissolved unions and associations of all kinds, establishing in their place obligatory and unitary corporate bodies. The Ordre des médecins, which mandated the membership of all physicians in a single organization, policed the practice of medicine and served as the policy conduit from the Vichy authorities to the medical profession. The officers of the order, medical doctors and civil servants, were appointed by the government.

With the Nazi defeat, French unions and associations were legalized in 1945, and the Ordre des médecins was reformed. Most important, the social security system established by the law of 1930 was replaced. The ordinance of October 19, 1945, instituted a new and expanded social security system in three parts: retirement, family allowances, and sickness. The political impulsion for this system came both from the widespread feeling that the prewar record of social services was dismal and from the suspicion, also widespread, that this state of affairs had a great deal to do with the 1939 defeat to the Nazis. A clear principle of social solidarity underpins these social security reforms.

The 1945 ordinances were originally designed by the Conseil national de la résistance to extend health care, retirement pensions, and family allowances in a unitary administrative system. The interwar system established between 1928 and 1930 covered only a small percentage of salaried workers, those below a relatively low wage ceiling. In the postwar politics of generalizing social security, however, miners, the merchant marine, functionaries, and employees of the national railroads fought to keep their own individual health care and retirement regimes. Initially, then, in addition to these specialized regimes, one general regime covered all other wage laborers, and another specialized regime covered agricultural workers. In subsequent years, social security protection was extended to students, writers, artisans, and independent shopkeepers. In the 1970s, the remaining margins of the population were covered: handicapped adults, widows, and divorced women in 1975, single parents in 1976, and all others theretofore not covered in 1978. This last category constituted little over 2 percent of the general population, including, ironically, physicians. As of 1985 only 0.4 percent of the French population (defined to include all citizens and residents) remained uncovered; these 0.4 percent are normally treated through public welfare funds.

French physicians generally favored the national health insurance of the new social security system, but there were numerous details of dispute. The first major conflict with the postwar government was over setting fees. Originally, the ministers of labor, health, and the national economy were to fix fee schedules independently. Organized medicine, which had not been consulted in the elaboration of the new social security and health care policies, objected. Michel Parodi, the minister of labor and chief proponent of a new comprehensive social security system, chose to accommodate physicians' demands in order to forestall further opposition to the implementation of his program. He agreed to establish tripartite commissions— composed of equal parts of state authorities, sickness fund representatives, and the medical profession—that would meet periodically to negotiate the fee schedules. The commissions would operate under the direction of the ministries of labor and the economy. Although in theory quasi-independent, in fact they were closely dependent on the government, for the law permitted the government to set overall contribution and expenditure levels of the system. Throughout the 1950s the deficits of the social security system grew, despite corrective measures as early as 1950. Successive governments believed that one essential way of grappling with these deficits was containing physicians' fees.

In 1946, the government wished to establish a fee system *opposable,* or binding, on all physicians. In the French system of *la médecine libérale,* patients paid physicians directly and were later reimbursed specified amounts by the sickness funds, usually from 75 to 80 percent of the scheduled fees. Hospitalization was covered 100 percent and paid directly by the funds. Because the scheduled fees were not binding, percentages of reimbursement of fees actually paid by patients varied widely—sometimes as low as 30 percent of the fee charged. Without a binding schedule, physicians could charge what they wished—and they did.

Responding to public discontent, successive governments sought, with the support of the sickness funds and both labor and management, a binding fee schedule. Two rationales advanced by the government proved to be equally compelling. First, the principle of solidarity was both widely shared in society and deeply perceived. This sentiment cut across traditional ideological cleavages and traditional economic class divisions. Second, as physicians raised fees beyond those specified by the schedules for reimbursement calculations, public pressures arose on the sickness funds and on successive governments to raise the fees specified by the schedules in order to reimburse a de facto 75 to 80 percent of what had become higher rates.

Throughout the 1950s, physicians fought these government attempts to establish binding fee schedules. In particular, the *project Gazier,* a comprehensive reform initiative of the minister of social affairs in 1956–1957, was barely stopped by the CSMF and, in the end, definitively forced French medical syndicalism into a highly reactive political posture. As the conflict developed, tensions and two tendencies within the medical profession became more apparent. The CSMF leadership moved toward a policy of relative conciliation as most realistic, but a large and growing dissident movement favored noncooperation with the government or the sickness funds in any new binding fee system. The difference between these two tendencies may be thought of as the difference between contestation from without versus contestation from within normal negotiating channels.

The controversy simmered, never too far below the surface, as the government persistently tried to circumvent organized medicine's resistance to reforming the health insurance system. The growing political crisis in France regarding the Algerian question, the fall of the Fourth Republic, de Gaulle's return to power, and the creation of the Fifth Republic, all in 1958, worked to distract the state authorities momentarily from domestic battles. But by 1960, the state had returned to business, and with a vengeance. The decree of May 12, 1960, imposed binding fee schedules negotiated at the departmental level on all physicians. Further, it provided for physicians to adhere individually to the negotiated agreements rather than through the mediating institutions of organized medicine. Individual physicians who did not sign agreements to abide by these fee schedules lost their patients' right to be reimbursed by the sickness funds. This development constituted an extraordinarily effective wedge driven by the state between, first, the patient and the physician and, second, the physician and organized medicine. In the face of this thorough defeat, the French profession formally splintered; several dissident movements broke off from the CSMF to form their own groups.

With the Decree of May 12, 1960, the Fifth Republic dealt the coup de grace to organized medicine as a voice in health care policy. The decline in organized medicine's influence had been well underway since the beginnings of the postwar period, when the state had not thought to consult organized medicine on how fees ought to be set. Only after vigorous protests from the CSMF was organized medicine reluctantly included in the process.

In the wake of the Decree of May 12, 1960, and in the face of the CSMF leadership's choice to contest from within in order to shape future policies, dissident movements that had long agitated for contestation from without broke off from the CSMF. Numerous departmental affiliates and some specialty associations left the CSMF to form the Union syndicale des médecins de France. Others left to constitute the Association médicale pour la recherche et l'union syndicale. The Fédération nationale des généralistes français was a third one. Each of these claimed a national membership among the medical corps. This fragmentation of organized medicine only accentuated the profession's reactive political posture in its relations with the state, further decreasing its influence in health care policymaking and by consequence strengthening the state's hand.

In 1967, the three dissident organizations joined together better to oppose the CSMF, still seen as having sold out to the state for having chosen to remain within the orthodox channels of politics. These groups formed the Fédération des médecins de France (FMF). From 1967 until 1985, a series of conflicts opposed the CSMF to the FMF over fee agreements, social benefits, cooperation with state authorities, and other matters. In 1971, the FMF was recognized by the state as officially representative of the entire medical profession, in addition to the CSMF. It thus became the second privileged interlocutor of the government and the second official negotiator for physicians with the sickness funds.

The split of French organized medicine into two competing national associations manifested itself in concrete ways over specific issues. In 1971, the CSMF signed the first negotiated National Convention fixing physicians' fees; the FMF refused to do so. In 1976, the FMF was the only party to sign the second National Convention, although both groups took part in negotiations. In 1980, the FMF alone negotiated and signed the third; the CSMF finally signed in 1981. Each time the state decreed that if one organization "representative" of the entire medical profession had signed, the provisions of the convention would therefore apply to all physicians. Only for the 1985 convention did both groups participate fully in the negotiations with the funds and approve the final product with their signatures. During the 1989 negotiations, matters were further complicated as three unions (now including MG France) sparred with each other over the terms of the convention at least as much as they sparred with the sickness fund itself.

The Fiscal Imperative and the Decline of Organized Medicine's Influence

Throughout its historical evolution, the character of the French national health insurance system has been critically influenced by two forces, and both have worked to reinforce state autonomy while diminishing the influence of the medical profession on health policy.

The first force, the concept of solidarity, underpins the development of social security since the nineteenth century. By solidarity, I refer to the agreement by all elements of an otherwise highly divided French society that social assistance was necessary to the strength and well-being of France—both to its internal cohesiveness and to its power internationally. This unity of purpose was focused around the concepts of mutual dependence and national obligation, and it was directed toward social welfare goals concerning unemployment, family allowances, retirement pensions, and health care. The theme of solidarity dates to at least the French Revolution and has historically attracted all shades of French intellectual thought. This sentiment was particularly strong in France at the close of World War II. It was a crucial factor in the coming together of all ideological factions in favor of a reformed social security system.

The second force, particularly important with respect to the financing and administration of the French health care system, is the corps of civil servants imbued with a strong sense of bureaucratic mission, or the sense that French high functionaries believe that they act with the authority to perform a special duty. This duty involves the constant definition and defense of the general interest in the face of all who would assert partisan interests contrary to the interests of the whole, or of France. This sense of mission is not unlike the preaching, teaching, and proselytizing of a religious order. It gives high functionaries the perception that the state has an interest that is both definable and defendable. It also shapes their understanding of where interests lie, which of these are compatible with the state's interest, and what types of conduct by decision makers and outside groups are appropriate to this administrative-political universe.

The overriding imperative that bound the principle of solidarity and bureaucratic mission together as a cohesive force against organized medicine in the postwar period was the financing of national health insurance. As early as 1946, bureaucrats fretted about the cost of health care. These worries were accentuated by rising expenditures throughout the 1950s. As early as 1949, the French social security system ran increasing deficits, due almost entirely to increasing health care expenditures. Corrective measures were instituted as early as 1951: increased fiscal controls, stabilizing administrative costs, and raising the contribution levels of employers and employees to the health care regime. Rationalizing the fee-setting structures of the system was increasingly important.

Increasing health care expenditures were also due, in part, to a persistent expansion of health care insurance, in terms of both populations covered and benefits provided. But the fiscal imperative in health care also was due in part to medical technology and more active treatment patterns on the part of the medical corps. The history of relations between the state and the medical profession that I have explored in this chapter shows a continuous decline in organized medicine's ability to set physicians' fees. Even in the immediate postwar period, the principle of solidarity, the overarching ethos of a strong, committed bureaucratic corps, and the imperatives of postwar social and economic reconstruction combined to place the French medical corps and its organizations in a reactive posture in its relations with the state. The postwar history of organized medicine in France is one of increasingly important challenges from the state.

In response to the fiscal imperative, the French state has consistently followed a strategy of severe income containment for providers, strict prospective budgeting for hospitals, and very low prescription drug prices. However, it has not chosen to attack vigorously the clinical autonomy of providers—that is, the freedom to treat, diagnose, prescribe to, refer, and admit patients—although it has controlled the kinds of facilities and equipment at their disposal. In this respect, the fiscal imperative combined with the French variant of national health insurance that I have described has not severely diminished the professional autonomy or dominance of the medical corps, but it has definitely reduced the socioeconomic status of doctors—their incomes and their prestige—thus proletarianizing the medical corps.

Acknowledgment

I wish to acknowledge the assistance of Frederic W. Hafferty in constructively critiquing the content and style of this chapter. It is better for it, though he bears no responsibility for remaining weaknesses.

11

The Power of
Organized Medicine in Greece

John Colombotos and Nikos P. Fakiolas

Half a century ago, the American Medical Association (AMA) was a dominant force in health care in the United States. One source considered it to be "the most powerful legislative lobby in Washington. . . . [It] holds a position of authority over the individual doctor, wields a determining voice in medical education, controls the conditions of practice, and occupies a unique position of influence in shaping government health policies" (Hyde et al. 1954). Although the AMA has lost a good deal of its power since then, it is still one of the dominant medical associations in the world.

This chapter examines organized medicine in another country, Greece, with a view toward better understanding the factors that enhance and restrict the power of organized medicine in different countries and over time. Factors that might be considered in such an analysis include those that are unique to organized medicine, as well as those that affect professional associations and interest groups in general. In the case of organized medicine, they fall into two broad categories. The first are characteristics of the health care system and the medical profession, such as how physicians are paid and the setting in which they practice, the amount and types of professional differentiation, the extent and intensity of colleague networks among physicians, the number of medical associations and whom they represent, the extent to which these associations are perceived to represent their constituents, the resources of these associations, the number and proportion of potential members who are members of each association, the social composition of the medical profession, including their social origins and gender, and the status and income levels of members of the profession. The second category refers to characteristics of the political system, such as the type of government and the political party system, and of the political culture that affect the power of all professional associations in a society (Eckstein 1960:37–38; LaPalombara 1963; Truman 1971; Altenstetter 1974; Grant 1989:113–32).

In this chapter, we examine two features of the health care system in Greece—the overlapping of salaried and private practice by the majority of physicians and the rapidly expanding oversupply of physicians—and two features of the political

138

system that affect the power of all professional associations and many interest groups—their legal relationship and domination by the state and the penetration of political parties into the affairs of these associations. Finally, we consider features of the political culture of Greece that emphasize personal connections in achieving personal goals, thereby undermining reliance on collective action.

In comparing this with other case studies, it is useful to locate these investigations in a framework of related questions; for example, different medical societies representing different segments of the profession (e.g., specialties versus general practitioners, academic physicians versus practitioners) may exercise power over different domains (e.g., entry into the profession, professional training and licensure, discipline over members of the profession, and organization and financing of health care) using different methods (e.g., by influencing health care legislation and the administration of programs affecting the profession and by setting standards for training and practice) in different countries.

Since Greece gained its independence in 1828, following four hundred years of Ottoman rule, its history commonly has been characterized as turbulent. Wars, including several civil wars, and continuous foreign intervention have been interleaved with political instability, including monarchies, dictatorships, and military juntas. A parliamentary democracy was restored in 1975, following a military dictatorship (1967–1974). The analysis in this chapter is set against a backdrop of dramatic changes in Greek politics and health care legislation over the past decade, including the election of the first Socialist government in 1981 and the subsequent passage of the National Health System Act (NHS) in 1983.

The current population of nearly 10 million has been remarkably stable over the past several decades. It is homogeneous ethnically and in the religious affiliation of its residents (96 percent are Greek Orthodox). Although its standard of living has steadily improved since World War II, Greece's gross national product per capita is higher only than Portugal's among the countries in the European Community (Organization for Economic Cooperation and Development 1991:26–27).

The Health Care System: Overlapping of Salaried and Private Practice and Physician Oversupply

The organization of health care services in Greece is best characterized as mixed. Although over 90 percent of the Greek population is covered by some form of health insurance (Yfantopoulos 1985:116), it is estimated that 25 percent of the cost of personal health care services is paid for in cash, out of pocket, mainly for private medical care. (The latter figure is an estimate based on studies of family expenditures, cited by Niakas, Skoutelis, and Kyriopoulos 1990.)

The country's population is covered by more than a hundred health insurance funds, most of them organized along industry-wide lines (e.g., banks, communications, and public utilities) and financed through compulsory contributions by employers and employees and subsidized by the government. Nearly three-fourths of the total population, however, is covered by two plans: the Agricultural Insurance Organization (OGA), established in 1961, which covers the rural population (34% of the total population), and the Social Insurance Institute (IKA), established in 1934, which insures salaried workers not covered by a specific industry plan (40% of the total population) (Yfantopoulos 1985:116). The National Health System Act, passed in 1983 and implemented in 1986, provided for the eventual absorption of OGA, IKA, and the industry-based health insurance funds into a unified system, but resistance from these funds has blocked this change. All but a small proportion of the ambulatory medical care covered by these funds, excluding NHS, is currently provided by physicians on a salaried, part-time basis.

The NHS employs about 9,000 of the 35,000 physicians in Greece on a salaried, full-time basis, most of whom are hospital based. Most of the remaining physicians work part-time for IKA (about 9,000 physicians) or for one of the health insurance funds (about 12,000). Fewer than an estimated 15 percent of all physicians (about 5,000) are engaged exclusively in private practice.

A large portion of out-of-pocket cash payments is for care in private practice. An estimated 90 percent of the country's salaried physicians, including the full-time NHS doctors, for whom it is illegal, carry on a private practice. Much of this income is not reported by physicians for tax purposes, a situation characterized by analysts as an "underground economy of health" (Niakas, Skoutelis, and Kyriopoulos 1990).

The high consumption of private care, despite insurance coverage of over 90 percent of the population, reflects patients' dissatisfaction with the technical and personal quality of services covered by insurance, including complaints about crowded facilities, long waiting time, and hurried care (Yfantopoulos 1985:119–20; Fakiolas 1988:217). Physicians foster and exploit these conditions. They show little interest in patients in their salaried practices and invite them to visit them in their private offices, or they may even openly treat them as private patients in the health center or hospital where they are employed.

Another major source of cash income for physicians—and out-of-pocket expenses for patients—is illegal payments to salaried physicians, the *fakelaki* ("little envelope"), essentially a bribe to facilitate services covered by insurance. The practice is all but universal in cases of surgery. Otherwise, patients experience long waits for an available hospital bed. The amount proffered depends on the resources of the patient and the reputation of the physician. Medical professors command the largest *fakelakia*.

Doctors' salaries are relatively low. In 1992, full-time salaried physicians in the NHS earned an annual salary of between $9,500 and $19,000 (U.S. dollars). IKA physicians, who work five and a half hours a day, earned between $3,800 and $6,300 annually. For most physicians, however, cash earnings from their private practice and *fakelakia*—an estimated $30,461 in 1992 U.S. dollars annually per physician—make up a major portion of their income. (We calculated this estimate by assuming that 70 percent of the total amount of out-of-pocket medical expenses in 1987 [105 billion drachmas] was for private medical fees and *fakelakia* and dividing that figure by the total number of 33,200 physicians at that time. We converted that figure into 1992 U.S. dollars by adjusting for the increase in the cost of living in Greece between 1987 and 1992 and by applying the exchange rate in 1992.) For comparative purposes, in 1992 high school teachers earned approximately $10,000 and midlevel civil servants about $15,800. These figures emphasize the importance of a salaried position to physicians. It provides a modest salary and, more important, a source of recruitment of private patients and an income, much of which is not taxed.

Although medicine is not regarded as rewarding financially or as prestigious as it was a few decades ago, it is still considered one of the most desirable careers in Greece. The proportion of university graduates of the total population in Greece is among the highest of those in Europe (Tsoukalas 1976), and career opportunities are limited. A university education, including the six-year course of study leading to a medical degree, is contingent on passing national examinations but is free of charge at one of the seven medical schools in the national university system. (There are no private medical schools in Greece.) Moreover, many students who do not pass the national examinations gain a medical education elsewhere and enter practice when they return to Greece. Consequently, Greece lags behind only Belgium and Spain among countries in the European Community in the number of physicians in relation to its population (Organization for Economic Cooperation and Development 1991:46–47). The number of doctors is rising rapidly; it nearly doubled from 18,000 in 1974 to 35,000 in 1991. The Ministry of Education is under intense public pressure to maintain the large number of positions in the country's medical schools. Physician oversupply is an issue that no group, including organized medicine and the political parties, has confronted.

Organized Medicine and Its Relationship to the State

There are two main types of medical societies: official medical societies, created by national law to perform official, public functions and to negotiate as trade unions on behalf of all physicians, and unofficial organizations representing special groups of physicians, in which membership is voluntary.

Official Medical Societies

The governance and duties of the fifty-eight official local societies and of the national confederation of local societies, the Panhellenic Medical Society (Panellinios Iatrikos Sillogos [PIS]), were defined by law in 1923 and codified in 1939 during the Metaxas dictatorship. Membership in the local society is mandatory. Similar official organizations represent the other professions (Legg 1969:98–124).

Like the *ordini* in Italy formed during Mussolini's regime (Krause 1988*b*), the national and local medical societies are legally defined as public institutions. Among the functions of the national society, decreed by law, are to coordinate the activities of the local medical societies; to maintain and administer the medical profession's code of ethics; to advise the Ministry of Health, Welfare, and Social Insurance on matters affecting the public's health and the medical profession; to encourage the development of medical science and to advise on medical education, postgraduate training, and the scientific and professional development of physicians; to publish a medical journal; and to represent the country's physicians in the World Medical Association. The local societies are charged with a wide range of administrative functions on behalf of the state. All doctors are required to register annually in their local society and to list their salaried position.

The internal governance of the medical societies is decreed by law in great detail. This includes the number, composition, and functions of the executive and disciplinary committees, the precise methods of voting and balloting, and the frequency of meetings and the quorums of the local societies and of the General Assembly of PIS. Voting and attendance at meetings are mandatory. The disciplinary committees of the local societies are presided over by a layperson. Even the size and design of the official seals used by PIS and the local medical societies are decreed by law.

The deliberations of the executive committee and general assembly of PIS are under the surveillance of the state. Sitting in on their meetings (without voting) is a representative of the minister of social services. Although none of our informants could recall such an instance (with the exception of the junta's action in 1967), the minister of health, welfare, and social insurance has the power to remove officers and members of the executive committee of PIS and of the local medical societies for just cause.

Although their advisory role is legally acknowledged, the official medical societies have little or no formal voice in such important matters as the number of physicians to be trained (medical faculty are consulted, but their advice is generally ignored by the Ministry of Education, which makes the decisions), undergraduate medical education and specialty training, which are the responsibility of the Ministry of Education and the Ministry of Health, Welfare, and Social Insurance, respectively, and the licensing of physicians, which is pro forma, without examination, after graduation from medical school.

Before the junta (1967–1974), the medical societies negotiated contracts between the health insurance funds and groups of physicians. This arrangement was abrogated by the junta. Its reinstatement has been discussed recently in the parliament.

The Unofficial Organizations

The main unofficial organizations are the Union of Hospital Physicians, Athens-Piraeus (Enosis Iatron Nosileftirion, Athenon-Piraeus [EINAP]), established in 1976 and representing about 8,000 salaried physicians below the rank of departmental director employed in hospitals in Athens-Piraeus, and the Society of Professional Health Personnel of IKA (Sillogos Epistimonikou Igionomikou Prosopikou, IKA [SEIPIKA]), established in 1972 and representing about 6,000 salaried physicians employed in the IKA health centers in Athens-Piraeus. Both were formed, according to their leaders, because their constituencies felt that their interests were not being represented by the official medical societies of Athens and Piraeus. Each of these organizations has regional counterparts outside the Athens-Piraeus metropolitan area, forming loose federations.

According to its president, EINAP has had a history, albeit short, of successful strikes to improve the working conditions of hospital doctors, including shorter hours, higher pay, better meals and sleeping conditions, improvement in learning situations, and grievance procedures that removed departmental directors' dictatorial power over junior physicians. EINAP was identified by others as a strong, militant organization with growing power.

Unofficial organizations also include specialty societies, which do not play any political role or have any official function in establishing standards for specialty training programs or in admitting or examining candidates. Their activities are mainly scientific (seminars, meetings, and journals).

In many other countries, the academic medical community is represented by an organization, official or unofficial, such as the Association of American Medical Colleges in the United States. This is not the case in Greece. Academic physicians are reputed to be a powerful influence on the government's personnel appointments and health policies, but that influence is expressed informally and personally, on the individual level, rather than formally, through an organization. Although their power is reputed to have declined recently, academic physicians are still considered a potent force in medical politics. "Their roots run deep," we were told by an informant.

In sum, the official and unofficial medical societies have complementary strengths and weaknesses. Official societies derive strength from their inclusivity and their legitimacy. Their recognition by the state as the official representative body of physicians supports their claim as "the voice of Greek medicine." But with respect to matters that count, their power is tightly limited by the state.

The unofficial organizations are less encumbered by legal restrictions in their principal role as trade unions, and because of the greater homogeneity of interests among their members, they can present a more unified and more militant stance than the more inclusive official societies. They are, however, limited by their restricted constituencies.

Penetration of Political Parties

The penetration of political party politics into the affairs of secondary organizations is pervasive in Greece. It appears in trade unions and professional associations, university student organizations, women's groups, environmental groups, and even village societies, which are social clubs in urban areas of persons from the same village or rural area (Legg 1969). With respect to organized medicine, the penetration of party politics is expressed in two ways: in the laws that define election procedures and the internal structure of the official medical associations and in the influence of the political parties on the policies of both official and unofficial associations.

Elections and Internal Structure

Although the specific election procedures of the executive committees of the official and unofficial medical societies vary, candidates are explicilty identified with a political party. Another example of the influence of party politics is the partisan-inspired national law under which the larger, official local medical societies (Athens, Salonika, Piraeus) are underrepresented in PIS's General Assembly. Passed in 1977, when the conservative New Democracy party was in power, the law effectively limits the influence of the larger medical societies, whose leadership was then left of center politically, and increased the influence of the smaller, rural medical societies, whose leadership was more likely to be loyal to the New Democracy party.

Policies

Following the collapse of the military junta in 1974, there have been two major proposals for reforming the health care system: New Democracy's Measures for the Protection of Health (MPH), introduced in the fall of 1979 but later defeated in parliament, and PASOK's (Panhellenic Socialist Movement) National Health System (NHS), which was passed by parliament in 1983 (Tsalikis 1988; Kent 1989). The politics of these proposals exemplify the penetration of party politics into the affairs of organized medicine.

New Democracy's plan provided for a national and regional health planning council representing health providers and consumers, the decentralization of health care services to make these services more accessible to the rural population, the promotion of primary care, the restriction of entry into speciality training based on competitive examinations, and a system of full-time hospital doctors prohibited from engaging in private practice. How the medical societies responded to the plan depended on the party loyalties of their leadership.

PIS, EINAP, SEIPIKA, and other organizations controlled by opposition parties argued that the plan did not go far enough and called for a national health service. Other organizations, controlled by the New Democracy party, were equivocal. In early 1980, only a few months after the initial announcement of the plan, EINAP staged a one-day strike against its introduction in parliament and demanded its withdrawal. The strike was interpreted by its opponents as a PASOK-directed tactic to embarrass the New Democracy government. Later in the spring, the PASOK-controlled Executive Committee of PIS missed, by one vote, voting in favor of a national strike to protest the MPH plan, demanding its withdrawal. The gingerly and equivocal response of the official medical society of Athens, controlled by an Executive Committee loyal to New Democracy, stood in sharp contrast.

The MPH bill was defeated in parliament a few months before the national elections in 1981, in which PASOK won control of a coalition government. Two years later, Parliament passed the PASOK-sponsored National Health System Act (Law 1397/1983), which was implemented in 1986. Like the New Democracy–sponsored MPH, it prohibited private practice by full-time salaried NHS doctors. Unlike the MPH, it provided for the absorption of the health insurance funds into a unified system.

Again, the responses of the medical societies to NHS were dictated by party politics. The opposition of the PASOK-controlled medical societies to New Democracy's MPH bill in 1980–1981 was consistent with both their own party loyalties and their members' interests, which were to continue to combine a salaried practice with a private practice. When NHS was proposed by PASOK in 1983, however, it was the turn of the PASOK-dominated societies, which included PIS and the three largest local official medical societies of Athens (which had switched from New Democracy control), Piraeus, and Salonika, as well as EINAP and SEIPIKA, to walk the tightrope between their loyalty to their party and the interests of their physician constituents. Party loyalties won out. The PASOK-controlled medical societies either supported NHS or remained silent. None opposed it.

In the 1984 elections of the executive committees of PIS and the official local societies of Athens, Piraeus, and Salonika, control shifted from PASOK to New Democracy. This shift was due in part to physician members' expressing their opposition to NHS by voting for the New Democracy candidates. These societies then turned against the PASOK-backed NHS. Conversely, EINAP and SEIPIKA, still controlled by coalitions of PASOK and other leftist parties, continued to support NHS.

Clearly, medical societies' responses to health care legislation are influenced by party politics, often more than by a concern for the interests of their constituents. Party loyalty is exchanged for party-controlled patronage, which includes positions in the NHS, the public hospitals, and other government posts. (Many physicians in Greece are active in general party politics; for example, 42 of the 300 members of the 1992 parliament were physicians, second only to lawyers.)

Influence also flows from profession to party. Passage of the NHS by the PASOK government in 1983 was followed by a protest vote in 1984 that elected majorities of New Democracy candidates to the executive committees of PIS and most of the local official societies. The New Democracy amendments to the NHS in 1991, providing physicians with the opportunity to work for the NHS part time and engage in private practice and loosening restrictions on the opening and expansion of private clinics, were also instances of professional influence on the New Democracy party. Serving as conveyor belts of mutual influence between profession and party are the branch committees of the political parties, each branch committee representing an interest group, for example, physicians, lawyers, and labor.

The net effect of the penetration of party politics into medical politics, however, is to fragment organized medicine along party lines and to compromise collective professional interests.

Discussion

The power of organized medicine, as is true of all professional associations in Greece, is limited by two features of the political system. First, like all other official professional associations in Greece, the official medical societies are muzzled by the state. They perform many administrative functions on behalf of the state, but they have little control over their own affairs. Legally defined as public institutions, their structure, governance, and functions are explicitly dictated by national law, their meetings are under the surveillance of a representative of the state, they are in the vulnerable position of negotiating on behalf of their physician-constituents with a ministry that may dismiss their leadership for just cause, and their right to strike is legally questioned. The restoration of their right to negotiate contracts between physicians and the NHS and the health insurance funds would add considerably to what little power they possess, much as the national health services in the United Kingdom and in Italy strengthened the hand of organized medicine in those countries (Larkin 1988; Krause 1988*b*). Nonetheless, they have little voice in such important matters as the entry, training, and credentialing of physicians. The unofficial medical societies are less restricted legally in their role as trade unions and pressure groups, but they represent only limited segments of the profession.

Second, the intrusion of political parties into medical politics splits the profession along nonprofessional lines. Medical societies' responses to health legislation, for example, are influenced less by its collective consequences for physicians than by party loyalty. Party influence works because party loyalty is exchanged for patronage for the party faithful.

The power of organized medicine is also affected by two factors, one positively and the other negatively, specific to the medical profession. While organized medicine in Greece is fragmented by diversity originating outside the profession in the form of conflicting political party loyalties, it is relatively free of differentiation originating from within the profession. In other countries, the medical profession has had to deal with the problem of balancing the collective interests of the profession as a whole against the conflicting interests of its segments: academics versus practitioners (Kendall 1965), general practitioners versus specialists (Stevens 1971), and salaried versus private practitioners (Honigsbaum 1979). Fragmentation between any of these segments is not yet a serious problem in Greece, as it is, for example, between the capitation-paid, community-based general practitioners and the salaried, hospital-based specialists in the British system. The overlapping of activities of the majority of physicians, who combine salaried and private practice, has prevented the development of distinct segments—one of exclusively full-time salaried practitioners and another of exclusively full-time private practitioners. The profession's solidarity and, consequently, its political power, modest to begin with, to be sure, are not threatened by this source of diversity and conflict.

The poor quality of care provided in the health insurance plans and by the NHS and the thriving underground health economy feed on each other. A salaried position in a facility delivering poor care provides both a modest salary and a source of private patients. The poorer the coverage is and the worse the quality of care in that facility, the larger is the market for private care. Physicians have a vested interest in maintaining that system.

One scenario, however unlikely, is that pressure for reform would create a system providing for a large full-time NHS cadre of salaried physicians who would be effectively prohibited from engaging in private practice. This would be followed by the emergence of two distinct segments: one of full-time salaried NHS doctors and another of full-time fee-for-service practitioners working outside the publicly funded system. As these distinct segments become more homogeneous internally, medical societies representing their conflicting interests, mainly in the form of competition for patients, are likely to clash with each other and with the umbrella official medical societies, fragmenting the profession and thereby further weakening it.

The second factor is that the expanding oversupply of physicians in Greece is likely to continue unchecked. As a result, the effectiveness of the official medical societies as bargaining agents with NHS and the health insurance funds will be increasingly compromised.

Little in Greece supports a strong, organized medical profession. Organized medicine in Greece has not lost power during the past two to three decades as has, for example, organized medicine in the United States (Tierney 1987). It did not have much power to begin with. This weak power arose not so much because of characteristics of the health care system (except for the worsening physician over-supply) but because of both the formal political system and enduring, historically rooted features of the Greek political culture, formed in large measure during the 400 hundred years of Ottoman rule. (*Political culture* refers to the pattern of orientations and attitudes toward political action in which the formal political system is embedded [Almond 1956]. It stresses the informal aspects of a country's politics, distinguishing them from the formal aspects of political systems, such as govern-mental institutions and laws.)

Organized medicine in Greece is formally controlled by a paternalistic state and fragmented by the penetration of political parties, and it is undermined by a political culture that emphasizes the following (Legg 1969:98–124; Diamandouros 1983):

• Suspicion and mistrust of public authorities and secondary organizations, especially if, like official professional associations, they are associated with the state.

• Lawlessness. Since the law is viewed as arbitrary, the objective is to ma-nipulate and evade it. For example, failure to report their cash income for tax purposes is not unique to physicians. A large volume of financial exchange in Greece, often involving large amounts of money, is carried out on a cash basis and is undeclared (Tsoukalas 1986).

• A system in which people pursue individual goals for themselves or their kin through personal influence and exchange of patronage for loyalty rather than through collective action. Often referred to as political clientelism, the significant social unit in this pattern of influence is the family rather than the community or the secondary organization. (For an excellent collection of readings on the broad concept of political clientelism, see Schmidt et al. 1977.)

The overarching theme of this political culture is that the use of personal con-nections in pursuing individual goals overrides the use of collective means in pursuing collective goals. This pattern flourishes in societies, such as Greece, characterized by social mistrust and weak secondary organizations. It feeds the cynicism that leads to mistrust, and it inhibits the development of strong interest groups, including professional associations.

Recent studies of the professions emphasize the role of the state in conditioning both the power of the professions as corporate bodies and the autonomy of individual professionals at work. Krause (1991) suggests a continuum of profession-state relations, ranging from the essentially private professions with limited state in-volvement in the United States, to the state-involved professions of Western Europe, to the primarily state-located and state-employed professions of Eastern Europe (p. 4).

Greece highlights the significance of the informal political culture, as distinct from the formal political system, in comparing profession-state relations in different countries. In this context, the similarities in the status of organized medicine, the health care systems, and the political cultures of Greece and Italy are striking (Krause 1988*a*, 1988*b*). State-dominated official medical societies, the penetration of political parties and political patronage, an oversupply of physicians, and illegal overlapping of salaried and private practice by most physicians are common to both countries, as are public mistrust of government and an emphasis on personal influence and connections to achieve individual goals.

Macridis (1983:12–13, 435–76) describes a "Mediterranean profile" of countries that distinguishes the political systems and political cultures of Greece, Italy, Spain, and Portugal from those of the rest of Europe. They are the poorest countries in the European Community, they have large numbers of peasant farmers with small landholdings, there are large gaps between the elites and the masses in terms of literacy and wealth, they are the most unstable politically (they currently have parliamentary democracies, but all four have experienced lengthy dictatorships since the 1930s, along with frequent interventions of the military into their politics), there are sharp cleavages in terms of social class, region, and church versus lay divisions, and political patronage and personal ties are dominant features of their political cultures. Also, economic modernization came late to these countries, after World War II, and has proceeded rapidly since then, with its familiar effects of clashes between traditional and modern values and massive migrations from village to city and to other, more advantaged countries.

A challenging question for future study is how the political systems and political cultures of Mediterranean-type societies are linked to their health care systems and to the power of organized medicine and how these clusters of characteristics differ from those of other types of societies.

Abbreviations

EINAP   Union of Hospital Physicians: One of the two largest unofficial medical societies. (The other is SEIPIKA.)

IKA   Social Insurance Institute: National health insurance program covering salaried workers not covered by an industry plan.

MPH   Measures for the Protection of Health: National health plan proposed by the New Democracy government in 1981 but defeated.

ND   New Democracy party: Conservative political party, in power between 1974 and 1981 and since 1990.

NHS   National Health System Act: National health plan proposed by PASOK and enacted in 1983.

PASOK   Panhellenic Socialist Movement: Left-of-center political party, in power between 1981 and 1989.

PIS   Panhellenic Medical Society: The official national medical association.

SEIPIKA   Society of Professional Health Personnel of IKA: One of the two largest "unofficial" medical societies (the other is EINAP).

Acknowledgements

This research was supported by a senior international fellowship to John Colombotos from the Fogarty International Center of the National Institutes of Health. We thank the National Center for Social Research and the Fulbright Foundation office in Athens for providing facilities and collegiality to John during the academic year 1979–1980, and the director of the Fulbright office, Dr. David Larsen, for his valuable comments and criticisms on several drafts of this chapter; and David Abramson, Sally Cohen, Lambros Comitas, Mary Duncan, William Glaser, George Kent, Elliott Krause, Mata Nikias, and George Tsalikis for their comments on earlier drafts. We also thank Fred Hafferty for his invaluable help in seeing through to completion what seemed like an endless stream of drafts.

This chapter draws from interviews we conducted in 1979–1980 and 1990–1991 with officers and leaders of medical societies, government officials, and others active in health affairs in Greece. We thank them for their participation.

12

The Medical Profession in the Nordic Countries

Elianne Riska

Parsons's (1951) seminal work on the role of the physician and the characteristics of modern medical practice gave rise to a new field of research, the sociology of professions. This genre of research has tended to view, in the same way as Parsons did, physicians as forming an archetype of a profession. The sociological interest in the medical profession is, however, not only due to the profession's unique, sheltered position, which yields it considerable autonomy and control over its work. The interest is also related to the kind of work physicians do, which among other things reflects the values and broader structure of the social order of a society (Parsons 1958, 1963). Hence, a study of the medical profession illuminates both the work of this particular occupation and the broader function of health care in society.

The early functionalist approach to the study of professions was based on a consensual model, but sociological research since 1970 has brought attention to the social and political factors involved in the creation, maintenance, and decline of a profession's position in the occupational matrix of a society. The neo-Weberian and Marxist approaches have been foremost among the new theoretical frameworks (Saks 1983). Both were represented in the debate waged in the 1980s about the implications for the professional power and autonomy of American physicians as they increasingly practice in corporate settings.

The concerns of the impact of a bureaucratic setting of medical practice on the power of American physicians do not at first glance seem to be a novel issue for physicians in the Nordic countries. The role of the state in securing the work setting of the traditional professions—physicians, clergy, and lawyers—is a shared characteristic of the Nordic countries. The relationship between the medical profession and the state and the changes in this relationship will be illuminated in three ways in this chapter. First, I will describe the crucial role of the state in facilitating the emergence of a modern practice of medicine and how the medical profession cooperated in this venture with the state to secure its privileges. Second, I will show that the rise of the modern welfare state has led to a loss of control over medical work in many respects. In particular, public support of a primary care system has

Table 12.1. Population per physician in the Nordic countries, 1860–1988

Year	Denmark	Finland	Norway	Sweden
1860	4,362[a]	18,472	4,808	8,674
1890	2,244	10,012	2,875	5,937
1900	1,824	7,093	2,517	4,542
1930	1,425	3,449	1,586	2,743
1950	962	2,005	985	1,440
1960	811	1,573	884	1,053
1970	629	964	684	763
1980	460	531	522	499
1985	392	482	452	398
1988	384	332	378	338

Source: Berg (1980:24), Ito (1980:58), *Statistical Yearbook of Finland 1972* (1973:316), Nordic Medical Statistical Commission (1980:34), *Yearbook of Nordic Statistics 1986* (1987:329), Finnish Medical Association 1991.
[a]The data are from 1850 and derived from Rørbye (1976).

created a dual labor market among physicians: one high-technology and specialized area of medicine and another characterized by high social interaction areas practiced in primary care settings. This internal division of labor has tended to follow gender lines. Finally, I will discuss the impact of plans to introduce elements of a market economy in Nordic health care on physicians' professional position.

The Rise of the Medical Profession in the Nordic Countries

The Nordic countries are often viewed as very similar in terms of their social, political, and economic structure. Although they share many common cultural features, both their past and present societies differ considerably (Flora 1986). A similar picture emerges from an examination of the rise of the medical profession and its position in the modern health care system. This is vividly portrayed in the availability of physicians since 1860 until today and the projected future. In terms of population per physician, the Nordic countries can be divided into two groups (Table 12.1). During the late nineteenth century and most of this one, Denmark and Norway had a higher ratio than Sweden and Finland. Historically these two sets of countries have been tied politically to each other, but distinction nevertheless remain.

Denmark: Organized Medical Market

The numerical strength and concomitant professional power of physicians in Denmark was related to the early organization of the medical profession. When the Danish medical profession founded its national medical association in 1857, one of its agendas was the establishment of sickness funds to guarantee reimbursement for the services of private physicians (Ito 1980:50–52). For Danish physicians, an organized market of clients was nothing new. Craft guilds had secured the provision of medical coverage for their members by contracts with physicians. As the guilds were to be dissolved, by a law enacted eventually in 1861, the medical profession was eager to guarantee reimbursement for the services of private practitioners with the social groups that represented the new free market society. Although most physicians in the other Nordic countries were public employees, 65 percent of the Danish physicians were private practitioners in 1880, a feature that persisted until the 1950s (Ito 1980:54–56). The Danish medical profession managed to maintain its professional control by transforming the prior health care delivery arrangements of the craft and guild society into a modern context and thereby remain protected from the consequences of a free market of health care. The local Danish medical associations negotiated the financing of their services directly with the federation of local sickness funds, which consisted of local consumer cooperatives (McLeod 1975). In this way the public medical officers never received the same role and power as links between a centralized national medical association and the state, as occurred in the Swedish and Finnish health care systems. The relatively weak role of the state, a well-organized medical profession, and state-subsidized local sickness funds have led to a characterization of the Danish health care system as collective voluntarism (Ito 1980:65).

Norway: Public Sector Dominance

In Norway the rise of the medical profession was dependent on physicians educated abroad, mainly in Denmark and Germany, well into the nineteenth century. The first three professors of medicine were appointed only in 1914 at the newly established university in Christiania (Oslo). Although a domestic education of physicians had been started, the number of physicians grew slowly, hampered by two inter-related circumstances—a widely dispersed population and confidence in folk medicine that remained higher than in scientific medicine—both of which led to a small market for the regular physicians. The government did, however, provide possibilities for a career in medicine, in the armed forces, in municipal health care as medical officers, and in academic medicine (Berg 1980; Elstad 1987). So channeled, a majority of the physicians in Norway were tied to the public sector as employees during the nineteenth century, and their professional power was tied to their affiliation with the state and public authorities rather than with the private market.

Following World War II, medicine in Norway increasingly came to be practiced within publicly owned health care facilities, and a majority of the physicians remained public employees (Elstad 1987:292). The Norwegian Hospital Act of 1970 made the municipalities responsible for hospitals and nursing homes (Stevens 1989), a role that was strengthened by the Municipal Health Act of 1984 (Elstad 1990).

Sweden and Finland: Cooperation between the State and the Medical Profession

In Sweden and Finland the modern profession of medicine was slow to develop. Unlike Denmark, there was no organized medical market stemming from the preindustrial era, nor were there any large middle and working classes in the nineteenth century that would have provided a clientele and market for the emergence of a profession consisting of private practitioners. In both countries the public sector provided the infrastructure for the rise and expansion of scientific medicine (Anderson 1972; Garpenby 1989; Pesonen 1980). During the nineteenth century, medical practice in Sweden and Finland, as in Norway, was made possible through the establishment of salaried positions within state and local governments. Examples included district physician, municipal or city physician, prison physician, and chief ward physician at the state or municipal hospitals. Hence, entering public service was the surest way to secure clients. It is estimated that about 90 percent of the Swedish physicians were public employees in 1880, but the proportion of private practitioners increased to a third in 1900 and remained so until 1970 (Bergstrand 1963:156; Ito 1980:56).

Their status as public employees seems to have retarded the professional organization of both Swedish and Finnish physicians. Compared to the establishment of the Danish Medical Association in 1857 and the corresponding Norwegian Medical Association in 1886, the Swedish Medical Society (founded in 1807) and the Finnish equivalent one (founded in 1835) were primarily learned societies of academic and scholarly oriented physicians. When the Swedish physicians founded their national professional association in 1903 and the Finnish physicians in 1911, the national associations acted primarily as an interest group to influence public decision making (Kock 1963; Garpenby 1989; Pesonen 1980). Up to that time, the Swedish physicians had been more interested in improving their salary and pension as civil servants than in defending professional interests or professional autonomy, which had been the goals of the medical profession in France (Herzlich 1982) and the United States (Starr 1982).

The Swedish situation was paralleled in Finland. When the Finnish medical profession founded its professional organization, it lacked a cultural heritage or dominant market position as independent practitioners from an era of economic liberalism. The Finnish medical profession has therefore never appealed to any "sacred trust" (Harris 1969) or "ideology of liberal medicine" (Herzlich 1982) as a strategy to defend the position of a profession of independent practitioners. Instead, the statutes of the Finnish Medical Association stated explicitly that its purpose is to "defend and promote the social and economic interests of the physicians" or, in today's language, to act as a union in the collective bargaining process within the public sector (Kauttu and Kosonen 1985:36).

The late organization of the Swedish medical profession hampered its ability to influence legislation enacted for the regulation of the medical market. The first sickness fund law was enacted in 1891 in Sweden (later laws in 1910 and 1931), more than a decade before the profession organized itself. By contrast, the Danish medical profession took an active role in both the initiation and further implementation of the sickness funds. This move was replicated by the Finnish Medical Association, which had as a major item on its agenda the enactment of a national health insurance (Pesonen 1980). This legislation was not perceived as a threat to the Finnish medical profession but rather as a consolidator of its position in health care delivery. As in most other countries with a national health insurance (NHI), this system has not only guaranteed a set fee and reimbursement for a service but also confirmed the existing medical division of labor since only services by formally authorized health care occupations are reimbursed. Hence, NHI has been an effective way to reduce competition from rival medical sects or to prevent subordinated health care occupations from encroaching on the domain monopolized by the medical profession.

The elite of the medical profession in Finland and Sweden worked in top positions, although as public employees, in government-controlled hospitals or universities. In this position they almost automatically became part of the state bureaucracy and power elite. From the turn of the century to the early 1960s, there was a close working relationship between organized medicine and the National Board of Health in Finland. The relationship was characterized by interlocking membership in various organizations and by a "cosy brotherhood" (Kauttu and Kosonen 1985:122). Similarly, the Swedish medical profession had to cooperate with the state, embodied in the National Board of Health, which granted the profession its privileges (Garpenby 1989:48).

Since World War II, the relationship between the state and the medical profession in Sweden has not always remained as harmonious as in Finland. Immergut (1989) challenges the conventional notion that a tradition of local responsibility and patriarchal values (Anderson 1972) would have supported public provision of health care in the modern Swedish welfare state. Instead she points to the political conflicts surrounding government involvement in health care and suggests that major advancements in health care have been shaped by the legacy of interest group representation to create a consensus for Social Democratic policies. For example, national health insurance legislation was not a top priority of the trade unions or the Social Democratic party at the beginning of this century, as was the case in most European countries. Nor was the Swedish Medical Association (SMA) particularly interested in such a venture at that time. Instead it was more interested in rationalizing the voluntary health insurance system. This was done through the Sickness Fund Law of 1931, which established a national network of sickness funds and increased state subsidies for the funds (Immergut 1989:150–54).

Garpenby (1989:83) has called the period between 1945 and 1950 in Swedish health care policy one of hesitation. No single public body was an advocate for a public health policy because of the uncertainty of the economy and the implications of increased public spending. The hesitancy is exemplified further by the fact that although a national health insurance law was passed in 1947, it was not implemented until 1955. Meanwhile a controversy evolved around the reorganization of ambulatory medical care. At issue was the so-called Höjer report of 1948, a government commission that proposed the establishment of a national health service. This system would have made all physicians state civil servants and eliminated the physicians' right to have private patients and charge private fees at hospitals. The proposal stirred up a controversy around the issue of private practice, and it was not adopted for fear that physicians would transfer all their work from public to private hospitals.

The issue of private practice was readdressed in the hospital law of 1959 and in the so-called Seven Crowns reform of 1969 in Sweden. The hospital law eliminated private hospital beds and private fees in public hospitals. The Seven Crowns reform established a fee schedule for hospital stay and physicians as salaried employees responsible for both inpatient and outpatient care and with no rights to have private patients in public hospitals (Immergut 1989:158–59). Furthermore, the government, spurred by the Social Democrats, increased admission to state medical schools, which resulted in an eightfold rise in the number of physicians between 1940 and 1985. These measures considerably weakened the physicians' market position and created an oversupply of physicians, estimated to be about 4,000 physicians by the year 2000 (Nordisk Medicin 1984:164).

Garpenby (1989:85) has labeled the period from 1950 to 1975 in the Swedish health system one of creation; it was a process of strengthening of public funding of and control over health care. The Swedish Medical Association (SMA) did not, however, passively accept the health policy of the Social Democratic government. In the 1950s, it pursued a conservative policy directed by its chairperson, Dag Knutson, who wanted Swedish physicians to become more conscious of the values of professional freedom and autonomy as a response to the increasingly state-planned and -regulated policy of the Social Democrats. Since the 1960s, the SMA has pursued a strategy of collective bargaining as a white-collar union (Heidenheimer 1980; Carder and Klingenberg 1980:158). As Immergut (1989:154–65) notes, the association's political strategy is an accommodation to the political context of Swedish domestic policy, which is formed by interest groups and the so-called *remissystemet,* whereby interest groups are heard before government enacts legislation. One of the major interest groups in Sweden is an umbrella organization of the organized interests of professionals, Sveriges Akademikers Centralorganisation (SACO), a member of which the SMA has been since the end of the 1940s. Membership in SACO has implied participation in collective bargaining and threats of industrial action determined more by professional groups subordinated to the physicians than by the medical profession.

The rise of a modern medical profession in Norway, Sweden, and Finland was bolstered by the resources provided by the state and local government in the endeavor to develop a public sector of health care. A majority of the physicians in these countries have been public employees and part of a larger corporate public system. The national medical association in Sweden and Finland has formed a centralized and unified body, which contrasts with the broader role played by the local medical associations in the Danish health care system. Moreover, the role of the state in the Danish system has been one of a benevolent subsidizer of the contractual relation between the locally organized consumers and physicians. In the 1980s, however, there was a decentralization of health care—a shift from a state-planned to a locally run health care and a move toward an increasing freedom for both patients and physicians in all the Nordic countries.

From State Planning to Local Administration of Health Care since the 1970s

The 1950s and 1960s were characterized by an increased planning and regulation enforced by the state government in the Nordic countries. The objective of this centralization was, in line with the adopted welfare ideology, to reduce inequality in health among citizens. During these two decades, the primary emphasis was on an expansion of the hospital system; the challenge for the next decades was to

Table 12.2. Distribution of active physicians by activity, Nordic countries

Main Activity	Denmark (1988)	Finland (1988)	Norway (1986)	Sweden (1989)
Hospital health service	59.9%	52.6%	50.5%	70.8%
Nonhospital health service	30.6	37.0	39.0	25.0
Administration	1.4	1.7	3.3	NI
Medical research, education, etc.	4.6	7.0	4.2	1.2
Other medical work	3.5	1.7	3.0	2.9
(*N*)	13,679	9,177	9,443	24,000

Source: *Yearbook of Nordic Statistics 1989/90* (1990:323, 1991:328).

develop a public primary care system. The objective of these endeavors, at least in Norway, Sweden, and Finland, was to reduce differences in access to ambulatory care among regions and thereby to address the issue of regional differences in morbidity. The agenda never contained any explicit effort to reduce social class differences in health. Hence, although regional differences in health have diminished, social inequities in health have remained, at least in Sweden (Lundberg 1991) and Finland (Lahelma and Valkonen 1990).

Since 1970, a trend toward a decentralization of the health care systems in the Nordic countries can be discerned. In the first phase, it implied a shift from state to local government responsibility. In the second phase, it has been reflected in the support for a deregulation of health care and an introduction of free market strategies. What has been the impact of these reforms on the power and professional freedom of the physicians in the Nordic countries? In order to address this question, we have to examine the distribution of physicians in different sectors of the health care system in the Nordic countries. The reforms have had and will in the future have a different impact on different segments of the medical profession.

Table 12.2 shows that almost half of the active physicians worked in hospital health service in the Nordic countries in the late 1980s. This circumstance reflects the long tradition of the state to develop modern hospitals and secure access to hospital services in various regions. The position of hospital physicians has changed very little as the state government has shifted the responsibilities for health care to local government. Hospital physicians in the Nordic countries have always worked as salaried employees of the municipal or state government (only a few private hospitals have existed). Hence, it is more the advancements in medical technology that have changed hospital physicians' work than the reforms in health care.

Recently, a more liberal policy toward private practice has allowed hospital physicians, who tend to be specialists, to work as part-time private practitioners in Finland and Sweden (Jäättelä 1990:232; Rosenthal 1989). In Finland the national social insurance system reimburses patients for services provided by private practitioners. In 1989, 7 percent of the physicians in Finland worked as full-time private practitioners, a majority of whom were specialists; additionally, 37 percent of all physicians had a part-time private practice (Jäättelä 1990:232). Private practice is generally pursued as a group practice and tends to be located in urban areas (in 1989 there were 180 private group practices in Finland). Nevertheless, this pattern does not signify any broader trend toward privatization of health care; of all patient visits to physicians in ambulatory care in 1989, 19 percent were to a private practitioner (Jäättelä 1990:232).

About a third of the physicians in Denmark, Finland, and Norway and a fourth in Sweden work in ambulatory care (Table 12.2). In Denmark the position of physicians in the primary care sector has remained relatively unchanged. The general practitioners work as independent family physicians on a contractual basis, a system regulated by the sickness fund system. The general practitioners refer patients to hospital-based specialists (Nordic Statistical Secretariat 1990:79–80; Weiner 1989). The 1980s witnessed a debate about providing patients with more freedom to choose a specialist, but no major changes have yet occurred (Brogren and Brommels 1991).

Municipal Health Center Physicians in Finland

In Finland the Public Health Act of 1972 established municipal health centers, with free primary care services. At the same time, municipal government was given the primary responsibility for ambulatory care and hospital health care in the municipality. The Public Health Act created a new group of physicians: municipal health center physicians who are full-time salaried general practitioners. Work at these centers is characterized by two central features. First, it resembles closely the features of "proletarianized" medical work portrayed by McKinlay and his colleagues (McKinlay and Arches 1985; McKinlay and Stoeckle 1988). A recent study conducted by the Finnish Medical Association showed that physicians working at municipal health centers perceived their work as stressful, and they suffered from burn-out more often than other physicians (Strid et al. 1988). Another study of the job satisfaction of primary care personnel in Finland showed that doctors were the least satisfied among various health professionals and that the willingness to change to another work setting was lowest among nurses but highest among the primary care physicians (Piri and Vohlonen 1987).

Another central feature of physicians' work at municipal health centers in Finland is that it is performed primarily by female physicians. In 1991, 21 percent of the physicians in Finland were working at municipal health centers; 54 percent of them were females. This figure has to be viewed in the general context of the gender composition of the medical profession in Finland. In 1991, women constituted 42 percent of the physicians in Finland. Comparable figures for the other Nordic countries were 31 percent in Sweden, 24 percent in Denmark, and 19 percent in Norway in 1985 (SNAPS 1986). The Finnish figure for 1985 was 39 percent.

The influx of women into the medical profession grew after the reform in primary care in 1972. A new category of physicians had been created, municipal health center physician, and women entered this structural niche in the health care system that had not been annexed as a male domain. Practice at the centers does not require specialization; hence, the low rate of specialization of female physicians in general might be both a reason for and a consequence of this circumstance. During the past two decades, the rate of specialization has increased only among male physicians; whereas 38 percent of the female physicians and 42 percent of the male physicians were specialists in 1960, only 36 percent of the female but 62 percent of the male physicians were specialists in 1991 (Official Statistics for Finland 1962; Finnish Medical Association 1991). This gender difference might be partly due to the age structure of the current physician population: 41 percent of the female physicians were under thirty-five years old in 1991 in comparison to 22 percent of the male physicians (Finnish Medical Association 1991). The female specialists are clustered in pediatrics, child neurology, child psychiatry, dermatology, and ophthalmology, in which a majority are females. By contrast, only 7 percent of the surgeons were female in 1991. Furthermore, a fourth of the physicians working in medical education research or administration were female in 1991; 12 percent of the professors of medicine at Finnish medical schools were female in 1990 (Räty 1991).

Women work within fields that are characterized by high social interaction with patients (pediatrics, psychiatry, municipal health centers) and low pay. This type of medical work entails skills in "emotion work" (Hochschild 1983), whereas male physicians tend to work in areas that demand technical skills and emotion control (see also James 1989).

In short, the entry of women into the medical profession has not made them colleagues of equal standing with the male physicians. Instead, a dual labor market for physicians has developed in Finland, one that displays the features of the traditional privileged social position of the physicians and another in which the physicians have lost professional control over their work. This gender-based division of labor in medicine has also been documented in Great Britain (Elston 1980) and the United States (Lorber 1984, 1991; Butter et al. 1987).

The Growth but Differentiation of General Practitioners in Norway

In Norway the Municipal Health Act of 1984 shifted the responsibility of the central government in funding and decision making to municipalities (Elstad 1990). As in Finland, this reform mainly influenced the work of the general practitioners and left unchanged the work of salaried hospital physicians. The reform of 1984 implied for general practitioners a closer tie to the public sector. Previously general practitioners had been a small group of independent practitioners; now they were provided a publicly financed structure for an expansion of their services. This implied a structural opportunity for a numerical growth of the general practitioners who wanted to separate themselves professionally from hospital physicians (Romøren 1989:183). One move in this direction had been to create general practice as a specialty. Hence, the new law provided a structural context and a guaranteed income for this new group of specialists.

The Municipal Health Act created two new types of general practitioners in addition to the general practitioner as an independent entrepreneur of the past. One was the employment of general practitioners as salaried municipal workers, a category called municipal physicians. Between 1979 and 1988, this group grew from 3 percent to 41 percent of all general practitioners (Elstad 1991b:122). The second category was composed of general practitioners who work for the municipality on a contractual basis. The latter group of physicians can, additionally, provide services to patients on a fee-for-service basis, for which the physicians are reimbursed by the state through the local social insurance agency. This system has considerably advanced the possibilities for increased incomes; in 1989, 42 percent of the contract physicians' income came from this system (Elstad 1991*a:*58). In addition, the general practitioners' position in the overall hierarchy of the health care system changed. Previously they had enjoyed professional autonomy; now they are formally subordinated to the directors of the municipal bureaucracy. Today physicians seldom occupy leading administrative positions in the primary care system, as was the case in the past (Elstad 1991*b:*125–27; Romøren 1989:184). This means that they have the same status as other semiprofessional groups, such as nurses and physiotherapists, in the administrative hierarchies of the primary care system in relation to municipal bureaucrats and directors (Berg 1991:160–61; Elstad 1991*b:*125–27). The old medical hierarchy has been replaced by a professional hierarchy in which each profession is represented in the decision making.

In short, the Municipal Health Act of 1984 in Norway has strengthened the hand of general practitioners by providing them with positions that guarantee them clients and a stable income. The reform has been a mixed blessing for this group, however. Although it has advanced the professional position of its members, it has tied them to the public sector. The municipal physicians have lost a considerable part of their professional autonomy because they are subordinated to and regulated by other groups occupying the top administrative positions in the public sector.

Municipally employed physicians in Finland have resisted this kind of administrative subordination. There, physicians still control top administrative positions in hospitals (Saltman 1987) and in the primary care system. In the fall of 1990, half of the physicians working at the municipal hospitals and health centers in Helsinki, Finland's capital, resigned, and more threatened to do so if the city implemented new directives concerning the appointment of the heads of the seven health districts of the city. The new directives stipulated that any person with a university degree, such as nurses, qualified for the positions; physicians, backed by the Finnish Medical Association, insisted that only a physician could qualify. The mayor finally worked out a compromise: only physicians were to be appointed, but as untenured, until new directives were enacted in 1993 (Pekkarinen 1990*a,* 1990*b;* Äärimaa 1990; *Nordisk Medicin* 1991). The physicians who had resigned were reinstalled in their previous positions in the city health care system. Hence, the medical profession won the first round in the battle of the autonomy of the profession. Physicians have accepted a salaried status within the public sector, and historically this circumstance has guaranteed them a clientele and reimbursement for their services. But the subordination to, and thereby regulation of their work by, nonmedical groups seems to be the last bastion of the professional control, and the Finnish medical profession seeks to maintain its traditional position.

Deregulation of Health Care in Sweden by 2000?

The Dagmar reform in 1984, aimed at curbing private practice, represented the last in the long line of efforts by the Social Democrats to regulate the medical profession. This reform required that physicians who wanted to establish private practice had to apply for permission from the Landsting, the local government. Despite this measure, an increasing number of physicians began to pursue part-time practice in the 1980s (Rosenthal 1989). By the end of the 1980s, an interest among the major political parties and the SMA to deregulate the Swedish health care system was evident. During the era of the Social Democrats, new ideological hybrids were introduced under slogans such as "freedom within the public sector" (Rosenthal 1989) and "planned markets" and "public firms" (Otter and Saltman 1991; Saltman 1991). Yet even more market freedom was envisioned by the Liberal and Conservative parties and the SMA. The Liberal party advocated a system of family physicians along the lines of the British and Danish general practitioner models (Garpenby 1989:113). This endeavor was given high priority as the Conservatives and the Liberal party formed the government after the defeat of the Social Democrats in the fall 1991 parliamentary elections. The current government has promised that "all Swedes will have a family physician by 1995," but no concrete measures have been taken. A parliamentary commission will provide a recommendation by 1993 (*Läkartidningen* 1991*b:*3873). A number of competing models have already been presented and reviewed. One of the models, offered by the SMA, introduces a family physician system. The original plan recommended that doctors would be free to locate their practices wherever they like, and the City Council and the national Social Insurance Institution would reimburse them for their services. A later plan recommended that the SMA model be financed through the establishment of a national sickness insurance (*Läkartidningen* 1991*a:*470–43, 1991*c:*3968–69). This new plan is understandable because it entails no involvement with the City Council, which has regulated the professional freedom of the medical profession in the past.

The SMA has touted its system as introducing "choice and efficiency" in health care (*Läkartidningen* 1991*c:*3968); the patient will have a choice of physician, the physicians will have the right to establish themselves as private practitioners, and it is assumed that competition will increase the efficiency of health care delivery. This model would give general practitioners more professional freedom than they have had in the past. Nevertheless, the increased competition for patients might create a new situation of economic insecurity for general practitioners. Temptations to "overtreat" patients to generate higher incomes have been debated, and plans to introduce a diagnosis-related group system has been proposed even by the SMA (*Läkartidningen* 1991*a:*472). Whatever model the government finally introduces as the plan for a national policy might ultimately be a symbolic gesture. A prior measure to decentralize health care, enacted in 1981, entitles local governments to organize health and medical care as they desire. This circumstance will most likely introduce regional variations in the implementation of the drive toward a deregulation of health care.

Conclusions

The prevailing economic conditions in the Nordic countries determined the early position of the medical profession. In the absence of a market for independent practitioners, the state and municipalities in Finland, Norway, and Sweden established hospitals and salaried positions for medical officers in the public sector. Hence, in the nineteenth century, physicians in these three countries were public employees and professionals, a status that in those days was prestigious.

Denmark, a small country with a higher population density and a middle class of craftsmen and merchants in the urban centers, provided a different starting point for its physicians. Danish physicians were professionally organized before the mid-nineteenth century, when the regulated medical market of the guild society ended. The Danish medical profession reached an agreement with the new social classes of the emerging market and industrial society to extend the contractual arrangement of the past. Hence, the medical profession in Denmark has been relatively well sheltered from both the threats of a free market and the regulating power of the state.

The state had a crucial role in the development of a modern hospital system well up to the early 1960s in all the Nordic countries. Over the years, the position of salaried hospital physicians, most of them specialists, has not changed much. By contrast, efforts to develop a public primary care system have significantly changed the position of general practitioners in Norway and Finland. In Norway, efforts to improve primary care delivery bolstered the growth of general practice as an occupation but differentiated this group of practitioners professionally. Those who work in the public sector seem to have lost some professional control and autonomy, whereas contractually based general practitioners seem to have won increased professional control through a secured access to clients.

In Finland, the efficient network of municipal health centers providing free primary care services has left almost no market for independent general practitioners. Most general practitioners work as municipal health center physicians, a field dominated by women, in contrast to hospital-specialist physicians, most of them men. In the major urban areas, a private market of services by specialists has grown, as is also the case in Sweden.

The public sector has and will continue to dominate health care delivery in the future in the Nordic countries (Rhode and Hjort 1986; Häkkinen 1987; Sosialde-partementet 1987–1988). Nevertheless, a growing interest in market strategies for health care in these countries will characterize health policy in the rest of the 1990s. In this sense, the health care delivery systems in the Nordic countries seem to be converging toward the Danish model of primary care delivery but allowing more consumer choice, as in the Finnish model. The changes will have different impacts on different groups of the medical profession. The profession will most likely introduce campaigns designed to bolster the autonomy of its weaker groups, perhaps by professionalizing general practice and maintaining top positions in the medical hierarchy for physicians. Furthermore, demands for increased efficiency in care might provide a stronger position for the medical profession, which can appeal to its specialized knowledge, and thereby consolidate its position in administration and decision making in health care.

13

The Physician in
the Commonwealth of Independent States:
The Difficult Passage from Bureaucrat
to Professional

Mark G. Field

Soviet socialized medicine was a creature of the Soviet regime, and it reflected in practically its every aspect the ideology, political culture, and organizational forms of that regime. Thus, the deconstruction of the Soviet Union cannot but profoundly affect the provision of health services to the population and alter the status, role, and work conditions of the physician. To understand these potential changes, it is important to have a purchase on the situation of the physician before the fall, shaped by seventy-three years of Soviet history.

A Bit of History

There was little in 1917 that distinguished the Russian doctor's position from that of his colleagues elsewhere. Physicians saw themselves as professionals charged with important responsibilities and enjoying a high regard and status among the population. They were members of the intelligentsia, a Russian term that denoted those with a higher education. Most of them probably would have considered themselves among those who were hoping, or working, for major reforms or even revolution. Many Russian physicians, particularly those in community medicine and public health, inspired by their social hygienist German colleagues, were convinced that the health and well-being of the population depended not so much on clinical care but resulted from social and economic conditions. Changes in these conditions implied political reforms of the type that the tsarist autocracy was unwilling to contemplate (Frieden 1981:231–311). Although a high proportion of

This paper is a revised and updated version of "The Position of the Soviet Physician: The Bureaucratic Professional," published in *The Milbank Quarterly* 66(Suppl. 2):182–201, 1988.

Because of the recent events in the former Soviet Union and the fluidity of the situation, I use the word *Soviet* (as in "Soviet physician") to denote the situation both before and after the collapse of the Communist regime.

Russian doctors were private practitioners, others served in salaried positions, particularly those who worked for the Zemstvo, or local rural boards, and who provided a modicum of health care to the largely impoverished peasant population. Zemstvo physicians were seen as dedicated individuals who sacrificed their comforts for the sake of those more unfortunate in the countryside and symbolized what was the best in the populist tradition—unselfish service to others. The revolution was to bring major changes in the role and the position of the physician and a loss of the personal dedication characteristic of the Zemstvo doctor.

The Revolution and the Medical Profession

Most physicians, who were liberals in their ideology, viewed with distaste, distrust, and sometimes hostility the coming to power of the Communist regime (Krug 1979). They were concerned that their roles as experts and specialists would be looked upon as bourgeois and that they would be placed under the control of ignorant or unqualified, but politically acceptable, subordinates.

Specialists, trained under the old regime, remained under suspicion in the first years of Soviet power. As Hutchinson (1987) has pointed out, "Physicians were usually perceived as the enemies of Soviet rule, and the majority of them had refused to recognize that the Provisional Government was dead, and that the Soviets were in power" (p. 27). There were cases when nurses or *feldshers* (physician assistants) were appointed as directors of hospitals and began giving orders to physicians. Physicians also rejected the ideologically determined class approach that members of the proletariat and the peasantry should receive medical care ahead of others as a simple case of retributive justice. They claimed it went against their ethical universalism that held that a sick or wounded individual deserved care regardless of current or past class membership. This the Bolsheviks rejected as pure hypocritical cant, arguing that under the tsar, most physicians had catered primarily to the elites.

The new regime, and Lenin in particular, did not, at first, want to mount a frontal assault on the medical profession and associations and sought a modus vivendi with these physicians (Krug 1979). The Bolsheviks wanted either the benevolent neutrality, if not the collaboration, of physicians' associations or control of these associations. But the physicians would have none of this, and eventually the old-regime medical associations were dissolved on the familiar ground that they were "counterrevolutionary." This was the death knell of the medical profession, if by *profession* we mean an association of practitioners who constitute a corporate group and have some political autonomy. A corporate group represents political power; its members can influence decisions concerning practically all aspects of the practitioner's occupational life. It can propose, shape, and sponsor legislation, and often it controls the number of students admitted to the medical schools, and hence the future of the profession. It can claim that the work of the professional is so complex that only its members are capable of passing judgment on the qualifications of new entrants into the profession, as well as on the misdeeds of peers. It can proclaim and enforce a code of ethical behavior that it says ensures the highest standards of care and protection for the public. It can threaten to go on strike, in an effort to wring concessions. It was this kind of power that the Soviet regime would not tolerate. It also abolished the oath that physicians took because of its "bourgeois" character. It was only in 1971 that an oath was reinstituted, and it emphasized not only the duties of the physician toward patients but also toward the Soviet government and Communist society.

Although the ground is now beginning to shift under the feet of physicians in the West, beginning to erode their autonomy and political power (McKinlay and Stoeckle 1987), this position of power and dominance has existed during the first three quarters of the twentieth century in democratic-pluralistic societies. The American Medical Association and the British Medical Association are prototypical and thus serve as a good contrasting medium when looking at the Soviet doctor (there was no Soviet counterpart to these associations).

The fall of the Soviet regime has led to discussions about the creation of independent associations of physicians, and the formation of an association of physicians of Russia has recently been reported ("Rossiiskoe zdravookhranenie" 1991). Under the previous regime, the nearest and quite inappropriate equivalent would have been the Union of Medical Workers, in essence a company union (the company being the state). It included all those who worked in health—not only physicians—and was a major means of control over health personnel. Politically it was inert.

The Doctor as a State Employee

The Soviet doctor was a salaried state functionary, educated at state expense. At graduation, the Soviet physician did not owe a sum of money or have to worry about establishing a practice. On the other hand, he or she was beholden to the state. Physicians could be assigned to areas that were underdoctored and unattractive because of their isolation and lack of cultural amenities. Conditions were primitive and the quality of medical institutions abysmal. Only 35 percent of rural district hospitals had hot running water, 27 percent lacked a sewage system, and 17 percent had no running water, according to former health minister Evgeny Chazov (*Sovetskaia Rossia 1987*). Most young physicians assigned to these areas, terrified at assuming responsibility for patients when they had had so little clinical experience, managed in one way or the other to escape such postings (Field 1967:108ff.). Moreover, an unacceptably high proportion of medical graduates were unqualified to perform the simplest tasks, like delivering a child or reading an electrocardiogram (*Pravda 1987c*).

There was also an economic factor that accounted for the fact that physicians might prefer driving taxicabs rather than report to the countryside: there was not much forgone income, given the very low salaries paid to physicians. Thus, whereas before the revolution Zemstvo physicians were motivated to serve the people, this dedication seemed to have largely disappeared under the Soviet regime.

The Economic Status of Doctors

Most Soviet doctors (except the medical elites) were poorly paid, not only by comparison with their colleagues abroad but also within Soviet society. Of all occupational groups in the Soviet Union, those in health occupied the lowest level in terms of official salaries (about 70–75% of the national average).

The fact that the majority of Soviet doctors are women (close to 70%) (Ryan 1990:37–48) may be the result or the cause of the relatively poor income of physicians, at least officially. The feminization of the medical corps, particularly in the light of a sexist society in which menial jobs seem to be reserved mostly for women, has not benefited the physician's official economic status in general. As we shall see, some physicians have other ways of supplementing their income.

Bureaucratization

An examination of the bureaucratic nature of medicine in the Soviet Union cannot be adequate without some consideration of the type of society that evolved there over the past seventy-four years or so. It is a system dominated by bureaucracies. It remains to be seen whether the new society (or societies) to emerge from the collapsed Soviet Union will be able to reverse that trend.

The bureaucratization of medicine and the transformation of the physician into a state functionary allowed the regime to use physicians often as agents of social control. The abuse of psychiatry for political purposes has become notorious (Bloch and Reddaway 1972, 1984; Grigoriants 1988; Field 1991a), but there were other aspects in which physicians exercised such control, the most important being the delivery of certificates of sickness. It did not occur to most Soviet physicians or psychiatrists to disobey orders from the authorities. In this respect, the absence of a profession as a countervailing power made physicians captive practitioners. But— and this was the paradoxical aspect of the role of the practitioner (and the Soviet bureaucrat in general)—the Soviet physician exercised over the patient and subordinates the kind of absolute "totalitarian" power that would hardly be possible now in more pluralistic settings, and it reflected the totalitarian aspect of the political system. This was, in no small part, due to the jurisdictional authority of the physician as a state functionary or officer, as an agent of social control. This bureaucratic power, it may be surmised, compensated for the subordination the physician felt in a hierarchic and autocratic structure. If to this we add the traditional power that derives from the authority of the doctor as a specialist and the regressive tendencies often found in the state of illness because of its association with dependency and death, we can see that in the clinical situation itself, the physician dominated the patient.

An examination of the Soviet doctor-patient relationship is thus akin to a time warp. It goes back to a situation in the West present some years ago. Now, however, there is a growing rebellion against the dictatorial style, sparked first by the feminist revolt against the insensitivity of physicians. A more egalitarian and informal relationship has emerged, one in which there is some degree of parity between the authoritarian-paternalism of the physician and an inquisitive, challenging, and increasingly better informed patient. And in the background there lurks the threat of malpractice suits. In addition, specialization and subspecialization and the proliferation of allied health professional have decreased both the charisma of the physician and the unity of the profession, as well as its near monopoly in the practice of medicine. Now, many of these functions have been taken over by other health professionals.

Practically none of these trends was visible in the Soviet Union. While Western physicians are slowly losing ground to a host of forces they cannot control, including the corporatization of medicine, which is turning them also into bureaucrats, the already bureaucratized Soviet doctor remains strongly and firmly in charge of patients. Articles and letters to the editors of the Soviet press have frequently complained about the officiousness and the lack of compassion shown by physicians; investigative journalists have been rebuffed by health authorities lest their reporting undermine the authority of doctors. There are no equivalents in the Soviet Union to the Boston Women's Health Collective, which published *Our Bodies, Ourselves,* the Canadian feminist health quarterly *Health Sharing,* the decentralized caesarean support groups in the United States, or La Leche League. As in other countries of the (former) Soviet bloc, childbirth and breastfeeding, for example, are under undisputed medical monopoly (Heitlinger 1987:100). In most instances, patients cannot choose their primary care doctor. A survey of Soviet medical professionals, whose average age was 38.5 years, and who had been practicing over twelve years, showed that the majority of doctors—70 percent—opposed the idea of free choice, 28.1 percent had no objection, and 2.4 percent, no opinion. They believed that patients lack medical knowledge and therefore cannot correctly evaluate physicians' qualifications. Free choice, physicians concluded, would "not serve society's interests." This view, however, sharply contrasts with that of the population itself. In other surveys, 25 to 49 percent of individuals questioned wanted to change their assigned doctors, and 55 percent favored a free choice of medical specialists. Patients' main complaints were insufficient attention paid to them during the examination and the general hastiness (Trehub 1986:5) in the provision of treatment, as well as the insufficiency of the information given to them by doctors regarding their illness, problems in getting sick leave, and other issues (Antipenko and Nesynova 1983). To some degree, the training of doctors is at fault. As Beilin (1977) complained some time ago, medical students are taught little medical psychology and how to deal with patients and their emotional problems.

Soviet physicians may have been under no pressure to satisfy patients, but they did have to please the managers of the health care system. One of the perennial complaints of Soviet physicians, usually expressed in letters to the editors of newspapers, was that their work was assessed in quantitative terms. In this respect, the Soviet health system, just like industry, operated on the gross output principle with its emphasis on quantity. Physicians were expected to see about eight patients per hour at the outpatient clinic or about one patient every seven and a half minutes (Trehub 1986:2–3). Most of that time was consumed by paperwork; indeed, some Soviet studies show that five of these seven minutes were spent filling in forms. Given the powerful position of physicians over patients and the press of work, it is not surprising that physicians were often criticized for their rudeness.

In another context, three Soviet authors wrote that although there were more than 1 million physicians in the Soviet Union, "almost one-third of them do not conform to contemporary professional, socio-psychological and moral demands" (Shchepin, Tsaregorodtsev, and Erokhin 1983:357). Recently, there have been more calls to physicians (and others) to display more compassion, more charity, and more kindness toward patients and to replace the impersonal responsibility of the physician who is on duty from a specific hour to another with the more universal medical ethic of providing assistance whenever needed to anyone. "What Soviet doctors lack most," declared the former health minister, "is humanity" (D'Anastasio 1987). Moreover, the power of physicians (and the temptation to abuse it) is inherent in their role of providing official excuses from work or manipulating psychiatric diagnoses either for personal gain (to escape legal sanctions) or to silence dissidents at the behest of the authorities. These factors not only tend to alienate patients from physicians but to emphasize the general trend toward depersonalization evident in medical care the world over, often exacerbated by a constant division of medical labor and the increased use of technology. The term *veterinarism* crept into Soviet discussions of the matter, underscoring the growing tendency to look upon patients as physiological and passive entities to whom something should be done rather than sentient human beings with their shares of emotions and anxieties (Bilioni 1968).

The Commercialization of Soviet Medicine

In the past few years, as the economic situation deteriorated, the Soviet health system became increasingly starved for funds and corrupt. In order to obtain care or more personal attention, patients increasingly were under pressure to give money to health personnel under the table, sometimes known as "envelope-passing medicine," since this was the way in which money discretely changed hands.

About three-quarters of a sample of population polled on the subject said that they had given money to health personnel to ensure better service or to ensure it at all (Makeyenko and Mariukan 1987). Apparently the situation in hospitals was so poor that patients or their relatives had to come armed with sheafs of ruble notes to secure the smallest service, be it medication, a change of linen, or a bedpan. In 1987, journalists investigated the situation in Baku and found that

> an operation here . . . costs the patients' relatives roughly 500 rubles now. . . . No one at the hospital comes right out and demands money but . . . you understand. No one will come near you, and the necessary medicine or whatever won't be found. (Makeyenko and Mariukan 1987)

At that time, the average physicians monthly salary was in the vicinity of 200 rubles. Nurses earned much less—probably under 100 rubles. It is thus paradoxical that in a system designed to remove the cash nexus from the doctor-patient relationship, it was reintroduced with a vengeance. The traditional professional ethic of placing the interests of the patient first disappeared in large part. Apparently, at least from stories reported in the press, in many instances a physician will not consider operating on a patient except with money up-front. In a specific case reported by the highly respected writer Daniil Granin, a surgeon was approached by an engineer whose mother needed an operation. The engineer, knowing that one had to "give something" but embarrassed in giving what was essentially an illegal bribe, offered the physician 25 rubles, ostensibly to buy medications, perennially in short supply. The physician rejected the offer, demanding 250 rubles, which the engineer managed to raise by borrowing. When the patient died, the surgeon explained to her son that she died not as a result of the operation but because she had "a weak heart," and therefore he was keeping the money. Granin adds that the doctor was convinced of his own decency: if he had determined that the mother had died because of something he did, he would have returned the money. Granin says that he told the story not because it was uncommon but because it was so commonplace (Granin 1987).

The widespread nature of such practices suggests how far from professional norms the doctor-patient relationship has deviated. The center of that ethic is that the professional must place the interests of the patient before his or her own, and the nature and quality of the professional service must be independent of the remuneration. Indeed, it is that obligation not to exploit the client's powerlessness that permits professionals to claim they are a breed apart. At the same time, this professional obligation cannot be seen simply as the expression of altruistic personality traits that separate the professional from, say, a businessperson or sales representative (Parsons 1958). In other contexts—for example, in purchasing or selling property—a professional may be legitimately expected to maximize self-interest. The disinterestedness of the professional is an institutionalized social norm, the transgression of which would expose him or her to social and collegial opprobrium. At the same time, it is functional in that it permits the establishment of a fiduciary relationship between doctor and patient, without which the medical task would be more difficult or impossible to perform (access to the body or to confidential or embarrassing information). The deprofessionalization of medicine, as was the case in the Soviet Union, removed many of these ethical safeguards and opened the way to commercial practices. Moreover, the miserable salaries assigned by the regime to health personnel may have been rationalized by the regime because of the existence of these additional sources of income.

The fine point, and one that cannot be determined, is whether these payments, whether solicited, requested, extorted, or hinted at, should be regarded as bribes for preferential treatment or tokens of gratitude, or both. Nevertheless, more than anything else, they perhaps constitute a countervailing power at the disposal of the patient to exert some control over the physician. It meets "the drive to have a choice, to gain some sense of control over the care received to manipulate the bureaucracy, instead of the other way around" (Shipler 1983:219).

But that countervailing power depends on the availability of money. Those who are too poor or destitute must throw themselves on the dubious mercies of an often indifferent service and personnel. Although there are surely many dedicated and devoted personnel, such widespread practices do not strengthen the professional status of medicine.

The Prestige of the Soviet Medical Profession

It is difficult to assess with any accuracy the general prestige or the relative desirability of the medical occupation in the Soviet Union. Physicians are well thought of (Jones and Grupp 1987), but they certainly lack the visibility of the more technical and military or space occupations. One study, published in 1985, reported that the prestige of medical doctors for urban male youths had fallen by 10 percent over the previous two decades and by 5 percent for rural youths, though it increased slightly among girls, by 3 and 6 percent, respectively (Cherednichenko and Shubkin 1985). Another study noted that a declining proportion of Soviet youths wanted to become doctors (Kosarev and Sakhno 1985).

With the exception of a small group of elite physicians, most Soviet doctors' incomes are very modest. (This finding does not take into account the monies paid under the table to some physicians best placed to request or extort such payments.) Thus, the general financial position of Soviet doctors hardly resembles that of their colleagues in the West. On the other hand, the position of the medical occupation in the Soviet Union does not necessarily reflect the financial position of the occupation, as it does in the West. The Soviets seem to regard income as relatively secondary in judging the attractiveness of an occupation. Nevertheless, there is well-recognized dissatisfaction with what the Soviets call the material conditions of life for health workers (Meditsinskie 1986). In interviews, the former health minister declared he was hoping that "good" physicians would attract more patients and that they would be better paid than poor ones. Income differentiation would undermine the usual bureaucratic style of work and perhaps improve the work, if not the image, of physicians.

Recent Trends

After the breakdown of the Soviet system, certain trends that began under *perestroika* are likely to gain momentum. One of them is the belief that Soviet physicians have been silenced long enough and that now is the time to lay the foundations of an articulate medical profession as a corporate group that essentially would resemble the status of the medical profession in democratic industrial societies. Doctors in a number of cities have urged the creation of an association of physicians, "an organization that would be outside the control of government and which would represent the needs and interests of medical practitioners" (Powell n.d.). As one physician put it in 1989, "At the present time, our practicing physicians find themselves in complete professional isolation from doctors the world over. . . . It is all but impossible not only to travel abroad in order to work or study, but even to subscribe to most medical publications" (ibid.). Closely tied to the idea of a medical profession free of governmental strings is the private practice of medicine. In fact, private practice was never formally forbidden in the Soviet Union, though it was heavily taxed, administratively restricted, and subject to ideological attacks as a "bourgeois" practice bound to disappear when the public (and free) service became more widely available and of higher quality. As physicians emancipate themselves from the dictates of the medical bureaucrats and begin to practice privately and independently, the ground is laid for what might be called the reprofessionalization, or the deproletarianization, of the medical occupation in a direction that is common in most industrial democracies. It is, however, interesting to note that in the West, physicians increasingly are concerned with the reverse phenomenon of the bureaucratization of health and hospital services, with the myriad of regulations that eventually will affect their clinical autonomy and their fear of becoming "employees," as pointed out by McKinlay, Stoeckle, and others. Thus, in comparing the situation of physicians in the West and the former Soviet Union, one may well think of a convergence in the status of doctors but from different starting points.

Conclusions

In this chapter I have touched on the major aspects of the position and role of Soviet physicians and examined that interesting combination of certain professional characteristics (derived from expertise and monopoly of that expertise), corporate powerlessness, and bureaucratic power. In trying to explain the general position of the average Soviet doctor to a Westerner, and particularly to an American, the nearest analogue (and a flawed one, at that) is that of an elementary or secondary American school teacher. Both the Soviet physician and the American teacher fulfill extremely important social functions—one in shaping capacity, the other in maintaining that capacity. Although the amount of training is greater for the doctors and the life-and-death responsibilities certainly more stressful than teaching, the conditions of work (salaried), the relatively poor compensation, the relative "cleanliness" of the work (as compared to factory work), the preponderance of women, the shortage of capital equipment, and so on make the resemblance interesting. At the same time, the increased bureaucratization of medical care in the West and the "proletarianization" noted by McKinlay and others suggest a degree of approaching convergence in the position of the former Soviet and the Western doctors. Although the percentage of women in Soviet medicine is slowly decreasing, it is increasing in the West, so that we can contemplate in the not too distant future a medical contingent in both cases made up equally of men and women.

One begins to wonder whether the Soviet situation was, to some qualified extent, a portent of things to come in the West as medical care becomes increasingly bureaucratized, corporatized, and feminized. Will the loss of the power of the medical profession then be compensated by an increase in the authority enjoyed by corporate physicians in the clinical sphere, or will their discretion in that sphere, as many think, also be increasingly constricted by the need to control costs? At the same time, parallels and convergence hypotheses are to be taken with great caution. In essence, the practice of medicine and the position of the doctor reflect at least two important and differentiated set of factors: the universal aspects of medicine as a type of applied knowledge valid in all settings and situations and the particular characteristics of the culture and the structure of the society in which this knowledge is applied. A physician is not simply any trained person who applies the universal knowledge of medical science uniformly. He or she is also the product of the culture, the tradition, the history, and the personal life course in the social setting in which he or she applies that knowledge.

The position of the Soviet physician thus reflects the corporate weakness of the profession under Soviet conditions and the power of the clinician as a bureaucratic employee. This created an intriguing form of status inconsistency that may well be gradually resolved as the profession acquires more independence and the political power to represent its interests and values before the larger society. And yet, given the nature of the health care system toward the end of the century, the increase in the administrative complexity of medical facilities in which physicians cannot operate as independent practitioners being members of a "liberal" profession, and as the technology (which is both labor and capital intensive) increases costs, physicians both East and West will find themselves dictated to by administrators and bean counters. As the former Soviet physician gains a measure of administrative and economic independence, his or her counterpart in the West is likely to lose some of that autonomy. At the same time, the Soviet experiment with socialized medicine shows that a blanket and universal guarantee of medical care by the polity is a difficult promise to keep under the best of circumstances. What is likely to emerge in the former Soviet Union is a system with more nuances, incorporating public and private initiatives. The position of the physician will reflect these trends. In the long run, the similarities in the East and West may become more and more apparent.

A Look into the Future

A historian is supposed to have said, "Don't ask me to predict the future, but when it happens, I shall be happy to explain why it was inevitable." The situation in what was the Soviet Union is so unstable that it would be foolish to try to predict what will happen to the medical profession in the different republics or states that constitute the Commonwealth of Independent States. But generally we can hypothesize that the fate, the status, and the role of physicians will be shaped by the nature of the societies that will evolve from those changes, as well as changes in the state of the art (particularly technology). If the evolution is in the direction of a democratic system, we may expect the emergence of independent physicians' associations, an increase in the legal incomes of doctors, and a constant (if sometimes latent) tug of war between physicians and those who are responsible for administering, managing, and financing medical services. Should the evolution go in the direction of authoritarianism and in placing (again) physicians at the service of the state as medical functionaries, then the independence of physicians and their associations may be curbed and controlled as they were under the Soviet regime. A third variant would be the creation of corporative associations mandated by the state, to which all physicians must belong, and which would serve the dual functions of representing their interests but also controlling their activities. But whichever the arrangements and the structures, the physician as an independent solo practitioner seeing patients privately and free of supervision and different forms of controls is not likely to be the dominant figure in the next century.

14

The Medical Profession in Czechoslovakia: Legacies of State Socialism, Prospects for the Capitalist Future

Alena Heitlinger

Czechoslovakia ranks third in Europe in the number of physicians and fifth in the number of hospital beds per capita, but its mortality rates for certain diseases are the highest on the continent (Pehe 1990). Since the early 1970s, Czechoslovakia has experienced rising rates of heart, circulatory, oncological, digestive, and muscular diseases; a growing proportion of the population has suffered from high blood pressure, diabetes, obesity, stress, and other health risks (Codr and Zelinka 1990). Between 1970 and 1985, morbidity among men increased by 30 percent and among women by 40 percent (Mozny 1990:178–79). Life expectancy—sixty-seven years for men and seventy-four years for women—is four to seven years below rates in Western Europe and as much as eleven years shorter in heavily industrialized and polluted northwest Bohemia (Codr and Zelinka 1990; Pehe 1990).

Czech health analysts do not blame the adverse morbidity and mortality trends on any one institution or specific factor. Instead, the worsening health of the Czechoslovak population has been attributed to the combined effects of environmental pollution, inadequate nutrition, ineffectual functioning of the health care system, lack of individual responsibility for health, and, above all, the totalitarian system of the Communist party-state (Ministry of Health, Czech Republic 1990: 3–4).

Since the November 1989 Velvet Revolution, which ended more than forty years of Communist rule in Czechoslovakia, pressure has been mounting to make changes in the health care system as quickly as possible, and a complete reorganization of the health care system is underway. The major goals of this chapter are to outline these health care reforms and assess the impact they are having upon medical prerogatives and the political influence of professional medicine as a corporate body. As in any other revolutionary transition, there have been both con-

This chapter was written well before the breakup of Czechoslovakia into two independent states. Although the current situation is still too new and ambiguous to address with any certainty, most of the issues and arguments raised herein reflect the situation in the current Czech Republic.

tinuities and discontinuities. Thus, my assessment of Czechoslovak medicine's prospects for the future will start with a brief review of the profession's recent state socialist past. We shall see that the medical profession under state socialism was neither fully proletarianized (in the economic and organizational sense) nor fully deprofessionalized (in the cultural and political sense), although it had relatively weak corporate political power.

The Legacies of State Socialism

The Health Care System

Traditionally, the Communist health authorities acknowledged, with considerable pride, that the socialist reorganization of the Czechoslovak health care system undertaken in the early 1950s was based "on the principles, experiences and achievements of the Soviet health care system" (Makovicky et al. 1981:285; Petro 1980). The current regime, however, regards the Soviet-based "principles, experiences and achievements" as a major source of the health care crisis. The main features of the health care system that state socialist Czechoslovakia shared with its Soviet counterpart included:

1. Separately organized primary care services for industrial, maternal, child, and general adult health.
2. A clear division of responsibilities between primary ambulatory care and the more specialized secondary outpatient and tertiary in-hospital care.
3. A centralized, top-down health care administrative pyramid, with a series of administrative levels serving as transmission belts for orders, directives, and policies from the apex, allowing little initiative among practicing medical personnel.
4. A system of special high-quality party and military clinics restricted to high party officials and their families.
5. A severe restriction on the right of patients to choose their own physicians.
6. Explicitly articulated priorities in the provision of medical services favoring industrial workers, expectant mothers, and children.
7. A system of unified, state-directed and -financed care (including dental care), free at the point of consumption, which since 1966 (1969 in the Soviet Union) has been based on citizenship rather than on insurance.
8. Low proportion of gross national product (GNP) spent on health care, reflecting the low priority assigned by the Communist elites to the "unproductive" service sector, which included health services.
9. Lack of sophisticated medical technology and shortages of drugs.
10. Weak corporate political power of professional medicine.
11. Low salaries of doctors and nurses.
12. Widespread practice of tipping and bribing medical and nursing personnel.
13. Doctor-patient and nurse-patient relationships in which patients are generally regarded as passive recipients of treatment.

The proportion of GNP spent on health care in Czechoslovakia rose from 3.6 percent in 1970 to 5.4 percent in 1988, well below the 7 to 10 percent generally spent in Western liberal democracies. (Only Great Britain was substantially below these levels, at 5.2 in the mid-1970s [Heitlinger 1987:94].) Until recently, nurses and other health care personnel, including many primary care physicians, were paid less than many manual workers (Pehe 1990:22).

Professional Prerogatives under State Socialism

The Communist party-state influenced through central planning both the definition of medical needs and the organizational framework of services to meet them. The state exercised tight budgetary control over medical facilities, technologies, drugs, and salaries and a high degree of administrative power over health norms and standards. With few exceptions (e.g., the health care services of the army and the railways), the entire health service was centralized under the federal and the two national ministries of health. At the top of the organizational pyramid was the so-called chief specialist (a physician by training), who was a full-time administrative official of the national Ministry of Health and was responsible for the expert direction and the improvement of standards of individual medical branches. The chief specialist gave direction to the officially designated regional and district specialists. Party membership was a requirement for these positions of authority in the administration of health services, though this was usually not necessary for the more directly medical work (as opposed to administrative paperwork) of chiefs of hospital departments.

In theory, the officially designated specialists, especially those at the national and regional levels, combined authority based on expertise with that based on office, and they played an important role in the centralized planning of health care. In practice, however, their influence was quite limited. The Czech and Slovak Ministries of Health were responsible only for setting policy on "expert" medical issues; the actual control of personnel and organizational matters in local health care centers was left to the national committees, the municipal agencies of the state administration. Thus, the Czech and Slovak Ministries of Internal Affairs, which controlled and coordinated the work of the national committees, rather than the Ministries of Health, functioned as the senior decision-making bodies in many areas of the health care system (Pehe 1990:22).

The influence of the health ministries and their chief specialists was also limited by the central economic plan, over which they had no control. The central plan not only specified the overall (low) budget for health care services but also provided detailed spending norms within that budget. Like its Soviet counterpart, the health system tended to use more of the resources that were relatively cheap—in this case, services of doctors and middle-level health workers, such as nurses, physiotherapists, hygienic assistants, opticians, and X-ray and laboratory technicians—and fewer of the resources that were expensive, such as imported pharmaceuticals or sophisticated medical technology. Nurses and even some physicians were paid less than some manual workers. Demand for many pharmaceuticals could not be fully met by internal production or by imports from the Western countries, resulting in substantial shortages and a highly visible health care crisis (Prochazkova 1990).

Unlike the private professions that have limited state involvement and employment (the American case) or the state-involved professions of Canada and Western Europe, state socialist professionals were primarily state located and state employed (Krause 1991). Socialist medicine was dependent on the state for financing, provision of workplace, medical supplies and technology, clientele, salaries, the license to practice, and an adequate supply of subordinate health workers. The party-state decreed by fiscal and legislative or administrative means the organizational framework of health services and who should receive them and in what order of priority. Individual doctors, however, were usually left free to choose how to treat their patients and how to practice their particular medical specialty, although there were important differences between primary care physicians and specialists in this respect.

Primary adult care involved physicians in assessments of a worker's fitness for a given job, a professional activity that stemmed from the socially approved monopoly and legitimate right of professional medicine to define illness. Absenteeism from work due to illness was rather high in communist Czechoslovakia (approximately seventeen days per year for each employee), as was compensation for wage loss due to sickness and injury. Moreover, workers taking sick leave were always required to see a doctor, irrespective of the seriousness of the illness. Many company physicians and general practitioners thus spent much of their time examining patients who might have recovered on their own within a few days, a practice that was tied to state-administered bureaucratic procedures rather than to professional medical guidelines and regulations. Weinerman (1969:68) estimated that the paperwork involved in issuing medical certificates for workers' disability occupied 20 percent of the time of a practicing general physician, a rather high proportion.

The low status of such work was reinforced by the administrative control exercised at each district level by a formal Work Assessment Service. The latter employed more than 2 percent of all practicing physicians in Czechoslovakia, an extremely high proportion by Western standards. Judging whether workers were fit to work—the sole professional responsibility of these doctors—also involved checking on how lenient individual primary care physicians were in declaring patients as unfit for work or visiting patients at home to ensure that they were genuinely sick (Syrova 1990).

External interference from the party-state was less visible among specialists, who maintained considerable control over discretionary clinical decisions. However, medical control over resources with which to implement these decisions was much more limited. As Pehe (1990:23) notes, "In recent years only 10% of all those needing heart surgery were actually operated on. Thousands of people died not because their diseases were incurable but because physicians were unable to provide the necessary treatment or life-saving medicines were in short supply." The severe restriction of diagnostic and treatment supplies meant that the discretion and control that physicians exercised in their clinical work translated into limited effective control over patients' treatment.

The low degree of de facto professional control over the conditions of medical work was further limited by an explicit rationing of medical services. Within the context of low overall health care expenditures, the party elites assigned the best care to workers in certain hazardous high-priority occupations in heavy industry (such as mining and steel work), followed by expectant mothers and children. As Knaus (1981:337) noted, "Fortunately young workers are, on average the least expensive population groups to keep healthy. In the United States we spend only $286 each year on medical care for each person under age nineteen and $764 for a person between the ages of nineteen and sixty-four, compared to $2,026 for each person over sixty-five." As a general rule, complicated surgical operations were not performed in Czechoslovakia once a person reached retirement age, with the exception of those eligible to attend the special party clinics.

The medical profession maintained some of its economic prerogatives, despite the salaried status of physicians (and of everybody else) under the Communist regime. As Freidson (1984:9) points out in a different context, relationship to the market is much more important than employment status:

> If one's goods or services are so highly valued on the market that consumers are clamouring for access to them, then one can exercise considerable control over the terms, conditions, content and goals of one's work. . . . Given a strong position in the market, one can be employed and "write one's own ticket" nonetheless.

State socialist economies have traditionally been consumer weak. Those who wished to obtain goods and services in short supply or to improve their quality frequently were forced to resort to bribes. There was little difference between a physician, a car dealer, or a plumber in this respect, although bribing a physician for a medically necessary treatment or life-saving drugs in short supply may be literally a matter of life and death and, as such, considered a high priority. Offering and accepting bribes is part of what Kemeny (1982) calls the shadow market, where providers of service (such as physicians) used bribes to adjust their low salaries imposed by the central authorities. The prevalence of tipping and bribing under communism for the officially "free" health services goes a long way toward explaining why the proposed partial privatization of health care has not been greeted by cries of indignation. The proposed two-tier provision of health care simply institutionalizes practices that were already established under communism.

Gender Inequality in the Medical Profession

Women physicians (currently 52 percent of all doctors) faced many problems not encountered by their male colleagues. Although the academic standards achieved by female medical students were often higher than those of their male counterparts, it was the male doctor who was most often considered to be the more talented and skillful when it came to clinical practice. Patients tended to prefer and trust male doctors more than female ones. The latter were not so much appreciated for their expertise as for their "human" (presumably "maternal") approach to patients (Heitlinger 1991).

Women doctors were further handicapped by their domestic responsibilities, which prevented them from acquiring further qualifications and the more prestigious and better-paid hospital jobs. Sociological research conducted in the early 1970s revealed that Slovak women doctors spent at most two hours daily on further study, while their male colleagues could afford at least three hours a day. Thirty-one percent of Slovak male doctors but only 10 percent of female doctors acquired a specialist qualification (the first and second degree *atestace*) at the expected age of thirty-four. Twenty-five percent of Slovak women doctors did not obtain the second degree qualification because of domestic responsibilities. This meant that a disproportionate number of women were found among primary care physicians, for whom the second-degree *atestace* was not required (Heitlinger 1991).

Post-Communist Agenda for Reform
Proposal for Reform of Health Care (PRHC)

Civic Forum, the Czech political group that, with its Slovak counterpart, Committee Against Public Violence, toppled in November 1989 the Communist regime, made health a high-priority issue for reform. In early January 1990, the Civic Forum's program committee of health care workers (composed largely of physicians) published *Theses Towards a Program of Health,* a document highly critical of the state socialist health care system and advocating major reforms. The document was published in a health weekly, *Zdravotnicke noviny,* which, like other newspapers, was by then free from state control and censorship. The theses were accompanied by a questionnaire asking readers whether they approved of the proposed reforms. People were encouraged to respond directly by sending letters with their own suggestions to the Czech Ministry of Health, which by then had a new minister, a new advisory Scientific Council, and several new committees, including the forty-five-member Working Group for Reform of the Organization of Health Care. Members of the working group—physicians, lawyers, economists, dentists, medical sociologists, and other credentialed professionals—were nominated by individual branches of Civic Forum. There were twenty-five physicians on the committee (55 percent), but neither nurses nor ordinary lay consumers were included.

The Working Group revised the theses and prepared a new consultative document, *Proposal for Reform of Health Care* (PRHC), offering several alternative strategies for reform and inviting individual and institutional responses from both lay citizens and health care professionals. The document was submitted for appraisal to France, Great Britain, and the Copenhagen-based European Section of the World Health Organization. At the conclusion of discussions in September 1990, the amended document was submitted to the Czech parliament. The *Draft of the New System of Health Care* was adopted by the Czech government in December 1990.

PRHC proposed a shift from a focus on disease and cure to health and prevention, greater individual responsibility for health, a compulsory national health insurance program, privatization of the pharmaceutical industry and of some medical services, patients' right to choose their own physicians, a more decentralized delivery and financing of health services and medical education, some minor modifications in the organization of primary care, integration of health and social services, greater humanization and increased standards of psychiatry, higher salaries for health employees, an independent self-governing professional medical association, and professional (as opposed to political) control of medical education and research. It promoted a two-tier health system, whereby all citizens will have access to standard care covered by medical insurance, with an additional "above-standard" form of care available through private medical services, which can be paid for directly by purchasing additional insurance or by contributions from municipalities, employers, and charities. In order to avoid major disruption in the functioning of the current health care system, it was proposed that the various reforms would be phased in in stages over three to four years, to be fully completed by 1995.

Breaking Up Party-State Control

The state socialist pattern of administratively centralized health care programs is now viewed as inefficient and excessively bureaucratic. Accordingly, the removal of "unnecessary barriers and deformations, and the freeing of hidden resources for health care development" was seen in PRHC as the first stage of the health care reform, "to be implemented by the end of 1990." In March 1990, all directors of the so-called Institutes of National Health were recalled and their positions refilled on a competitive basis. A whole administrative level of the organizational pyramid, the regional institutes of health (*KUNZ—Krajsky ustav narodniho zdravi*), was abolished by the end of the year, along with the positions of regional and district chief specialist (Pehe 1990:23).

Shortly after taking power, the Civic Forum government abolished the special party and military clinics, known as *Sanops,* but retained the central military hospital, the best in the country, for its exclusive use.[1] The requirement to see a doctor, irrespective of the seriousness of the illness, to obtain workers' compensation was also abolished. The new regulations allow workers to take up to ten to fifteen sick days a year, three to five days each time they are sick, without having to see a doctor (Pracovni skupina MZSV CR pro reformu zdravotnictvi 1990*b;* Tri kroky ke zdravi 1990). Government officials are assuming that workers, threatened by unemployment and increasing competition for jobs, will not abuse the new system (Pehe 1990:24).

When implemented in 1992, this reform had contradictory implications for physicians. On the one hand, it significantly reduced the high daily patient load of primary care physicians (which allowed on average only six to eight minutes per patient), thus potentially increasing professional standards. On the other hand, the number of doctors employed by the Work Assessment Service declined, thereby creating unemployment among doctors engaged in this type of low-status work. Although it is impossible to make any definitive predictions, it is fair to assume that these physicians will not find it easy to obtain other types of medical work.

By 1992, individuals were able to select their own physician. The right to choose one's physician has an important symbolic role in the current political climate because it visibly marks a fundamental break with the past, when no one was free to select one's own physician. Under the Communist regime, anyone requiring medical care had to see a particular doctor in the patient's place of residence or work. Patients could switch doctors officially only if they could prove that they had received inadequate care from their assigned physician, and then only after a lengthy bureaucratic procedure.

The proposed reform would enable patients to change doctors every six months, and the salaries of doctors and nurses would be scaled accordingly to reflect the number of patients registered with them. Reformers hope that as the health care field becomes more diversified, competition for patients among doctors working within the national health care and those practicing privately will improve overall standards of care (Pehe 1990:24).

Privatization of Some Medical Services

The new health care system will allow physicians to practice privately, but it is not yet clear how this will work. The Ministry of Health wanted to establish an experimental program of privatized medicine and run it for a year before introducing the new health insurance program; however, the Czech parliament refused to consider the proposal on the grounds that all legislative changes should be considered as a package.

It will take some time to develop professional guidelines governing standards, ethics, and fees with respect to private medical care. The medical professional associations—the Czech and Slovak Medical Chambers—will play an important role in these processes. The Slovak Medical Chamber has also been considering the possibility of creating a bank, controlled by the association itself, that would extend loans to physicians whose plans for their private practices are judged to be "progressive" (Pehe 1990:25). Very few Czechoslovak doctors currently have the capital needed to open a private practice. Officials at the Czech Ministry of Health expect that only psychiatrists, who do not require much technology, and a handful of physicians with relatives or friends in Western countries who are willing to send them some Western medical equipment will be able to establish private practices in the near future. There is apparently considerable naiveté among both doctors and patients about how privatized medicine works (interview, Czech Ministry of Health, May 21, 1991).

Thus, the national public health care system is likely to be preserved, with supplementary medical care provided in privately owned, voluntary, and church-run medical facilities playing only a marginal role. According to the Ministry of Health (1990:44), the boundaries between the standard and above-standard care will be subject to regular negotiations involving the health ministry, organized medicine (the Medical Chamber), and the health insurance company. The final balance between state- and privately financed medical care will depend on the general economic situation and the quality of the standard care covered by the compulsory national health insurance. Only widespread poverty and a completely ineffectual performance of the standard medical system would lead to an American-type health care system in which private medicine predominates and where only the relatively well-off can choose where to go for medical treatment.

Individual and Nonmedical Responsibility for Health

PRHC promotes greater individual responsibility for one's own health. It advocates greater reliance on lay self-care and care by one's family members and an increased sense of responsibility by the general public for the health of others. It argues that the general public

> must influence the development of health care not only by the free choice of health services, but also by public actions and interventions at both the municipal and the central state level, and by making contributions to health coverage in the independent mass media. The legislative guarantee of public participation in health care must be complemented by codes of ethics of individual health professions, which would respect a uniformly accepted code of patients' rights. (p. 8)

The proposed mobilization of members of a civil (as opposed to a totalitarian) society toward greater lay responsibility for health and illness is placed in the context of an open, democratic, and humanistic society and in the framework of an integrated system of health and social care. As the official English version of PRHC puts it, "The main motivation for participation of the public in health care are principles of personal responsibility for one's own meaningful life, civic virtues based on the ideal of assistance to fellow men in need and a democratic principle of control and participation. All these factors were undesirable during the late regime" (Ministry of Health and Social Affairs 1990:8). Thus, democracy and the transformation of the "totalitarian" doctor-patient relationship rather than deprofessionalization and demedicalization are the explicit goals of PRHC.

So far, there is little indication that either consumers or health paraprofessionals will mount any serious challenges to the medical profession's monopoly over health knowledge and technical medical skills. There were no nurses among the authors who drafted PRHC, and although PRHC offered several suggestions for reorganizing medicine, no such proposals were forthcoming for nursing. Health education and certain stigmatized categories of illness currently under the jurisdiction of psychiatry (e.g., drug addiction, alcoholism) were the only areas in which PRHC advocated demedicalization and transfer of jurisdictions.

The Corporate Power of Professional Medicine

The Communist party-state exercised through central planning tight budgetary control over the resources available to the health services (medical facilities, health care personnel, technologies, and drugs) and a high degree of administrative power over health norms and standards. The latter were typically planned by a handful of powerful physicians, the so-called chief specialists, who were members of the communist *nomenklatura*. They were more likely to defend the party interests than the professional and corporate interests of medicine.

The requirement for party membership normally did not extend to the clinical work of physicians practicing in ambulatory clinics or hospitals. Thus, throughout the state socialist period, the determination of clinical practice was left largely in the hands of the professionals themselves, though the resources with which physicians could make their clinical decisions were severely restricted. Muller and Kapr (1984:162), writing in the official journal of the Czech Medical Association, confirm that the dominant tendency has been "to view practically every situation connected with medical intervention as a situation closed to the evaluation and control·from the outside. This stand has led to the view that no one else other than the physician has enough expert knowledge and experience to control medical activity.''

Medicine had a high professional status in Czechoslovakia. Sociological studies on rank ordering of occupations conducted in the 1960s revealed a high occupational prestige for medicine, as high as in the United States (Heitlinger 1991:224–25). However, because of the Communist party's insistence on monopoly of power and doctrine, an independent medical profession free of party control could not emerge to campaign for higher salaries and better provision of medical technology. Thus, high professional status did not translate into corporate political power.

The situation in democratic Czechoslovakia promises to be quite different. PRHC envisages a powerful medical association, with wide-ranging legal powers and considerable professional and political influence. The Medical Chamber and its committees are expected to produce guidelines to govern medical education and clinical practice, formulate standards for evaluating professional performance, respond through disciplinary boards to consumer complaints, act as an employer, engage in salary negotiations with the national health insurance program, lobby Parliament and the Ministry of Health, and perform some unspecified other functions, possibly including the formulation and implementation of policies addressing acceptance of bribes, fixing of fees for private medical practice, or some other activities designed to prevent price competition among physicians.

An overall economic collapse, in contrast to economic growth and prosperity, would create a very different climate in which to sustain medicine's power and privilege. For the time being, the Czech government has made a formal commitment to maintain the existing health care budget and to adjust it every three months for inflation. Moreover, the various self-managing health institutions, freed from centralized control and able to save money, will be allowed to keep their surpluses to reward efficiency and discourage what currently is an enormous waste of resources (interview, Czech Ministry of Health, May 21, 1991).

As a result of the systemic discrimination against women, significantly more female than male physicians are likely to face unemployment. Patients tend to prefer and trust male doctors more than the female ones, despite the fact that the academic standards achieved by female medical students often have been higher than those of their male counterparts. Under the Communist regime, when patients could not freely choose their physicians, the impact of such prejudices on the livelihood of female doctors was quite limited. In the post-Communist economic and political climate, sexist prejudice may significantly disadvantage women doctors as they compete with their male counterparts for patients. The magnitude of the problem will also depend on how many women physicians choose to work part-time or are forced to do so.

In contrast, many of the predominantly male hospital-based and subspecialty-oriented physicians, with better diagnostic and therapeutic resources at their disposal, along with some of the privately practicing doctors, may become quite wealthy. As the 1990s unfold, it will be interesting to see how the Medical Chamber deals with questions of gender equity, unemployment, part-time work, bribes, privatized medicine, and the different interests of general practitioners and specialists. If it succeeds in maintaining professional solidarity, the corporate power of professional medicine will be greatly strengthened. However, if the divisions among different categories of physicians become so great as to threaten the formal unity of the Medical Chamber, the outcome may be different.

Much will also depend on what type of two-tier health care system eventually develops. The British or the Canadian models, in which the majority of patients and physicians remain committed to compulsory national health insurance and free medical care, provide a very different context for medical practice than the American system, where the standard of free medical care is of such low quality that most people turn to the second tier, governed by the market and private practice.

Conclusion

The prolonged and deep crisis in the Czechoslovak health care system was an important contributing element to the Velvet Revolution, which in November 1989 peacefully ended more than forty years of Communist rule. Reform of the health care system has been given a high priority by the new regime, and the medical profession is playing an important role in these reforms. With the abolition of the party monopoly of power and doctrine, medicine has considerably increased its political clout and its professional prerogatives.

The medical profession under state socialism was neither fully proletarianized (in the economic and organizational sense) nor fully deprofessionalized (in the cultural and political sense), although it had relatively weak corporate political power. Doctors now have a powerful independent self-governing professional association, whose mandate is to defend professional interests, as well as those of patients. It is quite unreasonable to expect that it can and will do both. Electing representatives to health councils, shopping around for their physician of choice, and paying extra for higher-quality care will give patients some degree of consumer power, but such highly dispersed forms of power will be no match for the organized power of professional medicine. The move toward a two-tier system of medical care seems to be broadly acceptable in the current economic climate because it simply institutionalizes existing widespread practices whereby physicians and nurses routinely accepted bribes for better care.

The extent to which medical care will become privatized is hard to predict at this time, as are changes in morbidity and mortality. Much will depend on the success of the national insurance program and efforts to eliminate corruption in the system. Above all, the outcome will depend on the state of the Czech and Slovak economies. Economic health will ultimately determine both the quality of medical care offered under the national insurance program and how many patients can afford extra payments for medical services.

Acknowledgments

Research for this chapter was generously supported by research grants from Trent University and the Social Sciences and Humanities Research Council of Canada.

Note

1. The government spokesperson argued that it would be quite unreasonable to expect overworked officials attempting to solve all that was neglected during the Communist rule "to wander countless hours in overcrowded community waiting rooms." He expressed confidence that ordinary people would allow these busy officials to jump the queue. It was also expected that the public would support some special arrangement to obtain prescribed drugs, so that these officials, or their assistants, would not have to spend their valuable time running all over Prague with a prescription for a drug currently in short supply. The journalists covering this story were not so sure that such priority treatment was justified. In their view, preferential treatment would delay the implementation of health care reforms because government officials who did not themselves have to experience the health care problems facing ordinary citizens would likely turn their attention to other serious problems facing the country. Thus, in the current political context, privatization of some medical services (and by analogy, market-based privileges) tends to be seen as preferable to the previous previous practice of administrative privileges enjoyed by the Communist party *nomenklatura* in its exclusive access to the special party clinics. The journalists also noted that most members of the Civic Forum government are former political dissidents who bravely struggled against the various privileges enjoyed by the Communist elites. By establishing a new health facility reserved for their exclusive use (and that of their families), the dissidents-turned-government-officials are suggesting (to the journalists and the general public) that what they disliked most about the special *Sanops* clinics was not their very existence but the fact that they were reserved for somebody other than themselves (*Lidove noviny,* June 13, 1990; *Respekt,* No. 16, June 27–July 3, 1990). This journalistic commentary is a telling illustration of the seductiveness of power and privilege, particularly in matters of health.

15

Physicians in China: Assessing the Impact of Ideology and Organization

Gail Henderson

In the early part of this century, the allopathic sect of American doctors gained control over a diverse occupation, eventually becoming dominant over other types of health care workers, as well as newly developing medical care organizations. This was a result of complex demographic, economic, and technological changes taking place in America and in biomedical science (Starr 1982). It was also part of a larger change in the relations between professionals and their clients occurring at this time in Western history (Johnson 1972). The theory of professional dominance (Freidson 1970a, 1970b) attributes the power of the medical profession to knowledge control, authority over other occupations, autonomy over the practice of their craft, and the resulting institutional power. It is only with the recent shifts in the organization and financing of medical practice (Madison and Konrad 1988) that the tenets of this theory have been challenged (Haug 1973; McKinlay 1977). The publication of comparative case studies of physicians in other nations has led to qualifications of this model. Thus, while in the American case, certain aspects of bureaucratization and government control over medicine have been viewed as a cause for the decline of professional autonomy, this has not been substantiated in other cases. In both Italy and Great Britain, for example, the dominance of the medical profession was achieved through and with the state (Larkin 1988:120; Krause 1988b).

An examination of physicians in China provides additional dimensions to our store of country cases. First, like many other countries in the developing world, China continues to maintain an indigenous traditional medical practice, which has persisted, in varying relations to the transplanted Western medical system, over this century. Second, during the first half of this century, two opposing models of state medicine were introduced to this predominantly agricultural nation by missionary physicians, philanthropists, proponents of Western medical education, and the League of Nations' health advisers. One focused on producing high-quality, well-educated leaders of medical research and education; the other promoted the development of rural-to-urban organizational networks to facilitate the distribution of modern services (Lucas 1982:9). As Freidson and others have observed, the first

184

model, associated with the rise of physicians in the West, has also been credited with maldistribution of physicians and the underservice of millions in need of care (Light and Levine 1988:12). Although the second model inspired the World Health Organization's primary care efforts, its extreme implementation in China during the 1960s and 1970s resulted in wasteful deterioration of hospital facilities and personnel.

Third, although Western-sponsored scientific medicine was the brand promoted by both the Nationalist and later the Communist regimes, most of the work of developing medicine and health care in China took place in the post-1949 era. This was a world in which physicians were not only employees in large bureaucratic organizations, but they and their organizations were subject to vertical as well as horizontal rule by Chinese Communist party (CCP) cadres. Fourth, during the Cultural Revolution (1966–1976), Chinese physicians experienced probably the most extreme experiment in radical deprofessionalization of the medical profession ever conducted. Doctors were stripped of all outward symbols of rank and prestige, and professional work that had been under their sole direction was either shared or redistributed to other, more proletarian health care personnel. Finally, in the post-Mao era, with the restructuring and depoliticizing of workplace organizations, we can observe the factors related to the status of physicians in state-run, medical organizations as they have regained control over many aspects of training, evaluation, and practice.

The China case enlarges recent challenges to the American theory of professional dominance in several ways. It reinforces the importance of examining not only the power of the state over physicians but of political parties as well (Krause 1988*b*). It adds evidence to the view that power of (even a very bureaucratic) organization can lend authority to those in responsible positions, while at the same time demonstrating the extent to which autonomy can be limited when employees are very dependent. Finally, it reminds us that the issue of the hegemony of Western scientific medicine is an ongoing dilemma. The position of Western medicine physicians in an Asian nation cannot be divorced from concerns about political and economic dependency nor can it be considered apart from the debate over which model of state medicine offers the best strategy to improve the public's health.

Traditional Medicine and the Challenge from the West

Confucianism dominated imperial rule in China from the second century B.C. During its renaissance (tenth to the fourteenth centuries), the government promoted learning through compiling and printing standard and new texts on mathematics, medicine, agriculture, and warfare, in addition to Confucian scriptures, histories, law codes, and philosophy. Official publications were supplemented by state-sponsored education at the lower levels, and a system of medical education, at its peak in the Northern Sung dynasty (960–1126), prepared a quota of three hundred students for posts in the state medical service (Elvin 1973:180). The codification of medical and pharmacological texts may have represented an attempt to exercise control over medical knowledge. However, in the face of a large and diverse occupation, this may be seen as an attempt to codify rather than legislate standards of care (Judith Farquhar, personal communication).

Despite state-sponsored compilation of medical texts, what is popularly called TCM (traditional Chinese medicine) did not have a single name or a unified school of practice in imperial China. Medical care was delivered by a variety of classes of practitioners, ranging from official Confucian physicians to Taoist priests and itinerant drug peddlers. It was the "commoner-doctors" who provided the bulk of medical care. Their medical knowledge and specializations were derived from various sources, including Confucian, Buddhist, Taoist, and spirit worship. Training was by apprenticeship. Many were specialists, basing their practices on secret remedies or treatments learned from masters or passed on from family members.

In contrast, Confucian medical practitioners were drawn from the gentry, a class whose social position derived from academic degrees in the government examinations, which often led to control over land and government offices. Although some gentry took jobs in the bureaucracy, most remained in their local areas, involved in education and public works (Chang 1962:Introduction). Records from the nineteenth century show that gentry doctors constituted only about 1 to 2 percent of all gentry, numbering between 15,000 and 30,000 in total, or 10 to 20 doctors per district (Chang 1962:121–22). They called themselves scholar-doctors to distinguish themselves from commoner-doctors. The term connoted both a service ideal and observance of Confucian ethics.

Literary and scholarly texts from imperial China reveal a long-standing rivalry between Confucian scholar-doctors and the commoner-doctors. Scholar-doctors were taught that medical knowledge should be part of the general education of a scholar, available free of charge (Unschuld 1979:18). In stories and essays, scholar-doctors are portrayed as adhering to ethical principles and to the service ideal, while commoner-doctors are characterized as unscrupulous, unskilled, or both. This denigration of commoner-doctors can be seen as an attempt by Confucians to assert to the public their trustworthiness as a class and, at the same time, reaffirm the virtue of the Confucian regime (Judith Farquhar, personal communication). Ironically, the gap between ideology and actual practice is revealed by studies of nineteenth-century gentry income, which found that scholar-doctors generated considerable profit from their practice; their incomes were a great deal higher than both commoner-doctors and gentry who relied solely on teaching (Chang 1962:121).

A far more serious challenge to Confucian rule appeared in the middle of the nineteenth century by missionaries, educators, and traders from the West. American and European missionaries first brought Western medicine to a number of coastal cities in the late 1800s. Gradually a small number of medical and nursing training schools were established, along with small hospitals, although the overall acceptance of Western medicine at this time was quite limited (Cheung 1988; Hillier and Jewell 1983; Bowers 1972).

By the fall of the Qing dynasty (1644–1911), contact with the West had created an intellectual and cultural crisis. Critics condemned the failure of the imperial system to modernize China. Some advocated wholesale adoption of Western political and educational institutions, while others, fearful of social and cultural disruption, pushed only for taking advantage of the scientific and technological advances that the West had to offer. Many Chinese scholars, including those who would later lead the nation, went abroad to study during this period, and many of those leaders studied medicine.

During the 1920s and 1930s, the development of Western medicine in China was guided by advisers from various Western medical schools and missionary and philanthropic organizations. The China Medical Board was established by the Rockefeller Foundation in 1913; in 1917 it founded the Peking Union Medical College (PUMC) in Beijing. This "American Transplant" (Bullock 1980) was based on the new Flexner model of medical education developed at Johns Hopkins University. With an eight-year curriculum, PUMC turned out 140 graduates in each class. These graduates, along with those from several other foreign-sponsored medical schools, exerted considerable influence over the evolution of medicine in China as heads of medical schools and leaders in the Ministry of Health.

Critics have noted the financial and intellectual dependencies created by such a program (Brown 1976; Bullock 1980). Americans dominated the faculty. PUMC graduates were criticized for learning about diseases prevalent in the West but not those most common in their own country. The Rockefeller presence in China has been attacked for its role in the promotion of a Western- and capitalist-dominated medical agenda (Brown 1976).

This kind of critique, however, fails to recognize the pluralism of views, both within the Rockefeller community and among Chinese medical and public health leaders of that era regarding the best road to improved health for the Chinese people (Lucas 1982; Bullock 1980). In the 1930s, the League of Nations' health advisers recommended a two-tiered physician training program, in response to concerns about unreasonable standards for physician training. It proposed national medical schools with eight years of training after approximately nine years of middle school, and provincial medical schools with five years after middle school (Lucas 1982:68). While medical schools implemented these recommendations, experiments in a community-based approach to public health and health services delivery, inspired by a model developed in Yugoslavia, were also carried out in various locations in China (Lucas 1982:71–80). John Grant, a member of the PUMC faculty, was one of the strongest advocates of getting out of the classroom and laboratory and into the community to do health work. He was instrumental in establishing a model training site for all levels of health personnel in Dingxian county, 100 kilometers from Beijing, where health and rural reconstruction work were addressed in an integrated program (Bullock 1980; Lucas 1982; Chen 1989). Many public health education programs initiated at this time emphasized the relationship between national health and national strength; pamphlets warned of the inevitable foreign domination that would result if disease depleted national vitality (Lucas 1982:48). These programs influenced policymakers in both the Nationalist (1925–1949) and the Communist (1949–present) regimes. The CCP would later become famous for implementing programs that directly linked health with rural development, using mass mobilization techniques and local paramedical personnel to combat health problems. These programs were carried out at great cost to the rising group of Western-trained physicians.

Medicine under the CCP

From the mid-1930s to 1949, China suffered first invasion by the Japanese and then four years of civil war. In 1949, there were 38,000 Western medicine doctors and 276,000 traditional medicine doctors. The numbers equalized in the mid-1970s (at about 250,000 each), and in the mid-1980s, there were twice as many Western medicine doctors as traditional (770,000 versus 341,000). Equally important was the greater than tenfold increase between 1949 and 1985 in the number of auxiliary health care workers, nurses, and basic-level paramedics (*Zhongguo Weisheng Nianjian* 1987:435). During this same period, the number of hospitals increased substantially, from 2,600 in 1949 to almost 70,000 in the mid-1980s (*Zhongguo Weisheng Nianjian* 1985:38).

In the initial years of reconstruction during the 1950s, the prestige of Western medicine remained high, and the CCP turned almost exclusively to the cohort of Western-trained physicians for advice and leadership (Bullock 1980). As the Soviet model of a centralized economy run by a Leninist party–dominated government was established, state-run medical organizations became the power base for a rising medical profession. During the 1950s, most of the leaders of the Ministry of Health (MOH), medical schools, and hospitals were both physicians and Communist party members (Lampton 1977). Initially this telescoping of political and expert roles did not produce conflict. Over time, however, the career backgrounds of physicians in the MOH "reinforced in these individuals a desire to resist complete Party political domination of 'professional' work. [They came to believe that professional] work should be controlled by Party members with expertise to carry out the work well" (Lampton 1974:66).

Curriculum at the newly organized state medical schools was set by MOH physicians, and not surprisingly, it was very similar to that of the pre-Liberation schools. The training of health personnel at all levels was a priority, but these leaders were concerned that in the rush to produce medical personnel, quality would be compromised. Ironically, this concern was echoed by Soviet advisers in China at this time, reflecting changes that had taken place in the Soviet system. In the 1940s, in response to international trends promoting scientific and technological solutions to health problems (such as vaccines and antibiotics), the Soviet Union had instituted lengthier and more specialized programs of medical study (Lucas 1982:92).

During the first decade of CCP rule, all urban workplaces, including medical institutions, were brought under state control. Private practice was gradually eliminated as medical practice was incorporated into the state-run hospitals and clinics. Doctors became salaried government employees, trained in state institutions, and allocated to jobs organized according to state plans (Henderson and Cohen 1984). In the countryside, state-supported medical care extended to the level of the county. In the mid-1950s, there were more than 2,000 county hospitals, and corollary institutions promoting antiepidemic disease work and maternal and child health work were also established at the county level. Mobile medical teams were often dispatched from higher levels to address epidemic and endemic health problems in rural areas. Nevertheless, the only clinics and practitioners at the village level were those with local financing or traditional physicians who had continued their practices.

To the Communist party, the MOH increasingly represented medicine's urban, Western bias. During the 1950s, the CCP's policies conflicted more and more with the priorities articulated by the MOH. From the perspective of the ministry, the most important problems facing China's new health care system were lack of trained personnel and the resources to expand them and major cost problems brought about by a sharp rise in the demand for care at urban hospitals (Lampton 1974:67). Until the cost problems were under control, the MOH did not want to enlarge health care delivery. But by the mid-1950s, the CCP was dissatisfied with the progress in expanding services and actively campaigned to undermine the ministry's authority.

The battle between the experts at the MOH and the antiprofessional CCP erupted when the CCP decided to form a national committee to work against parasitic diseases, which were endemic in rural areas. The Nine Man Sub-Committee (NMSC) was initially established to launch antischistosomiasis efforts by mobilizing county-level party committees to direct the work. Calling upon the legitimacy of the earlier community-based model of state medicine, which had been applied in the CCP revolutionary base of Yanan, the NMSC and rural party leaders effectively established their own health apparatus, responsive to the party, not the MOH, agenda. By the time of the 1958 Great Leap Forward and the creation of Commune Health Centers, the NMSC and rural health care delivery was dominated by middle-level, nonphysician party cadres. The MOH continued to oversee medical education, research, and the management of hospitals under its administration, but the attacks by the CCP seriously undercut the prestige of the MOH, as well as its ability to formulate and carry out policy in the overall health arena (Lampton 1977).

Coincident with these political and administrative changes, in 1955 Mao Zedong called for a reevaluation of traditional Chinese medicine as a "national treasure." One consequence was that traditional medicine was incorporated into the formal structure of medical education. Various schools of traditional medicine were encouraged to establish their own academies, and courses on traditional medicine were added in all medical schools. Departments of traditional medicine and of combined Western and traditional medicine were created in most hospitals, bringing many private practitioners into the state-run organizations. This elevation of the status of traditional medicine in relation to Western medicine reflected appeals to nationalist pride made earlier in the century. From a practical perspective, it immediately created an enlarged pool of practitioners, particularly for work in rural areas.

This formal incorporation increased the status of traditional medicine and brought previously unavailable resources to its practitioners. The resulting research, collaboration, and fruitful debate empowered what had long been a marginal occupation. More important, this was accomplished on party terms rather than those of the various leaders of traditional medicine. Mao's 1955 dictum forced the assimilation of traditional medicine into the Western medical framework, insisting on case records and the training of practitioners within medical universities. In essence, traditional physicians were required to accommodate to the Western mode of knowledge production in order to be recognized. Equally destabilizing, however, was the forced acceptance by practitioners of Western medicine of a different paradigm of medical knowledge. Above all, these efforts to combine Western and traditional medical practice in the late 1950s demonstrated the increasing success of the Communist party to control the definition of orthodox medical knowledge.

The economic setbacks suffered after the disastrous Great Leap Forward temporarily undercut the CCP and reinforced the power of the MOH. However, the pattern of conflict and competition continued until 1965, when, in a dramatic public message, Mao attacked the MOH as "urban Lords" who were running a "Ministry of Urban Health" (Lampton 1977).

Doctors under Siege: The Great Proletarian Cultural Revolution

The radical deprofessionalism of medical work during the Cultural Revolution was part of a much larger social and political movement that attacked the ideological and structural underpinnings of a new ruling class in China. Promoting egalitarianism and self-reliance, the Cultural Revolution was antiprofessional, antitechnological, antiurban, and antiforeign. Elitism, special privileges, and the channeling of resources to the already well-served urban population came under powerful criticism. No group, not even the Communist party, was free from suspicion.

During this period, medical schools were closed and research halted. Biomedical scientists were criticized for conducting research divorced from the needs of the masses; medical educators and practicing physicians were charged with arrogance and the promotion of their own interests above those of patients. Many of those working in urban settings were forcibly removed to locations in rural areas, to learn from the masses. In the countryside, many communes established their own hospitals and implemented collectively funded health insurance programs. A program to train local people in three to six months in county or commune hospitals to become village doctors (called "barefoot doctors") was popularized.

Within all workplace organizations, experts were replaced with those judged politically correct. Medical organizations were often taken over by party leaders who could demonstrate some connection to pre-1949, revolutionary health work, no matter how remote. Professional associations were curtailed. Journals stopped publishing. Anyone suspected of having a foreign connection or being a Western sympathizer was rounded up for criticism and punishment. Government budgetary allocations were shifted to provide a large increase in resources to rural (versus urban) areas (Liu and Yu 1984). The MOH was effectively closed down. "In the 1967–1969 period, not a single major health directive originated with the MOH. All directives were, instead, given the imprimatur of Chairman Mao, the Central Committee, the Cultural Revolution Group, or the Standing Committee of the State Council" (Lampton 1974:106).

In all medical institutions, ranks, salaries, and others signs of occupational prestige were abolished. Doctors were made to sweep floors and offer self-criticism of their elitist behaviors and attitudes; a number of nurses became surgeons and performed other tasks previously done by physicians, including rendering diagnoses.

Patients were encouraged to join in equal participation over treatment decisions. Although the extent to which this occurred is not known, it is clear that doctors were reluctant to offer unsolicited advice or supervision over patient care. Record keeping in general deteriorated, apparently because few were eager to take public responsibility for decision making. When schools and laboratories were reopened several years later, the curriculum was reduced to three years, material on traditional medicine was increased, and greater emphasis was given to rotations at grass-roots facilities. Research protocols were mainly focused on investigations of traditional therapies (Sidel and Sidel 1973; Horn 1969).

In no other time in recent history has Virchow's observation that "medicine is politics" been so completely realized. Every aspect of medical care and disease causation was politicized. This movement brought about the virtual destruction of physicians' control over knowledge and the regulation of their own work and that of other health care workers. They were not replaced with traditional practitioners, although this movement strengthened the legitimacy of these providers, and the antiexpert bias that dominated the times resonated with the moral view of Confucian physicians (Unschuld 1979:116). The party, and its newly created ruling committees within all workplaces, emerged in charge. It took control of the government; the state support that previously had bolstered the power of Western-style doctors was turned against them. Furthermore, because of the extraordinary extent of organizational dependency to which all employees in state-run organizations were subject, there were few countervailing forces available to break the authority of the party (Henderson and Cohen 1984; Walder 1986). Doctors, like other state employees, were assigned to jobs that were almost impossible to leave; the terms of their practice (salary, type, and number of patients seen) were set by the state; workplace leaders had considerable authority in personal as well as professional matters; and accountability and evaluation of work centered less on economic than political criteria.

Market Socialism and the Restoration of Physician Authority

The sweeping changes implemented after the death of Mao and the rise to power of moderate politicians reversed all major Cultural Revolution policies. Economics, not politics, was once again in command. The reforms decentralized state authority, demoted unqualified party leaders, introduced financial accountability in urban workplaces, and in the countryside abolished the collective and heralded a return to family farming. In education, entrance examinations were reinstituted. Curriculum was revised along pre–Cultural Revolution lines. Doctors at all levels who had received training during the Cultural Revolution were offered special review courses and subject to qualifying examinations in order to continue to practice. Scientists, educators, and other scholars were permitted contact with international colleagues. For the first time in many years, foreign technology was imported. Although some occupations have emerged as more prestigious (engineering, computer technology), the 1980s was the decade devoted to modernization, and medicine was a high priority.

Although the cultural authority of physicians probably was never entirely eroded during the Cultural Revolution period, the reforms certainly reconstituted their social authority. As in other sectors of the economy, the motives for this drastic reversal in the health sector were rooted in rejection of the radical Maoist model of social organization rather than associated with particular failures in health care delivery.

In the late 1970s and early 1980s, doctors working in hospitals and medical schools were given authority again. Expertise became a criterion for leadership at all levels of care. Ranks were reintroduced and salary increases implemented. Graduate programs were created. Many Chinese scientists and physicians went abroad for long- and short-term study. Western and international agencies and foundations appeared with advice, staff, loans, and outright grants. Medical equipment and pharmaceutical companies began to tap the China market; by 1985, for example, there were more computed tomography (CT) scanners in Guangzhou than in London (Henderson 1988). The mystique as well as the utility of the new technology reinforced the prestige of Western medicine.

Surprisingly, this focus on high-technology Western-style medicine has not eliminated interest in traditional medicine. In fact, much attention has been devoted to applying Western investigative techniques to understanding the underlying mechanisms of traditional therapy. A number of traditional techniques, such as acupuncture, and *qigong** have even been modernized with electrical or mechanical devices. Furthermore, hospitals at all levels continue to offer choices in both types of therapy, and part of the curriculum in medical schools remains devoted to traditional medicine.

For purposes of evaluating the extent to which physicians in this period have taken on the attributes of a profession, it is the changes in urban organizations that are the most relevant. In the past, state- or enterprise-run hospitals functioned with little attention to financial accountability. Prices for medical care were set by the state, and charges were well below cost. Expensive technology was generally unavailable, and physicians developed diagnostic and treatment skills that did not depend on extensive laboratory testing (Henderson and Cohen 1984:Ch. 8). The reforms have forced all workplaces, including hospitals at all levels, to balance their budgets. While constrained by continued state regulation of prices, this policy has nevertheless encouraged more careful attention to performance, efficiency in patient management, and the profitability of certain procedures. In rare cases, employees have actually been fired.

In the cities, demand for medical care continues to exceed supply; in rural areas, some small hospitals have occupancy rates of 20 to 30 percent and are consequently under financial pressure to attract clients. In both cases, however, the impact of the financial and organizational reforms on the authority and autonomy of the physician is complex.

On the one hand, programs to increase efficiency have been mandated for all hospitals and all health care workers, and in many cases these reforms have strengthened the authority of physicians. Doctors responsible for profit-generating procedures are able to push for the expansion of such care and in some cases will benefit from the income generated from the practice (in the form of gifts from patients or

*A series of exercises and practices by which one learns to control the power of *gi,* the vital force.

bonuses for overtime work). The cost-reimbursement insurance system available to many urban residents has promoted technology acquisition in Chinese hospitals in much the same way as it did in the United States during the 1970s.

On the other hand, Chinese physicians are not in private practice; they are salaried employees of state-run institutions. The context of medical care delivery is still highly bureaucratic. For example, the decision to purchase a new machine, although currently under the authority of experts, is still subject to many layers of committee review and to competing budgetary constraints of underfunded organizations (Henderson et al. 1988). In the same way that monitoring of physician outcomes in the United States constrains autonomy, the attention to profitability and efficiency in China has increased the intrusion of the organization into areas previously controlled by physicians, elevating organizational goals over those of patient care. Thus, although the overall impact of reforms on physicians has been to improve their status within health care organizations, these changes have also introduced more bureaucratic controls over their practice.

Ironically, it is at the lowest levels of care, provided by paramedics or middle-level practitioners, that there is the greatest autonomy over practice. In many parts of rural China, village doctors work (sometimes part time) in loosely organized private practices. In towns and cities, traditional medicine practitioners have opened private clinics, usually advertising a certain specialty, such as bone setting. The state regulates these clinics, particularly with an eye to prices charged for medicines, and county health departments are still able to mobilize village doctors to carry out less profitable prevention activities, such as childhood immunizations and infectious disease reporting. Nevertheless, under a new economic system that encourages private household production and announces that "it is glorious to be rich," pluralistic and private medical practices in rural areas may expand.

Conclusions

The China case demonstrates the remarkable power of the state, ruled by a single-party system, to confer authority on certain occupations and to remove it. This case also highlights the political as well as scientific nature of the complex interaction between two different paradigms of medical knowledge. Much like the controversy between Confucian and independent practitioners in imperial China, the conflict between Western and traditional medicine can be understood on several levels. It reflected debate over the virtue of two very different worldviews in China, identifying themselves through different responses to the models of state medicine, and it signified the struggle between two warring factions within the leadership of the country.

In the United States, the model of state medicine that advocates high-quality education and technical solutions to health problems has reinforced the dominant position of doctors. In China and many other developing countries, there is often more than one model, each with advocates from certain social positions and with certain political agendas. The diffusion of different models, and of medical knowledge itself, must always take account of these contextual factors. In China, the dominance of Western medicine physicians was limited by the politics of the worldview that they (rightly or wrongly) were held to represent and by the organizational dependency forced on them by the Soviet-style bureaucracy established in 1949. Today, under a very different economic system, these factors, within the constraints described, have contributed to their increased authority. Foreign technology, with the mantle of modern science, lends prestige and profit. Modernization is the order of the day. And the health care system that was developed in isolation from the West has now become the model for primary care for the rest of the world.

III

DISCUSSION

16

Some Problematic Aspects
of Medicine's Changing Status

Sol Levine

This book broadens and deepens our understanding of the changing circumstances of clinical practitioners and the medical profession in various national and cross-cultural contexts. Although there have been some excellent studies of the professions and professionalization in general (Freidson 1970a, 1970b, 1986; Larson 1977; Starr 1982), the perspectives of American students, at least, have been colored largely by accounts of the American experience.

The proletarianization or corporatization framework has served useful functions and has stimulated a good deal of deliberation and analysis (Oppenheimer 1973). It has called attention to the decline of control, prestige, and satisfaction of clinical practitioners (McKinlay and Arches 1985) and has inspired students in the field to ascertain the extent to which these changes obtain in different social settings and the reasons for them. The deprofessionalization perspective has also focused on interesting issues and developments within medicine and on the growing power and sophistication of the public, the influence of women, minorities, and consumer groups, and the growth of the holistic health movement (Haug 1973, 1976; Haug and Lavin 1978; Haug and Sussman 1969).

As the material in this book reveals, however, there is considerable variability, complexity, and dynamism within medicine and in medicine's relationships with business, the state, and other major institutions in different societies. We cannot assume that a uniform set of factors will influence medicine or that linear or one-directional trajectories will characterize medicine's fate in all countries. In her discussion of medicine in Czechoslovakia, for example, Heitlinger suggests that changes in Eastern Europe may herald an upsurge in organized medicine's influence and the individual physician's autonomy. In his analysis of the physician's changing status in a dramatically evolving Soviet society, Field also posits that physicians will enjoy greater professionalism and political autonomy.

The book provides rich accounts of the varying circumstances of the medical professions in different societies, as well as the influence of the state in forging and restricting the prerogatives of individual practitioners and the medical profession. In his review of medical dominance in the United Kingdom, Larkin testifies that the state acted to consolidate as well as constrain medical authority. Colombotos and Fakiolas are attracted to Krause's continuum of state-professional relations, ranging from the relatively limited role of the state in the United States to the Eastern European countries, where the professions are employed by the state. The pervasive role of the state is amply and thoughtfully illustrated and analyzed in Chapter 2 by Frenk and Durán-Arenas. Wilsford's comparison of the political power and effectiveness of the medical professions in France and the United States is especially instructive. He contrasts the professional histories, strategies, and modes of organization of the French and American medical associations (organizational particularism versus organizational universalism). He argues convincingly that the American mode of organization gave it an advantage in coping with efforts by the government and other bodies to control the medical professions. However, it is open to question as to how long a universalistic strategy may continue to be feasible in the United States as long as stratification increases within the profession.

A good deal of material in this book also underscores the need to pay more attention to the historical and cultural influences that impinge on medicine. Colombotos and Fakiolas, for example, raise the possibility that medicine in some Mediterranean countries may be influenced by a common cultural environment. It would be useful to explore more deeply the interplay of such cultural factors as the basic values that underlie the health system, images and perspectives of the healer, and the roles and trust assigned to governmental bureaucracies. We need more intensive information on cultural factors to balance the attention that has been given to organizational, economic, and political factors.

Studies and representations of medicine's predicament have often been obscured because it has not always been clear whether the unit of analysis is the clinical practitioner, the clinical specialist, the medical researcher, the medical administrator, the academician, or the profession of medicine as a corporate entity. Freidson and others in the field have explicitly distinguished between the circumstances of the practicing physician and the profession of medicine. We must be aware of different levels of analysis and differentiate among the various actors within medicine. Willis's discussion of the medical profession in Australia points up, for example, a tendency occurring in other countries as well for academically oriented specialists to take power from general practitioners and even private specialists. In tracing some of the inroads other health occupations have made in achieving legitimacy in Australia, Willis cautions us not to overstate the decline in medical authority. He reminds us that other types of health practitioners have been kept from entering the public or private hospital system. Similarly, Riska informs us that in Norway and, to some extent, in Sweden physicians stopped other health professionals from "taking over the administration of hospitals and public health agencies."

Nor has the dependent variable of the equation always been clear. Not only has the concept of dominance, for example, been used variably, but other dimensions such as autonomy and independence have been obscured. Willis's attempt to analyze medical dominance at three levels—autonomy, authority, and sovereignty dominance—is helpful. Especially welcome is the typology developed by Frenk and Durán-Arenas, which provides a more inclusive and systematic framework with which to assess the social organization of the medical professions, as well as medicine as a corporate entity. The four dimensions provided by the authors permit a more specific and discriminating analysis. It is thus easier to say, as the authors do, that "medicine can lose a substantial amount of control to the state regarding external economic conditions but still retain control over the internal process of production." In line with this perspective, they characterize the situation in Great Britain as one of high autonomy with low independence. Similarly, Light observes that medicine may be losing prerogatives and yet increasing its sovereignty. He asserts that the "American medical profession is losing dominance and even autonomy as its sovereignty expands. The latter is occurring as advances in pharmacology, molecular biology, genetics, and diagnosis uncovered more and more pathology and extend the range of problems the profession can treat."

The thrust of much literature in the field is on the forces constraining and shaping physicians. Students devote less attention to the varied and sometimes innovational adaptations that many physicians have made. Doctors are complaining vocally about their predicament, and some have even left the profession or abandoned clinical practice. Nevertheless, in nations such as the United States, Canada, Great Britain, and Australia, many physicians, particularly specialists and subspecialists, retain high social status, have maintained relatively high incomes, and have managed to adapt to and even circumvent the growing restrictions on their prerogatives. Coburn, for example, relates how Canadian physicians, in response to lower fees, increased the use and their mix of services. Even in Greece and Communist Czechoslovakia, where incomes have been low and the medical profession constrained by governmental policy, physicians have been able to use their salaried positions to supplement their incomes by taking advantage of culturally accepted bribes or gratuities.

One form of adaptation that should receive more attention is the ways in which physicians have made use of the services of other personnel. In view of how much many of the analyses of the medical profession have been stimulated by Marxist thinking, it is surprising that so little systematic attention has been given to the various ways in which physicians organize and utilize the labor of others in order to extract what some may designate as surplus value from them.

In understanding the status of the physician, we must recognize what is not explicitly stated in this book: the persistence and sometimes growing predominance of allopathic or Western "scientific" medicine, especially in the advanced capitalist societies. Even the Chinese experience cannot be viewed as an exception to the vitality of Western, or "scientific," medicine. Henderson vividly demonstrates the dependence and sometimes dramatic subservience of the medical profession to the state and points to the Cultural Revolution as the "most extreme experiment in radical deprofessionalization of the medical profession ever conducted." She indicates, however, that even during this extremely oppressive period, the cultural authority of physicians was "never entirely eroded." Moreover, with the passing of Mao Zedong, physicians and medical organizations regained some control.

Alternative health schools in various parts of the world have elected to adopt some features of allopathic medicine in order to improve their acceptability. Even in China when Mao vehemently promoted traditional medicine during the Cultural Revolution, it was necessary for traditional physicians "to accommodate to the

Western mode of knowledge production in order to be recognized.'' In turn, allopathic physicians in many parts of the world have had to incorporate some of the
popular features of holistic medicine and other alternative approaches, thereby
helping to avoid any threat to allopathic medicine's market dominance. What is
also conspicuous is that the services rendered by allopathic physicians are eagerly
and persistently sought by many consumers all over the world. People value health
services in general and medical services in particular, even as they vehemently
criticize problems of access, cost, dehumanization, and iatrogenesis.

Other health professions will continue to fight for and often win their right to
expand their domains and to operate as independent practitioners. It is not unlikely
that, as various health occupations become professionalized, they will make inroads
on some of medicine's historic domains. An enlightened and cost-conscious society
may compel medicine to relinquish some of its monopolies, particularly those that
involve the medicalization of normal life, such as childbirth. As research findings
enter the public domain and demonstrate that in many cases other health occupations
or professions may do as well as physicians—for example, psychologists and psychiatric social workers in place of psychiatrists and nurse-midwives instead of
obstetricians—the physician monopoly may be seriously dented. The current division of labor in the health field may be modified as the health picture changes
and as we look to the health care system for new types of services.

We have not given sufficient attention to the possible consequences of the
dramatically different health picture we face today in the highly developed societies,
at least in comparison with the situation at the turn of the century. Today we are
confronted with such major chronic diseases as heart disease, hypertension, various
forms of cancer, diabetes, mental illness, and arthritis that are not amenable to
cure. They can, however, be controlled or ameliorated, and the patient's health-
related quality of life or functional performance can be protected or improved.

Physicians will be pressed to pay more attention to the functional performance
and well-being of patients, a concern emerging as a major criterion by which to
assess the value of health care. How well is the patient doing on the job, at home,
with friends or relatives? Are medications making the patient depressed, sleepy, or
lethargic? What is the patient's perception of her or his health? Will other health
professions, such as nursing, social work, and clinical pharmacy, compete with
medicine to claim and address the health-related quality-of-life concerns of patients?
In addition, as Riska alerts us in her discussion of the medical profession in Nordic
countries, we have not yet seen the possible consequences of the increasing number
of women who are entering the profession of medicine, predominantly at the lower
rungs of the medical hierarchy. Will these women physicians eventually press for
more humanistic approaches to patients and greater attention to quality-of-life
concerns?

We must appreciate how dynamic and problematic the situation may be. Whether
physicians will continue to yield ground may be influenced by medicine's success
in overcoming growing public suspicion and disenchantment. Wolinsky calls attention to the efforts of organized medicine to retrieve the public trust it once
enjoyed. Medicine's future status may also depend on the types of new technologies
that emerge, the knowledge base the public believes the new technologies require,

and the ability of the medical profession to control the various processes in their deployment. For example, if gene therapies become practicable, the medical profession may argue successfully that this new class of important technologies should reside in its domain, to be controlled by medicine in all its phases, and surely to be dispensed only by physicians. Indeed, the medical establishment may be expected to favor the development of precisely those new technologies that promote its sovereignty.

Values underlie the work of scholars (Gouldner 1962). It is not completely clear whether the writers in this field are bemoaning the decrease in autonomy that the physician is experiencing or whether they think some form of justice is being served. Too little attention is given to the consequences of these changes for patients. If, indeed, were physicians to suffer a loss of income, power, and influence, becoming more bureaucratized, will it be possible to increase the quality of services, provide more humane health services, and attend to the patient's health-related quality of life? This question deserves more attention and should be reflected in our studies and deliberations about the changing status of medicine.

17

National Variations
on International Trends

Rudolf Klein

One of the occupational hazards of social science analysis is that of ethnocentric overexplanation. Conversely, one of the attractions of comparative studies is that they allow us to disentangle explanations or observations that are specific to one country, as against those that may be general across political systems or specific to particular groups like the medical profession. It is from this perspective that I shall discuss the case studies in this book. What do they allow us to say about the pattern of change? To what extent are there commonalities across frontiers? And to what can such commonalities be attributed? Is it something to do with the changing technology of medicine and the associated developments in its organizational structure? Does the nature of postindustrial capitalism dictate the trends, or do political systems play an independent role? What, in other words, can we learn from the differences and similarities between countries discussed in the previous pages?

Consider, first, the arguments about the proletarianization thesis. One immediate problem is the vagueness of the central concept. What would a "proletarianized" medical profession actually look like? Fortunately, comparative studies allow us to explore that question. We need only read the chapters on the former Soviet Union and Czechoslovakia. There we find, for example, that the average doctor's pay in the Soviet Union was equivalent to that of a qualified worker, which might suggest one benchmark against which to test the thesis in the United States and elsewhere. Interestingly, however, we also find that while Communist regimes did indeed proletarianize their medical professions in political and economic terms (apart from a professional elite that owed its prosperity and power to its party status), doctors continued to enjoy a surprisingly high degree of autonomy over the content of their work. Clearly, the various dimensions of the notion of professional dominance are not necessarily integrally related. Even a medical profession that has to take bribes in order to increase its income and that lacks any basis of organized power can still maintain its mystery. In short, the experience of Eastern Europe suggests that command over esoteric knowledge and the ability to maintain legitimacy for a monopoly of expertise is a sufficient condition for maintaining at least one dimension of domination, that of autonomy in the sense of control over the contents of their work. Even a "proletarianized" profession is sharply distinguished from the proletariat.

The East European case studies are instructive in other respects as well. They serve as a warning against being too ready to use changes in postindustrial capitalism as an explanation of wider movements in society. If such changes are also observable in Communist regimes (or what might be called backward state capitalist societies), then we have to look further for explanation. The "contradictions of the welfare state" literature (for example, Offe 1984) is a case in point. It was not the Keynesian welfare state societies that collapsed under the strain of dealing with the competing demands of capital accumulation, legitimation, and consumption. It was the East European command economies that disintegrated. Their political and economic systems lacked the flexibility and adaptability to cope with the competing demands; governmental authority collapsed as it became evident that they could deliver neither investment nor consumption. It is therefore much too facile to anchor explanations of changes in Western health care systems in some neo-Marxian diagnosis of a crisis in late capitalism or in the domination of the world economy by multinational firms. Indeed the only regrettable aspect of the collapse of the Communist regimes is that, in future, they will no longer provide counterfactuals against which theories can be tested.

The East European countries, however, will certainly offer an opportunity for testing theories of a different kind: those that seek to specify and predict the medical profession's role in the policymaking process in different political environments. The Czech case study strongly suggests that the move toward political pluralism has given the medical profession a very large—possibly dominating—role in the shaping of Czechoslovakia's new health care. In particular, the new health care system has created a powerful, monopolistic, professional medical association. This is all the more interesting given the medical profession's previous position as a creature of the party and the state. In one leap, the Czech medical profession appears to have achieved the kind of status in the policy process that the American Medical Association (AMA) and the British Medical Association built up over the decades. This would suggest that the ascribed expertise of the profession (and the need of states to rely on that expertise) explains its dominant position in pluralist societies rather than specific historical circumstances in individual countries.

Once again, however, comparisons can save us from drawing an overly simple conclusion too quickly. The various country studies in this book suggest that political variables matter a great deal when it comes to the role of the medical profession in health care policymaking, even in countries that can be described as pluralist. On closer inspection, it appears to be a function of the political system and may vary over time as political circumstances change (Immergut 1990). In other words, the monopolization of professional expertise does not of itself guarantee power in the political arena; technological determinism is not an adequate explanatory tool in this respect, however convincing it may be when it comes to explaining autonomy in the exercise of technical expertise. There is even a danger in assuming that there must be a logical link between the degree of political power and the degree of professional autonomy. It is quite easy to conceive of a strong state conceding a large degree of autonomy to a weak medical profession on grounds of self-interest—

that is, in order to disguise political decisions about rationing resources as clinical decisions about who should get treated. In other words, conceding medical autonomy may represent a sensible political strategy for diffusing blame rather than conclusive evidence of professional power.

To make this point is to underline the importance of conceptualizing the relationship between state and profession as a dialectic process, of identifying the resources over which the two parties have command, and of analyzing the institutional framework within which they operate. In adopting such an approach, one useful starting point is the distinction between diffuse and concentrated interests (Marmor 1983). In the case of the United States, a concentrated profession faces a diffuse state. Notoriously, the federal government finds it difficult to mobilize the political resources required to deal with the opposition of any intense, concentrated interest group—be it the AMA or the gun lobby. It is no wonder, then, that the thesis of medical dominance originated in the United States (although the case of the gun lobby does raise the question of whether this is a theory about the medical profession or about the role of group interests in the American policy process; if it is the latter, then much of what has been written about the special characteristics of doctors would seem to be redundant). A different model is provided by Britain, where a concentrated profession faces a concentrated state. The U.K. government normally commands an automatic majority for its policies in Parliament. The pattern that flows from this is one of mutual accommodation institutionalized in a corporatist relationship between the profession and the state, punctuated every few decades by a major confrontation (Day and Klein 1992).

A third model is described for France, where a diffuse profession faces a concentrated state. As in the case of Britain, this means that at critical points the state can get its own way. But unlike Britain, the relationship between the state and the profession does not appear to be institutionalized in quasi-corporatist arrangements (perhaps because the state does not actually run the health service and consequently is less dependent on the cooperation of the medical profession to keep the organization functioning). France may also provide an example of the importance of the prevailing public philosophy. The ability of the French medical profession to influence public policy, particularly in defense of its own autonomy, is perhaps greater than might be expected from its failure to match the state's concentrated power. This may in turn reflect the "normative framework" of French policymaking (Jobert 1989)—that is, the scientific bias of French political culture, which means that the elites of the civil service and the medical profession share the language of technocratic rationality. Finally, a fourth model is provided by the case of Greece, where a diffuse medical profession deals with a diffuse state, a recipe seemingly for incoherent policymaking.

There remains the question of whether it is possible to see across the different models any systematic changes over time in the role of the medical profession in shaping public policy. Godt (1987) has argued:

> In devising strategies to deal with overriding macro-economic concerns in an era of intense international competition, the French, British and West German states have come to view the medical profession as simply one interest group among many. There are still important aspects of health policy—clinical decisions and public health

campaigns—in which the physicians' technical expertise prevails. The overall patterns of national health systems have remained in place, in conformity as much with public as with professional preferences. But in those areas which are crucial to broader public purposes, professional power has had to yield. (p. 478)

How far is this contention sustained by the experience of the countries reviewed in this book? The evidence is mixed but, on balance, appears to point to an increasing assertion of state power in a period of rising expenditures on health care and a diminishing capacity to pay the costs out of the dividends of economic growth. Australia and Canada lend support to the argument that the medical profession's ability to shape public policy is diminishing. The case of Britain points in the same direction. The 1989 reforms of the National Health Service (NHS) were pushed through in the face of determined opposition from the medical profession (Day and Klein 1991); however, subsequent to the introduction of the changes, there has been a return to the "politics of the double bed" (Klein 1990): conflict contained within a consensual, corporatist framework. In New Zealand, as in Britain, there have been attempts to strengthen the role of management in health care and thus to restrict the scope of medical autonomy. In some other countries, notably the United States, the jury is still out. We are therefore still left speculating about whether the sense of crisis can overcome the characteristics of the political system: the built-in bias to pressure group veto.

So far the discussion has centered on the ability of the medical profession to shape public policy affecting the structure and finance of health care—macro policy, as it were. But what about micro policy, or decision making about priorities and policies within any framework? Here there is one striking omission cutting across the various contributions to this book: there is hardly any mention of the challenges to the intellectual hegemony of the medical profession. If most of the twentieth century can be characterized as a period during which social problems have increasingly been medicalized, the past decade or so can be characterized as a period during which medical problems have been redefined as social ones. For example, there has been the revival of the public health movement, ranging from Canada's Lalonde Report to Britain's Black Report. The new rhetoric is all about prevention, not cure; the limits of medicine are being stressed as increasing emphasis is put on social, economic, and behavioral factors. There is increasing recognition, in short, that most of the factors determining health, at least as measured by life expectancy, are outside the control of the medical profession.

No doubt many—probably most—of the exponents of the new rhetoric are themselves medical. But the policies they advocate represent a very different paradigm from the dominant biomedical model. They are a challenge to the existing distribution of resources within health care systems, a pattern of distribution that greatly favors precisely those sectors of the medical profession that hitherto have been dominant in terms of status, income, and power. In effect, the flag of revolt has been raised within the medical profession. The new paradigm threatens the established hierarchy of prestige among the medical specialties. The impact of this challenge has so far been limited, but if the British case is anything to go by, it is already beginning to shape the language of policy priorities, although the allocation of resources may lag behind the rhetoric (Secretary of State for Health 1991). For example, the new contract for general practitioners in Britain includes financial incentives to undertake health promotion and prevention activities. Whatever the outcome of this challenge, it serves as a warning against reifying the medical profession. In many ways, it is helpful to see the medical profession as a coalition of competing factions with a common interest in maximizing the resources invested in health care but perhaps sharp disagreements about distributional issues. It is far from self-evident that primary care physicians, hospital consultants, and public health doctors in Britain necessarily have the same interests. Indeed, they may well be competing for resources. One of the main issues for the future may well be the shifting balance of power within the medical profession, which in turn could affect the position of the profession as a whole. As various chapters indicate, there appears to be increasing emphasis cross-nationally on primary health care, which, if sustained, has considerable implications for the distribution of resources, power, and prestige within health care systems. So may the increasing "feminization" of the medical profession (Day 1982), to which many chapters allude, particularly when, as in the case of Scandinavia, the different sectors of health care are associated with the dominance of a particular gender.

The other challenge has come from quite a different source: the medical paradigm is under threat from the economic paradigm. Nothing is more striking—though hardly surprising, given the context of rising spending on health care—than the increasing role of economists in debates about health care (Fox 1979). What is significant is not so much that the economists have directly attacked the medical profession's claim to a monopoly of expert knowledge but that they have, in at least one important sense, bypassed it. They do not claim to know better than doctors about the treatment of individual patients, but they do claim that, in framing public policy, considerations about the treatment of individual patients must be subordinated to broader considerations. Contrary to the ethical individualism of the medical profession, the economists tend to take a utilitarian approach to policy issues (Klein 1977a; Mooney and Jensen 1990); instead of seeking to maximize the health of individual patients, they argue for maximizing the health of a given population. They thus join hands with the public health movement (Cochrane 1972) in challenging the medical profession to justify the efficiency and effectiveness of its activities. In short, managers seeking to control the expenditure-generating activities of clinicians now have an intellectual justification for what they are doing. They are not just trying to save money by preventing heroic doctors from doing their best. They are actually working to the benefit of the community as a whole.

Once again the implication seems to be that the hegemony of the medical profession—its ability to determine the language of debate in the health care policy field—may be eroding. It is far from clear, however, whether this is a cross-national phenomenon; most of the evidence to support my contention comes from the Anglophone countries, which have always been most susceptible to utilitarian doctrines and whose social policies have tended to diverge from those of other West European countries (Esping-Andersen 1990). If, as I suspect, we found considerable divergencies in this (as in other respects) between countries, then this would be a further warning against easy generalizations about the effects of contemporary capitalism on health care; national political, cultural, and social factors seem to be crucial in mediating and transforming international trends.

National factors also appear to be crucial when we turn to another issue thrown up by the debate about the changing position of the medical profession: that of the corporatization of the medical profession. The notion itself seems to be American in its origin (Starr 1982), the argument being that if the "corporate rationalizers" in the public domain failed to achieve their aims, then their counterparts in the private domain would step in. But the notion seems to have been widened to suggest that it is the increasing role of private industry (whether as purchasers or providers of care) that is the threat to medical domination in the sphere of clinical autonomy. The challenges posed to such autonomy—by way of reviews of clinical practice and the introduction of standardized forms of treatment embodied in protocols—is therefore seen as the product of this transformation in the medical marketplace. This conclusion follows, however, only if one ignores the fact that corporate rationalizers can be found in either the marketplace or in bureaucracies. Two definitions are elided into one, creating confusion. There are, therefore, very real problems about the interpretation that has been put upon this development in the United States, if it is advanced as a general thesis about what is happening to the medical profession cross-nationally as distinct from an explanation of what is happening in the United States.

First, it is not at all clear what significance should be attached to the increasing scrutiny of medical practice. Even if it limits the autonomy of individual practitioners, it does not necessarily limit the collective autonomy of the profession (Mechanic 1991). Doctors still determine the criteria to be used and the interpretation to be put on the data. Second, cross-national comparisons suggest that the new emphasis on medical accountability is not necessarily the product of corporatization in the American sense; that is, it is not necessarily linked with the emergence of for-profit providers or purchasers. Nor can bureaucratization be equated, without considerable qualification, with such corporatization. Traditionally the two terms have been treated as being the antithesis of each other, particularly if one defines the two terms strictly to use the former to describe the behavior of officials in public agencies and the latter to describe that of those working in for-profit firms.

When it comes to exploring the issue of bureaucratization in the strict sense, the British example is particularly instructive. Britain's NHS has always been held out as an example of bureaucratized medicine, and in the case of the hospital services (though not general practice) this characterization is accurate enough in the sense that hospital doctors are salaried employees of the state. Indeed, in terms of structure, the NHS is not very different from the model that was imposed by Communist regimes in Eastern Europe, with a strong emphasis on central planning and a large role for the central government bureaucracy. Interestingly, however, British doctors have always enjoyed more autonomy than their American counterparts. Their practices have never been scrutinized by review committees; their decisions about lengths of stay or form of treatment have never been challenged. Again, there are similarities in this respect with the East European systems, which, as noted in the chapters on the former Soviet Union and Czechoslovakia, allowed the medical profession considerable control over the contents of practice. Indeed, it can be argued that it is in the interest of the state to allow the medical profession such autonomy, since this means that political decisions about resource allocation can be disguised as clinical decisions about who should be treated. A health care system controlled by bureaucrats does not necessarily diminish medical autonomy; in the case of Britain, on the contrary, it is the move away from bureaucratic control in the traditional sense toward an internal market model that has led to an increasing challenge to medical autonomy. As part of the 1989 reforms, medical audit has been introduced, although the implementation of this change remains in the control of the profession itself.

The British example also raises a question mark about the general applicability of the model of development for America put forward in Chapter 5. The NHS has always been provider dominated; indeed the 1989 changes can be seen as an attempt to make it buyer driven (although the buyers will remain public servants spending tax-financed funds). In this sense, the direction of change appears to be consistent with Table 5.1. However, the pathologies of the two types of health care—buyer- and provider-driven systems—are very different in the British case than those suggested as being applicable in the American case. Thus, in Britain, cuts in services, undertreatment, and (in the view of the medical profession, at least) reduced quality characterized the pre-1989 provider-driven NHS. In contrast, the pathologies of Light's provider-driven model—overtreatment, unnecessary treatment, and high cost—were conspicuous by their absence. The explanation of this apparent paradox is simple: the producers in the two systems have quite different incentives. In the United States the incentive to producers has always been to maximize activity, whereas in Britain it has been to minimize activity. Similarly, the purchasers in the two countries are very different in kind, working within sharply contrasting financial and policy frameworks; most notably, British purchasers work within fixed budgets.

This contrast would seem to underline the importance, in cross-national comparisons, of analyzing with special care the different meaning of the same concept in different contexts. The significance of concepts like "buyer driven" or "corporatization" may be very different, depending on the institutional environment and organizational structure of health care. For example, much may depend on who the "buyer" is and how the purchases are financed. In this respect, it would be highly instructive to compare systematically the purchasing strategies—and their effects on medical autonomy—of different kinds of buyers: German social insurance funds, Swedish country councils, American insurers, and Britain's new-style health authority purchasers.

But even if we had more such studies, we would still be left with one puzzle, one that is inherent in all studies limited to the health care field. Logically, such a perspective cannot tell us whether what is happening to the medical profession is specific to medicine or whether it reflects a more general phenomenon. We need to know what (if anything) is special to the medical profession as distinct from being common to all professions. If we find that all professions are increasingly being called to account for the exercise of their autonomy—and in Britain this would certainly be true—then we might well conclude that we should be searching for explanations not in the particular circumstances of health care but in wider societal changes. In short, single-profession studies have the same limitation as single-country analyses. The latter lead to ethnocentric overexplanation, but the former may lead to profession-centric overexplanation.

18

Conclusion: Cross-cultural Perspectives on the Dynamics of Medicine as a Profession

Frederic W. Hafferty and John B. McKinlay

As is true for any contributed book, the structure of such a tome allows editors to avail themselves of a final opportunity to raise issues that they feel are of importance to the book as a whole or to particular chapters. We would like to do so here.

Support for a Professional Dominance Perspective

One issue of importance concerns the current status of professional dominance theory and its ability to extend our understanding of medicine as a profession. As was true for the original *Milbank* Supplemental Issue, the majority of the case studies presented in this book strongly support the continuing viability of a professional dominance perspective in comprehending the changing nature of the medical profession. Whether we consider the case of "high stateness" (France or the erstwhile Soviet Union) or "low stateness" (United States), the case studies stand as virtual testimonials to the continuing power and influence of medicine as a profession. Although at times that support may be equivocal (see Light's distinction between autonomy and sovereignty in the United States or Coburn's observations on the rise and influence of alternative providers in Canada), the "median" case study in this book documents a health care system undergoing significant change but one in which professional prerogatives still prevail.

Perhaps nowhere else is medicine's power, authority, and professional autonomy more showcased than in the case studies of Czechoslovakia (Heitlinger), China (Henderson), and the Commonwealth of Independent States (Field). In each case we see the amazing resilience of medicine's hegemony, particularly under the circumstance in which extended state control has faltered or weakened. Field, for example, argues that the presence of capitalistic forces, even when co-mingled with a massively entrenched bureaucracy, need not precipitate a decline in physician prerogatives. In turn, he characterizes the United States and the Commonwealth of Independent States as moving in opposite directions: one retreating from centrali-

210

zation, bureaucratization, and deprofessionalization and the other moving toward a system characterized by increased infringements on professional autonomy. Similarly, Henderson notes that the traditional presence of radical deprofessionalization in China has been reversed with the reemergence of capitalistically flavored medicine. For her, the rise of market socialism appears concurrent with a rise in physician authority. Accompanying this trend, she sees the emergence of economics in general, and the status of the expert in particular, as a new badge of legitimacy in this country. China also serves as an excellent example of how physicians in state-run medical organizations can regain control over many aspects of training, evaluation, and practice. Finally, in a less extreme example, Fougere illustrates how programs designed to increase the efficiency and availability of medicine in New Zealand ironically have enhanced the authority of physicians as they push to expand such operations and, in a certain limited fashion, profit from it. Certainly, the growth of a private insurance system in New Zealand not only raises questions about the irreversibility of forces toward centralization (particularly in the absence of revolution) but also the issue of how countervailing forces toward privatization may result in a reemergence of professional prerogatives.

In some instances, support for the professional dominance perspective arrives by somewhat indirect routes. For example, Larkin (Great Britain) criticizes the deprofessionalization and proletarianization perspectives for their implicit assumption that medicine must previously have occupied a dominant and autonomous status (without prior dominance and autonomy, the terms *deprofessionalization* and *proletarianization* are meaningless). In general, Larkin supports the characterization of medicine as a dominant profession, noting that over the past century, medical authority in Great Britain has been state sponsored as well as state circumscribed. Instead of positing an inherently antagonistic relationship, he notes that there can exist a form of partnership as the state both acknowledges and supports the monopolistic desires of organized medicine. Finally, because the British medical profession never acquired any of the statutory licensing forces with respect to related health occupations, Larkin's chapter raises questions about the necessity of licensure for professional status. Finally, we have Riska's multilayered analysis of Denmark, Sweden, Finland, and Norway, which highlights cultural traditions, such as independent professional employment, gender relations, and the existence of dual labor markets among physicians, to shed light on important variations in physician-state relations and the myriad of ways in which organized medicine seeks to establish and extend its hegemony. In contrast, encountering an example like Greece (Colombotos and Fakiolas), with its combination of high state control, the corrosive influence of party politics, and factors such as high physician supply, documents a situation of relative powerlessness for medicine that appears almost an anomaly.

On the Nature of Medical Work

With this consensus, it may appear that there is little left to say; we believe otherwise. One issue raised both directly and indirectly in many of the case studies is the relationship between the context and the content of medical work. In his early writings, Freidson (1970*a*, 1970*b*) drew some important distinctions between the terms and conditions of medical work versus the content of that work. For most of this century, particularly in low-stateness countries like the United States, it was relatively clear that physicians exercised substantial control over all three of these domains. More recently, however, it has become evident that medicine no longer is able to exercise exclusive control over the context and the conditions of its work (Freidson 1973). Nonetheless, the distinction made allows Freidson and others to claim that medicine remains in control of the content of its work, and, as such, physicians continue to maintain and enjoy their professional autonomy. For Freidson, the critical issue is that physicians, and physicians alone, retain a cultural mandate, as well as the exclusive and legally protected right (as established by transformation of a claimed exclusive and esoteric knowledge base into legal codifications), to render medical diagnoses and to undertake medical treatment. We certainly agree that only physicians may execute medical diagnoses and undertake medical treatments; nevertheless, we also believe that the territorial markers identifying things as exclusively medical are less well delineated today. Furthermore, what territory remains (and it is still considerable) faces meaningful challenges and inroads by competing groups. For example, in the United States, the introduction of diagnosis-related groups (DRGs), a payment scheme designed to impose controls over hospital charges for patients under Medicare, brought about several changes to traditional physician prerogatives. In certain instances, substitution of generic equivalents for physician-prescribed name brand drugs was made mandatory. More significant, hospitals were provided with length-of-stay provisions in which physicians' discretion over how long they could keep their patients in the hospital was sharply limited. Although medicine's continuing ability to manipulate bureaucratic structures may be evidenced in the complaints of physicians about the absurdity of having to "check out" a patient in order to "readmit" him or her under a different diagnosis in order to keep the patient in the hospital, such clinical charades also illustrate how such rules can and do change the flow and the content of medical work.

When we encounter entities such as nursing diagnoses, the push for independent treatment and diagnosis by physical therapists, or a concerted movement by pharmacists to allow for independent prescribing privileges (and thus indirectly undertake diagnostic work), we are witnessing more than skirmishes along the boundaries of territorial prerogatives. Rather, these are attempts to restructure what many consider to lie at the core of medical work: diagnosis and treatment. In an era of organizational schemas such as managed care, we believe it is important to analyze and understand the work of "occupationally enhanced" nurses (as well as a cadre of "retired" or "part-time" physicians, the latter considered to be something less than "real clinicians" by rank-and-file physicians), both of whom have been at least marginally empowered to review the diagnostic and treatment decisions of practicing clinicians (Gamble 1989; Zoldi 1992). Thus, although we agree with Freidson that the origin of clinical algorithms (and related devices) used in such reviews is an important issue (Freidson claiming that since physicians develop and design these algorithms, organizational power remains with medicine), it is not all determining. More important, we maintain, is how these codes are implemented in the workplace, not their origin per se. Furthermore, the amount and type of control exercised by organized medicine in the construction of such rules of practice has not been empirically established. Thus, Freidson's assertions, although provocative, remain at best a contention. Finally, we believe that even when physicians are engaged in the construction and implementation of devices intended to control the terms, conditions, or content of their work, it is not altogether clear whether these individuals are acting as extensions of medical culture or in the interest of other organizational entities. In this book, Heitlinger notes how shortages of critical medicines and technologies in Czechoslovakia can at least indirectly limit the discretion and control that physicians exercise in their clinical work. Nonetheless, she concludes that physicians in Czechoslovakia continue to exercise more control over the content that the conditions of clinical practice.

Finally, we believe that the control physicians exercise over the content of their work cannot be operationally (as opposed to analytically) separated from the terms and conditions of that work. One might argue, for example, that regardless of the particular structural restrictions (e.g., in countries of high stateness and low technological resources such as the former Soviet Union), physicians retain the exclusive privilege to utilize or prescribe that resource. Nonetheless, we believe that something meaningful has happened if other organizational sites of power, such as insurance companies, refuse to pay for a particular treatment *and as a consequence* physicians modify or drop this alternative from their clinical armamentarium. Thus, although it may remain literally true that physicians, and physicians alone, are able to order a particular treatment (the rationale for which may even have been established by current scientific knowledge or professional standards), their ability to utilize such a treatment option has been effectively limited or even eliminated. Like Dr. Seuss's Yertle the Turtle, King of Sala-ma-Sond, medicine may rule over all that it sees, but its throne is still dependent on its ability to convince others of its legitimacy. Medicine's hegemony may not be as fragile as Yertle's throne (which crumbled when a tired and hungry turtle named Mack burped) but medicine's position in the social order remains vulnerable and, thus, potentially limited. In the end we must consider a "So what?" question. So what if physicians retain the exclusive right to diagnose and treat, if the discretion they are able to exercise (a key criterion for Freidson in establishing professional dominance) is effectively muted? In advancing our argument, we need not claim that medicine faces restriction of choice within some range of currently acceptable alternatives. We do claim, however, that medicine faces a loss of discretion over what exists as a given range, something once solely established by claimed technical expertise and now facing the more explicit presence of economic or political considerations.

Along other dimensions, there is increasing evidence that forces other than medical-professional ones are influencing the physician-patient encounter. In the United States in 1991, the state ordered physicians not to mention certain legally available medical options (abortion) to a certain class of patients (those who seek care at federally funded family practice clinics, most often the poor), with this action supported by the Supreme Court (Federal Register 1988; *Rust et al. v. Sullivan* 1991; Ball 1991). Although congressional efforts have been made to loosen gag restrictions on physicians (while maintaining that gag for other less powerful, less culturally legitimate, and less well-organized health care workers), doctors continue to be restrained in counseling patients on abortion. In fact, the law not only requires physicians to *not advise* but to tell patients that abortion is not an appropriate method of family planning (Hilts 1992). In sum, physicians have become a legally mandated conduit for governmental policy. On any given day at multiple sites across the United States, we can find the federal government crowding into the examining room and sitting alongside (or more appropriately in between) the patient and the physician. Although a few changes have been made in the original legislation, these modifications have turned out to be more smoke than substance and actually document medicine's loss of hegemony as opposed to any evidence that organized medicine has been able to mount a meaningful counteroffensive. In anticipation of a loss of federal funding, Planned Parenthood, a national organization providing medical services to women around issues of pregnancy and birth control, has begun to close some of its clinics, thus leaving physicians unable to serve and patients unable to receive such services (Associated Press 1992).

But one might counter, "The issue is abortion!" (as if it could never be, for example, diabetes), or, "It's not that the government is prohibiting all physicians from mentioning abortion to patients; it's only when that physician works in a federally funded family planning clinic!" Moreover, the voice continues, "If the clinic does not want to accept federal monies or if the physician wants to work elsewhere, there is no ban and therefore no intrusion." All of this may be literally true, but such distinctions are basically irrelevant to the issue at hand. Medical work is rife with diagnostic and treatment options that have been established by medicine as science; if these options are not supported by critical resources (including money, political mandates, and cultural authority), they become unavailable for use and therefore outside the realm of physicians' discretion. If medicine is defined by what it does rather than what it can do, then the medicine we have today is meaningfully different from the medicine we had yesterday.

Ever resilient, a supporter of the professional dominance perspective might argue that although managed care and medical effectiveness research is beginning to impinge on the amount of discretion traditionally enjoyed by physicians in clinical practice, it remains true that physicians and organized medicine sit at the source of these changes. Medicine, the argument continues, drafts the rules and oversees their implementation. Several points are relevant. First, such claims have not been empirically established. Second, some of the case examples in this book provide evidence to the contrary. In Czechoslovakia "medical" authority is based on the combined conditions of technical expertise and office (party membership). Clinical work is shaped by a central economic plan controlled not by the health ministries and their chief specialist but by party functionaries. A similar state of affairs (somewhat modified recently) exists in China. In Canada, important decisions about the organization and content of medical work do not emanate solely from organized medicine, evidenced by the staffing (medical versus nonmedical) and important overseeing functions of the Review Commission in Ontario. Finally, and continuing with the abortion example, we question whether it is analytically neutralizing to argue that key elements in a doctor gag rule originated in the Surgeon General's Office, within a blue-ribbon panel of eminent physicians (most probably male) or within some subcommittee of the American Medical Association's House of Delegates known as Physicians for Life (fictitious). We think not, and thus stand at some odds to arguments Freidson raises in this book. The bottom line, we believe, is that a territory once considered to be the exclusive domain of medicine has been breached, and whether individuals with an M.D. degree were responsible for or participated in that breaching is largely irrelevant as a de facto argument in favor of a professional dominance perspective. What is relevant is the possibility that physicians have come to operate as agents of the state or other organizational interests, not as representatives of a professional community. This possibility of dual (and thus potentially conflicting) allegiances is one that Freidson has identified as threatening to professional hegemony in his past writings (1984, 1985, 1987) but not so here. On this point we may return to Heitlinger's observations on the role orientations of chief specialists in Czechoslovakia who occupy full-time administrative positions in the national ministry of health. Similarly, we find Willis (Australia) arguing that medical dominance has changed its form and become more subtle and indirect than previously. Among his examples, he cites the influence of corporate managers to not only increase productivity by speeding up seeing patients but otherwise to influence physicians to practice in a manner not solely based on their professionally derived judgment. Nonetheless, we would be less than complete (or fair) if we did not include Willis's conclusions about professional control and the distinctions he draws among among the concepts of autonomy (control over the content of one's work), dominance (authority over related health workers), and sovereignty (dominion over the matters of ill health), as well as Light's (United States) conclusion that although medicine is losing its autonomy, its sovereignty is increasing with advances in pharmacology, molecular biology, and pathology. Finally we note Levine's observations in Chapter 16 on the importance of delimiting one's level of analysis along with specifying the dependent variable (e.g., autonomy versus dominance) in question.

Physician Income

A second issue of concern in assessing the changing nature of medicine focuses on the relationship of physician income to that of physician status, prestige, and ultimately physician hegemony. In the past, claims about the source of physician incomes (employed versus independent practitioners), along with claims that physician incomes were leveling off or declining, have been used to support a proletarianization thesis (McKinlay 1988; McKinlay and Arches 1985). In turn, Freidson and others (see Wolinsky 1988a; Wolinsky, this book) have dismissively countered that the source of monies is irrelevant to the issues at hand and that conclusions about salary declines are based on faulty or misinterpreted data. Similar points have been made about the absurdity of asserting that anyone making more than six times the average blue-collar worker's salary is being proletarianized.

Around these points we structure the argument at a different level and stress, as did Marx, that a worker's position in society is located not with respect to his or her income per se but to his or her relationship to the predominant means of production. Our argument traces the reasons for any historical change in the social position of physicians to the historical changes in the means of medical care production during late capitalism. Thus, although physicians in capitalistic countries command high salaries on both an absolute and relative scale, these salaries must be viewed in relation to the total value created by a physician's labor for his or her employing organization (which includes, as Levine notes in Chapter 16, the ability of physicians to organize and utilize the labor of other health care workers in terms of their surplus value). Through the presence of sophisticated biotechnology, testing procedures, referrals, and other means, a physician can easily generate in excess of $1 million in value for an employer, thus rendering a $200,000 salary as less than a 20 percent return on the value created. Historically, the ratio of what is created (for an employer) to what is return (to a physician) is working against the doctor (there is an increase in the rate of exploitation).

In the United States, the means of medical care production has changed dramatically since the 1950s. As a consequence, the position of doctors has also altered. Changes in physician income may be related to the terms and even to the conditions of medical work, but it has much less to do with the content of that work. Witness the differences in salary, but not necessarily their clinical hegemony, between physicians in the Commonwealth of Independent States and the United States. Finally, it should be obvious that physician employers, whether corporations or the state, may raise physician income even as they take steps to reduce professional prerogatives, including physician autonomy. Money thus comes to function as a balm, masking the sting or perhaps even the reality of what is really going on. In this sense, rising incomes may generate a false consciousness, similar to the sense of control generated by specialization, in which physicians, feeling their pocket-books flush with cash, are rendered myopic to steps being taken by corporate and other interests to reduce their control over the context, terms, and even the content of medical care. Looking over the case studies in this book, it appears that while the infusion of free market capitalism into a previously "socialized" medical system may fuel increases in income as well as professional prerogatives (see Field, Heitlinger, and Henderson in this book), an alternative scenario—that an increase in physician income will promote an increase in physician prerogatives—is neither as direct nor as compelling. In short, physician salary per se, with respect to either its source or amount, is not an appropriate vehicle for viewing changes in professional status.

The Rise of a European Community

A third issue, and one not formally mentioned in this book, is the advent of a European common market. This movement raises important questions about the impact of increased economic homogeneity and/or symbiosis on professional forms of organization. Four of the twelve countries that will make up this new European Community are included in this book (France, Great Britain, Greece, and Denmark), and there exist considerable distinctions among these countries in terms of how health care is organized, including the relative degrees of professionalization and the nature of state-professional relations. In addition, there exist important differences in language, as well as cultural variations in physician preference for particular diagnostic categories and treatment options, including what is considered to be pathology and what is not. Whether medicine as a profession will be able to surmount these traditional barriers is an extremely interesting issue.

The prospects of a "single" medical profession operating across different nation-states warrants closer scrutiny. Some steps have already been taken to minimize a variety of potential stumbling blocks. Mutual recognition of medical diplomas has been established, and major steps have been taken to make the structure and content of medical education more uniform. Licensing reciprocity has also been accepted. Within this context, we are intrigued by observations made by Heitlinger (for Czechoslovakia) and Field (for the Commonwealth of Independent States) and wonder if a consequence of economic harmonization might be a weakening of control by individual nation-states and a subsequent unleashing of medicine's power and professional autonomy. Of course, all of this would be highly contingent upon organized medicine's within each of these countries having the interest, the re-sources, and the commitment to combat long-standing traditions of professional isolation and intercountry segmentalization.

Finally, and again with reference to the chapters by Heitlinger and Field, the emergence of a European common market alongside the conjoint dismantling of the former Soviet Union makes for a unique analytical opportunity. Sociologically, the movement of Western Europe toward a more unified economic (and perhaps even politicocultural) system, while countries in Eastern Europe begin to embrace the boundaries of diversity, presents social scientists with unparalleled opportunity to explore the diversity and texture of state-professional relations. As Levine noted in Chapter 16, relatively little attention has been given to cultural as opposed to organizational, economic, and political factors in exploring the nature of profes-sions. We often have cast Eastern European countries as a homogeneous counter to the socioeconomic-political systems of the West. The dismemberment of the Soviet Union may allow us to explore better the importance of cultural (and social) contributions to the dynamics of professionalism, effects that may have been masked under the structural delimiters of a single nation-state.

Some Thematic Similarities among the Case Studies

A fourth task we undertake briefly is to highlight a few of the many themes that make several appearances throughout this book. For example, Riska (Nordic coun-tries), Heitlinger (Czechoslovakia), and Henderson (China) comment on the rela-tionship between state control and specialty differentiation. Heitlinger notes that in Czechoslovakia, the state exercises more control over primary care adult medicine, particularly in the areas of workers' compensation and work exemptions, than do subspecialists, who enjoy more autonomy over their work. Riska finds that features of proletarianized medical work are best observed within the public primary care sector with its bureaucratized and gender-specific (female) medical practice. Hen-derson introduces the elements of geography and space and reports that the greatest practitioner autonomy is found at the lowest levels of care, in rural areas, where the possibilities of a pluralistic and private medical practice were very much in evidence.

Larkin (Great Britain), Wilsford (France), Colombotos and Fakiolas (Greece), and Freidson all comment on the relationship between physician supply and professional dominance, particularly the negative impact of a physician surplus on the professional status of medicine. Although not specifically mentioned in this book, it appears that physicians face an appreciable level of unemployment in several of the countries covered in this book, including the Nordic countries, France, New Zealand, and Australia. Recent claims in the United States and elsewhere that there exists a current or impending crisis of physician oversupply have generated contentions relevant to the professional dominance-proletarianization debate. One argument is that the presence of too many physicians will erode their market position. Others claim that physicians are able to create a demand for their services and therefore mute the market forces of supply and demand. The former position appears to support a proletarianization thesis, while the latter seems more in keeping with a professional dominance perspective.

Moving to the topic of gender and medicine, Field (Commonwealth of Independent States), Light (United States), Coburn (Canada), Riska (Nordic countries), Wilsford (France), and Heitlinger (Czechoslovakia) all focus varying amounts of attention on the relative roles of men and women in medicine. Field, for example, notes that women in the Commonwealth of Independent States constitute the majority of the rank-and-file physicians, while men disproportionately occupy the seats of power. Indirectly, this finding raises the possibility that power in medicine resides not so much within the legitimacy (and supposed sanctity) of the clinical (physician-patient) encounter but rather within the structure of gender relations and within the relationship of organized medicine to other organizational entities, including the state. These findings have implications for other countries, including the United States, particularly in terms of the positive significance routinely attributed to the increasing number of women entering medicine (often referred to as the "feminization of medicine"). It appears that neither raw numbers nor individual commitment to clinical practice and the care of patients is necessary or sufficient to ensure the exercise of influence within this particular culture of medicine.

Issues of trust and medicine also make several appearances throughout this book. Donald Light, in his chapter on the United States, explicitly relates the existence of professional autonomy to the phenomenon of trust, noting that claims of esoteric knowledge by medicine mandate that the public places its trust in either medicine's intentions or its skill and knowledge base. Light sees a transition in the United States from a provider-driven era, in which patients trusted doctors, to a buyer-driven distrust of physicians and their values, decisions, and even competence. Wolinsky appears to agree, arguing that medicine's status as a profession will be undercut by internal neglect—that is, if medicine fails to fulfill its fiduciary responsibilities. In an important qualification echoing Freidson, Wolinsky notes that medicine actually need not possess the trustworthiness it claims. All that is required is that the public believe that it possesses such an orientation. One consequence, Wolinsky argues, is that in the future, medicine's professional dominance may be contingent more on its ability to manipulate public opinion than on anything else. In this respect, appearances become more important than any tangible posturing of good intentions.

Continuing with our focus on trust, David Frankford (Law) asks us to rethink our assumptions about the nature of law and challenges us with the question of whether law should function to encourage patients and doctors to trust one another. Willis (Australia) raises the possibility that coalitions might emerge between doctors and patient groups to preserve social expenditure in the face of pressures to reduce it, thus invoking the specter of trust and the issue of why the public should believe in medicine to represent the public's interests rather than its own. Heitlinger notes that in Czechoslovakia, male physicians are often considered more talented and skillful than female doctors and that patients tend to prefer and trust male doctors more. Her observations raise the provocative question of whether trust in medicine is really so much a trust in technical expertise or whether it involves more a trust in fiduciary orientation (Barber 1983; Hafferty 1991).

Issues of trust and professionalism also appear in several of the case studies that describe what appears to be the fairly commonplace practice of patients bribing physicians with gifts or money in order to secure technically necessary services. Mark Field reports a shadow market in the Commonwealth of Independent States, Heitlinger a similar way of life in Czechoslovakia, and Colombotos and Fakiolas the *fakelaki* ("little envelope") in Greece. Similar practices have been reported in Japan (Wilsford 1992, personal communication).

While it certainly would be prudent to acknowledge the importance of cultural differences in interpreting such arrangements and it is certainly true that none of the case study authors claims that such practices are exclusive to medicine, the existence of such financial encumbrances raises serious questions about the ethical core of medical practice, including whether the normalization of such arrangements represents a direct assault on medicine's claims to service and, ultimately, its professional identity. Individuals as analytically diverse as Freidson (1970*a*, 1970*b*) and Coser (1961) have noted the self-insulating nature of professional autonomy, as well as medicine's tendency to place its own self-interests ahead of those of the public—and this in spite of medicine's continued claims that a service orientation stands at the center of its organizational values. When the more blatant examples of financial opportunism noted in the case studies are laid alongside reports of how physicians in public practice settings encourage patients to seek subsequent care in the physician's private (and more financially remunerative) practice (see the case studies of New Zealand, China, and the Nordic countries), we are left with a picture of physicians as economic animals, influenced more by the pocketbook than by any overshadowing commitment to service and espoused fiduciary responsibilities. In short, medicine appears to be passing from a status of *credat emptor* ("Let the taker believe in us") to *caveat emptor* ("Let the buyer beware").

But perhaps we are being too nostalgic or even summarily romantic. In this book Light (United States) notes that the image of the professional as an autonomous gentleman who renders good services to humanity based on a tradition of noblesse oblige is a decidedly Anglo-American concept. It is possible that we are witnessing a revamped notion of service in which the concept of a fiduciary orientation somehow stands divorced from the particulars of remuneration. On the other hand, we may be witnessing a replacement of medicine's service ethic by one stressing entitlement (Dubovksy 1986) and with trust no longer implying responsibility (see Coburn on Canada). In an age of corporate rationalization, medicine itself may be engaged in reshaping the meaning and nature of trust. For example, medicine has long argued that trust is critical to clinical efficacy by promoting an optimal physician-patient relationship. But where trust once existed as a medium of exchange, extended from the patient to the physician in return for medicine's promise of a fiduciary orientation, it now appears that trust functions more as a vehicle designed to ensure patient fidelity. Trust has been recast from something offered and received within a contingent, reciprocal relationship to something owed to medicine by patients in return for medicine's promise—not of service per se but of esoteric knowledge and technical expertise. As a profession finds its authority culturally legitimated and its autonomy legally enforced, professions may seek to divorce issues of fiduciary concern from issues of technical expertise by relegating the former to a subset of the latter (Hafferty 1991). In this light, perhaps we need to reexamine what we mean by the term *professional*.

Fifth and finally, we encounter in this book several different (but complementary) ways of characterizing state-professional relations. Freidson in Chapter 4 draws on the work of Heidenheimer (1989) and Wilsford (1991) in constructing a continuum between high and low stateness. Heitlinger (China) contrasts the "private" professions of the United States, with its limited state involvement and employment, to the "state-involved" professions of Canada and Western Europe, and finally to the "state-socialist" professions which are primarily state located and state employed. Frenk and Durán-Arenas (Chapter 2) offer a more detailed model, differentiating among the dimensions of state power, the organization of civil society, and the representation of physicians, with the last two dimensions further divided on the basis of corporatist and noncorporatist interest representation. Finally, case study authors such as Light (United States) and Willis (Australia) draw upon the concept of sovereignty in discussing the particular dynamics of professional-state relations.

Turning to the discussants, we find both considerable agreement and a diversity of opinion in Klein's chapter when compared to Freidson's. For example, although both discuss the shifting balance of power within the medical profession, Klein, unlike Freidson, concludes that this shifting balance may negatively affect the position of the profession as a whole. Similarly, Klein and Freidson both discuss alleged challenges to the intellectual hegemony of the medical profession. Klein concludes that the ability of medicine to determine the language of the health care policy debate may be eroding and cites the incursion of economists into both the language and the content of the health care debate as an example. Klein sees physicians as tending to preach ethical individualism while economists tend to take a more utilitarian position. Freidson concludes that the profession continues to exercise considerable influence over the way the media represent medical matters. Both address the issue of a shifting balance of power within the medical profession, but Freidson perceives strength in diversity, while Klein views the trend as being more toward segmentalization and fractionalization. In this matter of fractionalization, we find ourselves sympathetic to Klein's arguments. In the United States, it was once deemed both sufficient and entirely appropriate that organized medicine be represented by the singular voice of the American Medical Association (AMA). Today, less than 40 percent of all practicing physicians belong to the AMA. Although it would be incorrect to characterize the situation as one of "disorganized medicine,'' rank and file are turning with ever greater frequency to their specialty organizations for representation in areas of concern. These organizations do not always adopt similar positions on matters of common interest. In this context, we also point to the attention given by Frenk and Durán-Arenas in Chapter 2 to matters of physician homogeneity and internal stratification and the development of a new constellation of positions in the medical division of labor. Finally, we concur with Klein's parting criticism of single-profession studies and note the work of Abbott (1988), Heidenheimer (1989*b*), Wilsford (1991), and Jones (1991) as offering significant contributions to our understanding of the condition and status of professions in a changing world.

On Freidson

It is fitting that we end this chapter with some observations on Eliot Freidson's contribution to this book. It was the consensus of both case study and ''theory'' authors in the original *Milbank* Supplemental Issue that the professional dominance perspective was the most viable framework for understanding the changing character of the medical profession. In this book, Wolinsky's opening chapter summarizes the professional dominance, deprofessionalization, and proletarianization perspectives and reaches a similar conclusion.

With his latest essay, Freidson has chosen to extend his earlier arguments about the dominance and autonomy of medicine in several interesting but not altogether innocuous ways. Freidson appears to have stepped back from earlier claims (1985, 1987) that the professional dominance perspective represents an analytically superior approach to an understanding of medicine as a profession. He concludes that the appraisal of power or dominance is not unambiguously addressable, with answers to important questions necessarily containing arbitrary and stereotypical elements. One's conclusions, he argues, depend on to what segment of the profession one is referring, at what level of analysis one chooses to function, and in what arenas one chooses to focus. In this respect Freidson indirectly evokes McKinlay's (1977, 1988) analogy of athletic competition to illustrate how one's view of the game, and thus one's sense of what is going on, is dependent on whether one occupies the position of a spectator (patient), a player (providers), a referee (the state), or an owner (financial and industrial capital), an analogy also employed in this book by Willis for Australia. Ultimately, Freidson warns against phenomena he feels are too complex to be reduced to ''such simple and sweeping characterizations as 'dominant,' 'hegemonic,' 'proletarianized,' 'corporatized,' 'bureaucratized,' 'rationalized,' or 'deprofessionalized.' ''

In this book, Freidson presents a somewhat different medical profession, one that is relatively heterogeneous yet still unified. In previous essays he has drawn attention to what he perceived to be the increasing internal stratification of medicine and the negative consequence of such a trend for medicine's professional status (Freidson 1984, 1985, 1986*a*, 1986*b*, 1987). Here, Freidson envisions a viable profession not as a ''community of equals'' (Goode 1957) but as an organizational entity substantively and meaningfully divided by different specialty orientations, work settings, role obligations, intellectual orientations, the presence of rival associations, and different and often competing alliances with outside agencies.

Freidson uses this focus on heterogeneity to advance two major arguments. First, the body of knowledge and skill under a profession's jurisdiction is not being replaced by competing notions from outside the profession (particularly by lay knowledge and ideas). Instead, he claims, all such themes, ideas, or arguments, even those counter to what might be thought to be the position of organized medicine, can be found emanating from currently existing factions within the profession. As such, these contrary claims do not constitute examples of lay ideas displacing a professional voice. Freidson's second argument is that physicians continue to exercise considerable influence over the shape and direction of health policy issues by occupying key administrative positions (e.g., minister of health) or by forming a second echelon of authority in which they provide the technical expertise to laypersons who do hold such offices. Finally, bona-fide members of the profession can exercise an even more informal brand of authority by functioning as ministers without portfolios.

These arguments represent an extension of Freidson's previous position (summarized by Wolinsky in this book) that the introduction of computerized rules for clinical decision making, the use of clinical algorithms, and the growth of computer-based monitoring of physicians' clinical activities do not represent, in and of themselves, a loss of professional status for medicine. Complementing this argument, Fougere (New Zealand) points out that the growth of a hospital management hierarchy and the implementation of management information systems paradoxically has highlighted the reliance of managers on the cooperation of physicians for meeting their targets. Furthermore, Fougere notes that information technologies used to document work and practice costs are as likely to be used by physicians seeking to challenge management's goals as they are useful to managers seeking to control the work (and particularly discretionary activities) of physicians. For Freidson, what remains critical is that physicians establish the algorithms, select and operationalize the variables, and interpret the data. This argument has been adopted in this book by Klein and outside this book by Mechanic (1991). To this base, Freidson has added the argument that the ascendancy of views apparently antagonistic or antithetical to organized medicine and medical work (for example, issues of preventative versus curative medicine) should not be taken as a victory of lay versus professional positions but rather as an echo of voices emanating from within the profession. Thus, not only does Freidson have physicians creating the algorithms and interpreting the data, but now he appears to view all arguments and counterarguments as residing within the profession as well. Finally, in analyzing the influence of medicine under conditions of high stateness, Freidson concludes that even in the absence of formal associations independent of the state, the profession continues to play a decisive role in matters of state health policy through its members' formal and informal positions. According to Freidson, medicine continues to be a source of especially authoritative knowledge, and thus professionals are able to exercise influence policy even in the presence of an absolute state. Medicine, says Freidson, still calls the shots.

Freidson's assertions are provocative because they represent what appears to be an appreciable departure from his earlier writings on the increasing internal strat-ification and the declining solidarity and communality of professional groups. In these earlier writings, he expressed grave concern about the rise of a technical and administrative elite within medicine. Now, he notes, these same elites, once thought to be so potentially divisive, appear to facilitate the advancement of professional prerogatives and status.

Freidson's positions bring us to an important series of issues. First, and in the language of Freidson's chapter in this book, what makes a physician a "bona-fide" or a "qualified" member of the profession? The answer is critical, but it is not explicitly addressed in either his prior or recent writings. In the past, Freidson has hinted that it has something to do with a common educational background, but this appears to grant more salience to the importance of prior socialization (relative to the importance of current work setting) than he has otherwise seen fit to acknowledge (Hafferty 1988; Hafferty and Wolinsky 1991). In both this book and the earlier *Milbank* Supplemental Issue, Wolinsky suggests that the key issue is whether phy-sician-administrators, as a class, "fully and permanently divest themselves of all actual medical practice" (1988*a*:43). If they do not so divest, Wolinsky argues, they will continue to function as physicians, thus, supposedly, representing the interests of organized medicine. Conversely, any such a divestiture will result in physician-administrators' acting to advance the interests and issues of other players, say, the corporation.

This issue of physician membership touches on an important methodological point for Freidson. Freidson consistently urges us to ignore formal administrative authority and examine instead how policy is actually implemented and how influence is actually exercised. We agree with this methodological stand and therefore suggest that mere possession of an M.D. degree or clinical license is an insufficient basis on which to establish the identity and identification of the individual or individuals being so scrutinized. In this vein, the increasing trend of physicians to curtail their clinical practices and assume administrative responsibilities on some ongoing basis (as opposed to a rotating administrative position that clinicians begrudgingly tolerate for some relatively short and fixed period of time) cannot be used as a de facto argument that medicine is losing its professional prerogatives. Similarly, the mere presence of physicians' donning the administrative mantle does not stand as proof positive that medicine continues to exercise its professional prerogatives. Elemen-tary role theory holds that the adoption of new role responsibilities, particularly responsibilities that may be viewed by one or more of the parties involved as be-ing in conflict with previous norms, values, mores, or rationales, is fraught with structural tensions. As such, it is exceedingly problematic simply to assume that physicians who undergo training as administrators, who join administrative orga-nizations (e.g., the Association for Physician Administrators), or who function primarily as administrators in their daily work will retain the norms, values, and rationales of medical culture. Instead, we believe that the burden of proof should rest on those who claim that physicians retain their prior identity and show why this should be so. There is something more to being a professional than the command over some body of valued and esoteric knowledge. Correspondingly, there are important moral and analytical differences between someone with an M.D. degree who draws on a body of knowledge gained through medical training and who adopts a "pro-medicine" stance in seeking to advance the values and general ethos of the medical community and someone who intentionally uses that same background, skill, knowledge, and reputation for the advancement of political or corporate ends, some of which may be quite antagonistic to any "professional" concerns. The first individual is acting as an extension of the profession. The second is acting as a technocrat who brings a certain cadre of skills to bear on a certain issue or problem. Wolinsky's criteria imply that the key elements are not certification, licensure, or degree but instead some issue of identity or identification, or both. We concur. Whether the measure is the presence of patient contact (versus the mere possession of an M.D. degree), amount or type of patient contact, or some self-defined perception of allegiance or professional orientation is an open, and ultimately empirical, question. What is not so open to debate is the inappropriateness of determining professional identification and identity based simply on the presence or absence of an M.D. degree.

Finally, we are not persuaded (Freidson's arguments notwithstanding) that an understanding of medicine as a profession is meaningfully advanced by identifying factions within this group that may be associated with one point of view or another. If the group in question is large enough, and medicine certainly qualifies in this respect, then one can most likely find a cell advancing virtually any persuasion. What matters is not the mere existence of these cells (and here we return to Freidson's methodology) but how they function. For example, do we have a gaggle of voices or an organized group? If the latter, are they unified, well financed, and able to mobilize their membership for collective action? Are they at the vanguard of the issue at hand, or is medicine a solitary and distant voice emanating somewhere from within the herd? We certainly agree with Freidson's call to reject evidence of formal or administrative authority and focus instead on the concrete actions of the individuals occupying those positions. Where we apparently differ from Freidson is in his apparent unwillingness to subject this issue to the very methodological standards he so eloquently espouses in his broader writings on the professions.

Conclusions

The case studies sit at the heart of this book, and by and large these materials affirm the viability of a professional dominance perspective. Historically, and particularly with respect to Western industrialized countries, the accession of medicine to a position of professional dominance appears to have been relatively swift and reasonably nonproblematic. For the most part medicine's nineteenth- and twentieth-century marriage with science and laissez-faire capitalism resulted in a high degree of control for medicine over the content, and in many cases the context and the conditions, of its work.

What should not be overlooked, however, is the variety of ways in which the state is able to exercise control over professional prerogatives, particularly if the state is monolithic and market forces are missing or operating under considerable restraints. In Western industrialized countries, we observed important variations in the degree and type of state (or political party) involvement and thus in the particulars of professionalization. Even the recent introduction of capitalism or market socialism into countries with more of a socialist tradition illustrates not only the emergent strength of professionalism but also the ways in which the state has been able to exercise more subtle types of influence over this type of occupational entity. Finally, there exist examples such as China where state, political, and cultural controls established a decisive jurisdiction over even the content of medical work.

As a whole, the case studies in this book illustrate that professionalism is neither inevitable nor irreversible. These studies point toward, albeit indirectly, a dynamic of professionalization that ranges over three different phases: professional ascension, professional maintenance, and professional decline (the latter two captured by the similar, but not equivalent, concepts of deprofessionalization and proletarianization).

Of these three phases, the process of professional maintenance has received relatively little analytical attention. Too often, the steps taken by professional groups to consolidate or reinforce their gains are interpreted either as an extension of professional ascension or as evidence of professional decline. Neither interpretation is analytically satisfactory. Although the boundaries among these three phases can be quite amorphous, their dynamics are different. The growth of professional dominance follows a different process than does the maintenance of professional powers, with professional decline constituting yet a third dynamic. The successful attainment of professional prerogatives (to whatever degree) is always followed or accompanied by a stage in which the group in question seeks to solidify, further extend, and ultimately protect those prerogatives against encroachment from outside forces. These threats or countervailing forces (see Light, United States) can be found in the actions of other groups seeking to establish their own ''professional credentials'' or in actions taken by the state to control, restrain, or otherwise recapture some of the autonomy it once ceded to the group in question. In the case of rival groups, attempts to establish their claims may be made either in isolation, without reference to other groups currently in power, or in some countervailing fashion by attempting to usurp some of the territory claimed by those currently enjoying those prerogatives being sought. To the extent that these groups (or forces) are successful, there is a diminishment of the status of the group in question, but any such diminishment should not be viewed as a forgone conclusion and never proceeds unchallenged by the dominant group in question.

Perhaps the greatest drawback to an adequate understanding of professional decline is viewing it as the antithesis of profession ascension—a reversal of the path and a mirroring of the tempo of the preceding rise. In fact, professional decline is neither the inverse of professional ascension nor as quick, decisive, or clear-cut as any of the examples we have of professional ascension. The decline in doctors' status is a slow historical process and, as a process, something distinct from the rise of professional prerogatives. At minimum, the shift from professional dominance to professional decline is buffeted by a period of professional maintenance in which the group in question seeks to consolidate its gains, protect them from outside incursions, and, if possible, extend those benefits. However, we are not proposing a model of professional dynamics in which the processes of ascension, maintenance, and decline function in some stepwise fashion—whether linear (from ascension to maintenance to decline) or circular (from ascension to maintenance to decline, back to ascension, and so on). What we do claim is twofold. First, the attainment of professional prerogatives is always accompanied by some form of professional solidification and maintenance. Similarly, any claims of professional decline must differentiate between any "real" loss of professional prerogatives and what Freidson has so aptly characterized as "mere" skirmishes along the boundaries of professional powers. Whatever the case, activities directed toward consolidation and maintenance, proactive or reactive, cannot be taken as prima facie evidence of professional decline. Such actions and activities may extend over a considerable period of time, and they do not necessarily lead to the diminishment of professional prerogatives nor do they necessarily indicate the presence of imminent decline. In fact, maintenance activities may actually function to promote a subsequent period of professional ascendancy.

The second claim involves the relationship of these three entities. Although maintenance does not lead inevitably to either decline or ascendancy, it does represent a stage of transition. Both ascendancy and decline are accompanied (but not characterized) by the presence of maintenance activities. Although there is no strict timetable governing transitions among the three stages, it does appear that ascension is the most rapid, maintenance the most incremental, and decline the most enigmatic. Part of the difficulty in delineating ascendancy (or decline) from maintenance is that claims to professional prerogatives are often infused with rhetorical elements. For the group currently in power, a fundamental strategy in its maintenance effort is convincing other parties (including pretenders to the throne, the state, or the public at large) that situations of conflict do not exist as proof positive that its professional powers are on the wane. As such, it is to be expected that any dominant group will continue to claim control over critical domains, even if that control is no longer "real." Similarly, claims by pretenders attempt to influence both the public at large and the power elite that the group in question no longer enjoys or warrants the cultural authority and legislative protections previously established. These difficulties in differentiation notwithstanding, it is important not to interpret maintenance activities as indicative of either ascendancy or decline, nor should maintenance activities be interpreted as simply part of some other process.

If there is one central cross-cultural message to be gleaned from this book, it is that there are meaningful differences in the condition and status of medicine across different countries. These variations are shaped by political, cultural, and economic forces and are reflected in the way medical work is structured, carried out, and valued. There is not one profession of medicine undergoing some universal process of professional dominance or proletarianization. Depending on one's vantage point and level of analysis, at any given time one can identify instances of professional ascendancy, professional maintenance, or professional decline. Each example is shaped by a particular configuration of political, economic, and cultural forces, and each allows for a different vantage point on a continuing process of change in the character of medicine as a profession.

REFERENCES

Äärimaa, M. 1990. Helsingin johtosääntökiistassa sovinto (Editorial). *Suomen lääkärilehti* 45:3282.

Abbott, A. 1988. *The System of Professions: An Essay on the Division of Expert Labor.* Chicago: University of Chicago Press.

Alford, R. 1975. *Health Care Politics.* Chicago: University of Chicago Press.

Almond, G. A. 1956. Comparative Political Systems. *Journal of Politics* 18:391–409.

Altenstetter, C. 1974. Medical Interests and the Public Interest: Germany and the United States. *International Journal of Health Services* 4:29–48.

American College of Physicians. 1990. Access to Health Care. *Annals of Internal Medicine* 112:641–62.

American College of Physicians. 1991. Universal Health Care: A Plan for Change. Draft working paper circulated from Philadelphia, July.

American Medical Association. 1990. *Health Access America: The AMA Proposal to Improve Access to Affordable, Quality Health Care.* Chicago: American Medical Association.

Anderson, O. W. 1972. *Health Care: Can There Be Equity?* New York: John Wiley.

Anderson, O. W. 1977. Are National Health Service Systems Converging? Predictions for the United States. *Annals of the American Academy of Political and Social Sciences* 434:24–38.

Anderson, O. W. 1985. *Health Services in the United States: A Growth Enterprise since 1875.* Ann Arbor: Health Administration Press.

Antipenko, E., and R. Nesynova. 1983. Ob izuchenii mnenii patsientov o rabote vrachei polikliniki. *Sovetskoe zdravookhranenie* 112:16–18.

Armstrong, D. 1976. The Decline of Medical Hegemony: A Review of Government Reports during the National Health Service. *Social Science and Medicine* 10:157–63.

Armstrong, D. 1990. Medicine as a Profession: Times of Change. *British Medical Journal* 301:691–93.

Ashmore, M. 1989. *The Reflexive Thesis: Wrighting Sociology of Scientific Knowledge.* Chicago: University of Chicago Press.

Associated Press. 1992. 3 Planned Parenthood Clinics to Close in Wisconsin. *Duluth News-Tribune,* May 8, 2A.

Atkinson, M. M., and W. D. Coleman. 1989. Strong States and Weak States: Sectoral Policy Networks in Advanced Capitalist Economies. *British Journal of Political Science* 19:47–67.

Attewell, P. 1990. What Is Skill? *Work and Occupations* 17:422–48.

Australian Public Opinion Polls. 1986. *High Regard for Doctors.* Poll no. 04/8/86. Sydney.

Baer, H. A. 1984. A Comparative View of a Heterodox Health System: Chiropractic in America and Britain. *Medical Anthropology* 8(3):151–68.

Ball, J. R. 1991. Law, Medicine, and the "Gag Rule." *Annals of Internal Medicine* 115(5):403–4.

Barber, B. 1983. *The Logic and Limits of Trust*. New Brunswick: Rutgers University Press.

Barer, M. L., and R. G. Evans. 1986. Riding North on a South-bound Horse? Expenditures, Prices, Utilization and Incomes in the Canadian Health Care System. In *Medicare at Maturity*, ed. R. G. Evans and G. L. Stoddart, 53–163. Banff: Banff Centre School of Management.

Barer, M. L., R. G. Evans, and R. J. Labelle. 1988. Fee Controls as Cost Control: Tales from the Frozen North. *Milbank Quarterly* 66:1–64.

Barsukov, M. I. 1951. *Velikaia oktiabr'skaia sotsialisticheskaia revolutisiia i organizastia sovetskogo zdravookhraneniia: X. 1917–VII. 1918*. Moscow: Medgiz.

Beilin, P. 1977. Chelovecheskii faktor. *Literaturnaia Gazeta,* December 14.

Belgrave, M. 1991. Medicine and the Rise of the Health Professions in New Zealand, 1860–1939. In *A Healthy Country: Essays on the Social History of Medicine in New Zealand,* ed. L. Bryder, 7–24. Wellington: Bridget Williams Books.

Bensman, J., and R. Lilienfeld. 1991. *Craft and Consciousness: Occupational Technique and the Development of World Images,* 2d ed. New York: Aldine de Gruyter.

Benson, J. K. 1973. The Analysis of Bureaucratic-Professional Conflict: Functional Versus Dialectical Approaches. *Sociological Quarterly* 14:376–94.

Berg, O. 1980. The Modernization of Medical Care in Sweden and Norway. In *The Shaping of the Swedish Health System,* ed. A. J. Heidenheimer and N. Elvander. London: Croom Helm.

Berg, O. 1991. Medikrati, hierarki og marked. In *Mellom idealer og realiteter,* ed. D. Album and G. Midre. Oslo: Ad Notam.

Bergstrand, H. 1963. The Medical Profession and the Organization of Medical Services in Sweden. In *Medicinalväsendet i Sverige 1813–1862,* ed. W. Kock. Stockholm: Nordiska bokhandelns förlag.

Bilioni, A. F. 1968. Vrach-eto myslitel. *Meditsinskaia Gazeta,* October 25.

Birnbaum, P. 1988. *States and Collective Action: The European Experience*. New York: Cambridge University Press.

Björkman, J. W. 1989. Politicizing Medicine and Medicalizing Politics: Physician Power in the United States. In *Controlling Medical Professionals: The Comparative Politics of Health Governance,* ed. G. Freddi and J. W. Bjorkman, 28–73. London: Sage.

Bloch, S., and P. Reddaway. 1972. *Psychiatric Terror: How Soviet Psychiatry Is Used to Suppress Dissent*. New York: Basic Books.

Bloch, S., and P. Reddaway. 1984. *Soviet Psychiatric Abuse: The Shadow over World Psychiatry*. London: Gollancz.

Bobbitt, P. 1991. *Constitutional Interpretation*. Cambridge, Mass.: Basil Blackwell.

Boli-Bennet, J. 1976. The Expansion of Nation-States, 1870–1970. Ph.D. dissertation, Stanford University.

Bollard, A., and R. Buckle, eds. 1987. *Economic Liberalisation in New Zealand*. Wellington: Allen & Unwin Port Nicholson Press.

Boreham, P. 1983. Indetermination, Professional Knowledge, Organization, and Control. *Sociological Review* 31:693–718.

Bourdieu, P. 1977. *Outline of a Theory of Practice,* trans. R. Smith. New York: Cambridge University Press.

Bové, P. A. 1986. *Intellectuals in Power: A Genealogy of Critical Humanism*. New York: Columbia University Press.

Bowers, J. 1972. *Western Medicine in a Chinese Palace: Peking Union Medical College, 1917–1951.* New York: Josiah Macy Jr. Foundation.

British Medical Journal. 1928. (Suppl.):35–36.

Brogren, P.-O., and M. Brommels. 1991. Frå Plan Till Marknad i Nordisk Sjukvård. *Nordisk Medicin* 106:210–11.

Brown, E. R. 1976. Public Health in Imperialism: Early Rockefeller Programs at Home and Abroad. *American Journal of Public Health* 66(9):897–903.

Brown, H. I. 1990. *Rationality.* New York: Routledge, Chapman and Hall.

Bullock, M. B. 1980. *An American Transplant: The Rockefeller Foundation and Peking Union Medical College.* Berkeley: University of California Press.

Butter, I., E. S. Carpenter, B. J. Kay, and R. Simmons. 1987. Gender Hierarchies in the Health Labor Force. *International Journal of Health Services* 17:133–49.

California Court of Appeals. 1986. Wickline v. State of California. *California Reporter* 228:661–72.

Canadian Medical Protective Association. Various years. *Annual Reports.* Ottawa: Canadian Medical Protective Association.

Capron, A. M. 1985–86. Containing Health Care Costs: Ethical and Legal Implications of Changes in the Methods of Paying Physicians. *Case Western Law Review* 36:708–59.

Carder, M., and B. Klingenberg. 1980. Towards a Salaried Medical Profession: How ''Swedish'' Was the Seven Crown Reform? In *The Shaping of the Swedish Health System,* ed. A. J. Heidenheimer and N. Elvander. London: Croom Helm.

Carr-Saunders, A. M., and P. A. Wilson. 1933. *The Professions.* Oxford: Clarendon Press.

Chang, C. L. 1962. *The Income of the Chinese Gentry.* Seattle: University of Washington Press.

Charloes, C. A. 1976. The Medical Profession and Health Insurance: An Ontario Case Study. *Social Science and Medicine* 10:33–38.

Chen, C. C. 1989. *Medicine in Rural China: A Personal Account.* Berkeley: University of California Press.

Cherednichenko, G., and V. Shubkin. 1985. *Molodezh vstupaient v zhizn'.* Moscow: Mysl.

Cheung, Y. W. 1988. *Missionary Medicine in China: A Study of Two Canadian Protestant Missions in China before 1937.* Lanham, Md.: University Press of America.

Clark, J. A., D. A. Potter, and J. B. McKinlay. 1991. Bringing Social Structure Back into Clinical Decision Making. *Social Science and Medicine* 32:853–66.

Cleavoes, P. S. 1987. *Professions and the State: The Mexican Case.* Tucson: University of Arizona Press.

CNAMTS. 1985. Caisse nationale de l'assurance maladie des travailleurs salariés. *Carnets Statistiques* 20(Nov.).

Coburn, D. 1988. Canadian Medicine: Dominance or Proletarianization? *Milbank Quarterly* 66(Suppl. 2):92–116.

Coburn, D., and C. L. Biggs. 1986. Limits to Dominance: The Case of Chiropractic. *Social Science and Medicine* 22(10):1035–46.

Coburn D., G. M. Torrance, and J. Kaufert. 1983. Medical Dominance in Canada in Historical Perspective: The Rise and Fall of Medicine? *International Journal of Health Services* 13(3):407–32.

Cochrane, A. L. 1972. *Effectiveness and Efficiency.* London: Nuffield Provincial Hospitals Trust.

Cocks, G., and K. H. Jarausch, eds. 1990. *German Professions, 1800–1950.* New York: Oxford University Press.

Codr, G., and L. Zelinka. 1990. Zdravotnictvi-prusecnik ekonomicke, politicke i lidske dimenze. *Hospodarske noviny, no. 20.*

Coney, S. 1988. *The Unfortunate Experiment*. Auckland: Penguin Books.

Conrad, P. J., and J. M. Schneider. 1980. *Deviance and Medicalization*. St. Louis: C. V. Mosby.

Cope Report. 1951. Report of the Committees on Medical Auxiliaries. Cmnd 8/88. London: Her Majesty's Stationery Office.

Coser, R. L. 1961. Insulation from Observability and Types of Social Conformity. *American Sociological Review* 26:28–39.

D'Anastasio, M. 1987. Red Medicine: Soviet Health System, Despite Early Claims, Is Riddled by Failures. *Wall Street Journal*, August 18.

Davidson, A. 1968. *Antonio Gramsci: The Man, His Ideas*. Sydney: Australian Left Review Publications.

Davies, C. 1987. Things to Come: The NHS in the Next Decade. *Sociology of Health and Illness* 9(3):302–17.

Davis, J. 1977. *People of the Mediterranean: An Essay in Comparative Social Anthropology*. Boston: Routledge & Kegan Paul.

Davis, P., ed. 1992. *For Health or Profit?* Auckland: Penguin Books.

Day, P. 1982. *Women Doctors*. London: King's Fund.

Day, P., and R. Klein. 1991. Britain's Health Care Experiment. *Health Affairs* 10(13):39–59.

Day, P., and R. Klein. 1992. Constitutional and Distributional Conflict in British Medical Politics: The Case of General Practice, 1911–1991. *Political Studies* 40(3):462–78.

de Secondat Montesquieu, C. L. 1748. *De l'Esprit des Loix*. Geneva: Barillot & Sons.

Department of Health and Social Security. 1983. NHS Management Inquiry (The Griffiths Report). London: Her Majesty's Stationery Office.

Department of Health and Social Security. 1985. *Annual Review of Medical, Dental and Non-Medical Manpower*. London: Her Majesty's Stationery Office.

Department of Health. 1989. *Working for Patients*. London: Her Majesty's Stationery Office.

Derber, C. W. 1982. Managing Professionals: Ideological Proletarianization and Mental Labor. In *Professionals as Workers: Mental Labor in Advanced Capitalism*, ed. C. Derber. Boston: G. K. Hall.

Derber, C. W., A. Schwartz, and Y. Magrass. 1990. *Power in the Highest Degree: Professionals and the Rise of a New Mandarin Order*. New York: Oxford University Press.

Diamandouros, P. N. 1983. Greek Political Culture in Transition: Historical Origins, Evolution, Current Trends. In *Greece in the 1980s*, ed. R. Clogg, 43–69. London: Macmillan.

Donnangelo, M. C. F. 1975. *Medicina e Sociedade: O Médico e su Mercado de Trabalho*. Sao Paulo: Livraria Pionera Editora.

Dubovksy, S. L. 1986. Coping with Entitlement in Medical Education. *New England Journal of Medicine* 315:1672–74.

Durán-Arenas, L., and M. Kennedy. 1991. The Constitution of Physicians' Power: A Theoretical Framework for Comparative Analysis. *Social Science and Medicine* 32:643–48.

Easton, B., ed. 1989. *The Making of Rogernomics*. Auckland: Auckland University Press.

Eckstein, H. 1960. *Pressure Group Politics: The Case of the British Medical Association*. Stanford: Stanford University Press.

Elling, R. H. 1980. *Cross-National Study of Health Systems: Political Economies and Health Care*. New Brunswick, N.J.: Transaction Books.

Ellul, J. 1964. *The Technological Society*. New York: Vintage Books.

Elstad, J. I. 1987. Legene og samfunnet. *Tidskrift for samfunnsforskning* 28:290–302.

Elstad, J. I. 1990. Health Services and Decentralized Government: The Case of Primary Health Services in Norway. *International Journal of Health Services* 20:545–59.

Elstad, J. I. 1991a. Flere leger, større bruk? Artikler om bruk av allmenlegetjenester. *Inas-Rapport (Oslo)* 91:11.

Elstad, J. I. 1991b. En helse- og sosialarbeider? Profesjonsstrid og lagdeling i helse- og sosialsektorn. In *Helsevesen i knipe: En antologi om helsetjenesteforskning*, ed. Hroar Piene. Oslo: Ad Notam.

Elston, M. A. 1980. Medicine: Half Our Future Doctors. In *Careers of Professional Women*, ed. R. Silverstone and A. Warr. London: Croom Helm.

Elston, M. A. 1991. The Politics of Professional Power, Medicine in a Changing Health Service. In *The Sociology of the Health Service*, ed. J. Gabe, M. Colman, and M. Bury. London: Routledge.

Elvin, M. 1973. *The Pattern of the Chinese Past*. Stanford: Stanford University Press.

Esping-Andersen, G. 1990. *The Three Worlds of Welfare Capitalism*. Princeton, N.J.: Princeton University Press.

Evans, R. G. 1984. *Strained Mercy*. Toronto: Butterworth.

Evans, R. G. 1986. Finding the Levers, Finding the Courage: Lessons from Cost Containment in North America. *Journal of Health Politics, Policy and Law* 11:585–615.

Fakiolas, N. 1988. Health Insurance in Greece. In *Health and Greek Society*, ed. M. Madianos, O. Zarnari, A. Katouseli, G. Kotaridi, P. Pappas, E. Tsakiri, and N. Fakiolas, 183–239. Athens: National Center for Social Research. (In Greek.)

Federal Register. 1988. Rules and Regulations. 53 (12):2944–6. February 2.

Field, M. G. 1957. *Doctor and Patient in Soviet Russia*. Cambridge: Harvard University Press.

Field, M. G. 1967. *Soviet Socialized Medicine: An Introduction*. New York: Free Press.

Field, M. G. 1973. The Concepts of the "Health System" at the Macrosociological Level. *Social Science and Medicine* 7:763–85.

Field, M. G. 1987. Reflections on Medical Technology as a Special Type of Capital: Some Implications for the Hospital. *International Journal of Technology Assessment in Health Care* 3:275–80.

Field, M. G. 1988. The Position of the Soviet Physician: The Bureaucratic Professional. *Milbank Quarterly* 66:182–201.

Field, M. G. 1990. Noble Purpose, Grand Design, Flawed Execution, Mixed Results: Soviet Socialized Medicine after Seventy Years. *American Journal of Public Health* 80:144–45.

Field, M. G. 1991a. Soviet Psychiatric Abuse: Are Post-Mortems Premature? *Institute for the Study of Conflict, Ideology and Policy (Boston) Pub. Series No. 8.*, June, 12–33.

Field, M. G. 1991b. The Hybrid Profession: Soviet Medicine. In *Professions and the State: Expertise and Autonomy in the Soviet Union and Eastern Europe*, ed. A. Jones, 43–62. Philadelphia: Temple University Press.

Finnish Medical Association. 1991. *Physicians in Finland 1991* (Abstract).

Flexner, A. 1910. *Medical Education in the United States and Canada*. New York: Carnegie Foundation for the Advancement of Teaching.

Flora, P., ed. 1986. *Growth to Limits: The Western European Welfare States since World War II*. Vol. 1: *Sweden, Norway, Finland, Denmark*. Berlin: Walter de Gruyter.

Fortescue, S. 1987. *The Communist Party and Soviet Science*. Baltimore: Johns Hopkins University Press.

Foucault, M. 1970. *The Order of Things: An Archaeology of the Human Sciences*, trans. A. Sheridan. New York: Random House.

Foucault, M. 1972. *The Archaeology of Knowledge*, trans. A. M. Sheridan Smith. New York: Pantheon Books.

Foucault, M. 1975. *I, Pierre Rivière, Having Slaughtered My Mother, My Sister, and My Brother . . .*, trans. F. Jellinek. Lincoln: University of Nebraska Press.

Foucault, M. 1977. *Discipline and Punish: The Birth of the Prison*, trans. A. Sheridan. New York: Vintage Books.

Fougere, G. 1978. Undoing the Welfare State: The Case of Hospital Care. In *Politics in New Zealand*, ed. S. Levine. Sydney: George Allen & Unwin.

Fougere, G. 1984. From Market to Welfare State? State Intervention and Medical Care Delivery. In *In the Public Interest*, ed. C. Wilkes and J. Shirley. Auckland: Benton Ross.

Fox, D. 1979. *Economists and Health Care*. New York: Prodist.

Fox, T. E. 1956. The Greater Medical Profession. *Lancet* 2:799–80.

Frankford, D. M. 1989. Creating and Dividing the Fruits of Collective Economic Activity: Referrals among Health Care Providers. *Columbia Law Review* 89:1861–1938.

Frankford, D. M. 1993. Privatizing Health Care: Economic Magic to Cure Legal Medicine. *Southern California Law Review* 66(1):1–97.

Freidson, E. 1970a. *Professional Dominance: The Social Structure of Medical Care*. Chicago: Aldine.

Freidson, E. 1970b. *Profession of Medicine: A Study of the Sociology of Applied Knowledge*. New York: Dodd & Mead.

Freidson, E. 1973. Professions and the Occupational Principle. In *The Professions and Their Prospects*, ed. E. Freidson, 19–38. Beverly Hills: Sage Publication

Freidson, E. 1977. The Future of Professionalization. In *Health and the Division of Labour*, ed. M. Stacey, 14–40. London: Croom Helm.

Freidson, E. 1980. *Doctoring Together: A Study of Professional Control*. Chicago: University of Chicago Press.

Freidson, E. 1983a. The Reorganization of the Professions by Regulation. *Law and Human Behavior* 7:279–91.

Freidson, E. 1983b. The Theory of Professions: State of the Art. In *The Sociology of the Professions: Lawyers, Doctors and Others*, ed. R. Dingwall and P. Lewis. London: Macmillan.

Freidson, E. 1984. The Changing Nature of Professional Control. *Annual Review of Sociology* 10:1–20.

Freidson, E. 1985. The Reorganization of the Medical Profession. *Medical Care Review* 42:11–35.

Freidson, E. 1986a. *Professional Powers: A Study of the Institutionalization of Formal Knowledge*. Chicago: University of Chicago Press.

Freidson, E. 1986b. The Medical Profession in Transition. In *Applications of Social Science to Clinical Medicine and Health Policy*, ed. L. H. Aiken and D. Mechanic. New Brunswick, N.J.: Rutgers University Press.

Freidson, E. 1987. The Future of the Professions. *Journal of Dental Education* 53:140–44.

Freidson, E. 1989a. Industrialization or Humanization? In *Medical Work in America*. New Haven: Yale University Press.

Freidson, E. 1989b. The Organization and Control of Medical Work. In *Medical Work in America*. New Haven: Yale University Press.

Freidson, E. 1989c. Preface to *Medical Work in America*. New Haven: Yale University Press.

Freidson, E. 1989d. The System Surrounding Practitioners. In *Medical Work in America*. New Haven: Yale University Press.

Freidson, E. 1989e. *Medical Work in America*. New Haven: Yale University Press.

Freidson, E. 1990. The Centrality of Professionalism to Health Care. *Jurimetrics Journal of Law, Science and Technology* 30:431–45.

Frenk, J. 1990. The Political Economy of Medical Underemployment in Mexico: Corporatism, Economic Crisis and Reform. *Health Policy* 15:143–62.

Frenk, J., and A. Donabedian. 1987. State Intervention in Medical Care: Types, Trends and Variables. *Health Policy and Planning* 2:17–31.

Frenk, J., and M. A. González-Block. 1992. Corporatism and Health Care: A Comparison of Sweden and Mexico. *Health Policy* 21:167–80.

Frenk, J., J. Alagon, G. Nigenda, M. A. Munoz-del Rio, C. Robledo, L. A. Vasquez-Segovia, and C. Ramirez-Cuadra. 1991. Patterns of Medical Employment: A Survey of Imbalances in Urban Mexico. *American Journal of Public Health* 81:23–29.

Frieden, N. M. 1981. *Russian Physicians in an Era of Reform and Revolution, 1856–1905*. Princeton, N.J.: Princeton University Press.

Furrow, R. B. 1989. The Changing Role of the Law in Promoting Quality in Health Care: From Sanctioning Outlaws to Managing Outcomes. *Houston Law Review* 26:147–90.

Gai, D. 1988. The Doctors' Case. *Moscow News* 6. (In English)

Galbraith, J. K. 1956. *American Capitalism: The Concept of Countervailing Power*. Boston: Houghton Mifflin.

Gamble, S. W. 1989. Changing Roles in the 90's: Will RNs Manage MDs? *Hospitals* 63(22):42–44.

Garpenby, P. 1989. *The State and the Medical Profession: A Cross-National Comparison of the Health Policy Arena in the United Kingdom and Sweden, 1945–1985*. Linkoping Studies in Arts and Science, No. 39. Linkoping, Sweden: University of Linkoping.

Geison, G. L., ed. 1983. *Professions and the French State, 1700–1900*. Philadelphia: University of Pennsylvania Press.

Getzendanner, S. 1988. Permanent Injunction Order against AMA. *Journal of the American Medical Association* 259:81–82.

Ginzberg, E., E. Brann, D. Hiestand, and M. Ostow. 1981. The Expanding Physician Supply and Health Policy: The Clouded Outlook. *Milbank Memorial Fund Quarterly/Health and Society* 59:508–41.

Glaser, W. A. 1970. *Paying the Doctor: Systems of Remuneration and Their Effects*. Baltimore: Johns Hopkins Press.

Glaser, W. A. 1978. *Health Insurance Bargaining: Foreign Lessons for Americans*. New York: Gardner Press.

Glaser, W. A. 1987. *Paying the Hospital: The Organization, Dynamics, and Effects of Differing Financial Arrangements*. San Francisco: Jossey-Bass Publishers.

Godt, P. J. 1987. Confrontation, Consent and Corporatism: State Strategies and the Medical Profession in France, Great Britain and West Germany. *Journal of Health Politics, Policy and Law* 12(13):459–80.

Goode, W. J. 1957. Community within a Community: The Professions: Psychology, Sociology and Medicine. *American Sociological Review* 25:902–14.

Gouldner, A. W. 1962. Anti-minotaur: The Myth of a Value-free Sociology. *Social Problems* 9:199–213.

Gramsci, A. 1971. *Prison Notebooks*. New York: International Publishers.

Granin, D. 1987. O miloserdii. *Literaturnaia Gazeta*, March 18, p. 13.

Grant, W. 1989. *Pressure Groups, Politics, and Democracy in Britain.* New York: Philip Allan.

Gray, B. H., and M. J. Field., eds. 1989. *Controlling Costs and Changing Patient Care? The Role of Utilization Management.* Washington, D.C.: Institute of Medicine, National Academy Press.

Green, D., and L. Cromwell. 1984. *Mutual Aid or Welfare State: Australia's Friendly Societies.* Sydney: Allen and Unwin.

Grigoriants, S. 1988. Soviet Psychiatric Prisoners. *New York Times,* February 23, p. A31.

Gruber, L. R., M. Shadle, and C. L. Polich. 1988. From Movement to Industry: The Growth of HMOs. *Health Affairs* 7(3):197–298.

Habermas, J. 1970. Technology and Science as "Ideology." In *Toward a Rational Society,* ed. J. Habermas, 81–122. Boston: Beacon Press.

Habermas, J. 1988. Law and Morality. In *The Tanner Lectures on Human Values,* vol. 8, pp. 219–79. Salt Lake City: University of Utah Press.

Hafferty, F. W. 1988. Theories at the Crossroads: A Discussion of Evolving Views of Medicine as a Profession. *Milbank Quarterly* 66(Suppl. 2):202–25.

Hafferty, F. W. 1991. Trust, Ideology, and Professional Power. Presentation to the American Sociological Association, Eighty-sixth Annual Meeting, Cincinnati, August 23–27.

Hafferty, F. W., and D. W. Light. 1989. The Evolution of Eliot Freidson's Theory of Professional Dominance: A Twenty-Year Retrospective. Paper presented at the Fifty-third Annual Meeting of the Midwest Sociological Society, St. Louis, April 6–9.

Hafferty, F. W., and F. D. Wolinsky. 1991. Conflicting Characterizations of Professional Dominance. In *Current Research on Occupations and Professions,* ed. J. Levy, 225–49. Greenwich, Conn.: JAI Press.

Häkkinen, U. 1987. Terveydenhuollon talous sekä julkisen ja yksityisen sektorin suhde Suomessa ja muisa OECD-maissa. *Sosiaalilääketieteellinen Aikakauslehti* 24:93–104.

Hall, E. J. 1964. *Report of the Royal Commission on Health Services.* Ottawa: Queen's Printer.

Hall, E. J. 1980. *Canada's National-Provincial Health Program for the 1980's: A Commitment for Renewal.* Report of Health Services Review '79. Saskatoon, Saskatchewan.

Hall, M. A. 1988. Institutional Control of Physician Behavior: Legal Barriers to Health Care Cost Containment. *University of Pennsylvania Law Review* 137:431–536.

Halliday, T. 1985. Knowledge Mandates: Collective Influence by Scientific, Normative and Syncretic Professions. *British Journal of Sociology* 36:421–47.

Halmos, P. 1970. *The Personal Service Society.* New York: Schocken Books.

Hanson, E. 1980. *The Politics of Social Security.* New York: Oxford University Press.

Harris, R. 1969. *A Sacred Trust.* Baltimore: Penguin.

Harrison, S. 1988. *Managing the National Health Service in the 1980's: Shifting the Frontier?* London: Croom Helm.

Haug, M. R. 1973. Deprofessionalization. An Alternate Hypothesis for the Future. *Sociological Review Monograph* 20:195–211.

Haug, M. R. 1975. The Deprofessionalization of Everyone? *Sociological Focus* 3:197–213.

Haug, M. R. 1976. The Erosion of Professional Authority: A Cross-cultural Inquiry in the Case of the Physician. *Milbank Memorial Fund Quarterly* 54:83–106.

Haug, M. R. 1977. Computer Technology and the Obsolescence of the Concept of Profession. In *Work and Technology,* ed. M. Haug and J. Dofny. Beverly Hills: Sage.

Haug, M. R. 1988. A Re-examination of the Hypothesis of Physician Deprofessionalization. *Milbank Quarterly* 66(Suppl. 2):48–56.

Haug, M. R., and B. Lavin. 1978. Method of Payment of Medical Care and Public Attitudes toward Physician Authority. *Journal of Health and Social Behavior* 19:27991.

Haug, M. R., and B. Lavin. 1981. Practitioner or Patient: Who's in Charge? *Journal of Health and Social Behavior* 22:212–29.

Haug, M. R., and B. Lavin. 1983. *Consumerism in Medicine: Challenging Physician Authority*. Beverly Hills: Sage.

Haug, M. R., and M. B. Sussman. 1969. Professional Autonomy and the Revolt of the Client. *Social Problems* 17:153–60.

Havighurst, C. C. 1978. Professional Restraints on Innovation in Health Care Financing. *Duke Law Journal*, pp. 303–87.

Havighurst, C. C. 1983. The Contributions of Antitrust Law to a Procompetitive Health Policy. In *Market Reforms in Health Care: Current Issues, New Directions, Strategic Decisions*, ed. J. A. Meyer. Washington, D.C.: American Enterprise Institute for Public Policy Research.

Havighurst, C. C. 1985. Doctors and Hospitals: An Antitrust Perspective on Traditional Relationships. *Duke Law Journal*, pp. 1071–162.

Havighurst, C. C. 1986. The Changing Locus of Decision Making in the Health Care Sector. *Journal of Health Politics, Policy and Law* 11:697–735.

Havighurst, C. C. 1990. *The Antitrust Challenge to the Professional Paradigm of Medical Care*. Chicago: Center for Health Administration Studies.

Havighurst, C. C., and N. M. P. King. 1983. Private Credentialing of Health Care Personnel: An Antitrust Perspective. Parts 1 and 2. *American Journal of Law and Medicine* 9:131–334.

Havlicek, P. L. 1990. *Medical Groups in the U.S.: A Survey of Practice Characteristics*. Chicago: American Medical Association.

Health Professions Legislation Review (Toronto). 1988. Striking a New Balance: A Blueprint for the Regulation of Ontario's Health Professions.

Heidenheimer, A. J. 1980. Conflict and Compromises between Professional and Bureaucratic Health Interests, 1947–72. In *The Shaping of the Swedish Health System*, ed. A. J. Heidenheimer and N. Elvander. London: Croom Helm.

Heidenheimer, A. J. 1989. Professional Knowledge and State Policy in Comparative Historical Perspective: Law and Medicine in Britain, Germany and the United States. *International Social Science Journal* 122:529–53.

Heitlinger, A. 1987. *Reproduction, Medicine and the Socialist State*. New York: St. Martin's Press.

Heitlinger, A. 1991. Hierarchy of Status and Prestige within the Medical Profession in Czechoslovakia. In *Professions and the State: Expertise and Autonomy in the Soviet Union and Eastern Europe*, ed. Anthony T. Jones, 207–32. Philadelphia: Temple University.

Henderson, G. 1988. Issues in the Modernization of Medicine in China. In *Science and Technology in Post-Mao China*, ed. D. F. Simon and M. Goldman, 199–221. Cambridge, Mass.: Council on East Asian Studies, Harvard University.

Henderson, G., and M. S. Cohen. 1984. *The Chinese Hospital: A Socialist Work Unit*. New Haven: Yale University Press.

Henderson, G., E. A. Murphy, S. T. Sockwell, J. L. Zhou, Q. R. Shen, and Z. M. Li. 1988. High Technology Medicine in China. *New England Journal of Medicine* 318:1000–1004.

Herzlich, C. 1982. The Evolution of Relations between the French Physicians and the State from 1880–1980. *Sociology of Health and Illness* 4:241–53.

Hillier, S. M., and J. A. Jewell. 1983. *Health Care and Traditional Medicine in China, 1800–1982.* London: Routledge and Kegan Paul.

Hilts, P. J. 1992. Easing of Abortion Curb Is Disputed. *New York Times National,* March 31, p. A18.

Hochschild, A. R. 1983. *The Managed Heart: Commercialization of Human Feeling.* Berkeley: University of California Press.

Hodges, D., K. Camerlo, and M. Gold. 1990. *HMO Industry Profile.* Vol. 2: *Utilization Patterns, 1988.* Washington, D.C.: Group Health Association of America.

Holland, M., and J. Boston. 1990. *The Fourth Labour Government: Radical Politics in New Zealand,* 2d ed., ed. M. Holland and J. Boston. New York: Oxford University Press.

Honigsbaum, F. 1979. *The Division in British Medicine: A History of the Separation of General Practice from Hospital Care, 1911–1968.* New York: St. Martin's Press.

Horn, J. 1969. *Away with All Pests: An English Surgeon in People's Republic of China.* New York: Josiah Macy Foundation.

Hunter, D. 1991. Managing Medicine, a Response to the Crisis. *Social Science and Medicine* 32(4):441–49.

Hutchinson, J. F. 1987. The Bolsheviks and the Politics of Medical Reform, October 1917– March 1918. Paper presented at the meeting of the American Association of Slavic Studies, Boston, November 5–8.

Hyde, D. R., P. Wolff, A. Gross, and E. L. Hoffman. 1954. The American Medical Association: Power, Purpose, and Politics in Organized Medicine. *Yale Law Journal* 63:938–1022.

Illich, I. 1976. *Medical Nemesis: The Expropriation of Our Health.* New York: Pantheon.

Illich, I. 1980. *Toward a History of Needs.* New York: Bantam Books.

Immergut, E. M. 1989. Procedures for Conciliation: The Institutional Basis of Swedish National Health Insurance, 1930–1970. *Scandinavian Studies* 61:146–68.

Immergut, E. M. 1990. Institutions, Veto Points and Policy Results: A Comparative Analysis of Health Care. *Journal of Public Policy* 10(4):391–416.

Inkeles, A. 1954. The Totalitarian Mystique. In *Totalitarianism: Proceedings of a Conference Held at the American Academy of Arts and Sciences,* ed. C. J. Friedrich. Cambridge: Harvard University Press.

Ito, H. 1980. Health Insurance and Medical Services in Sweden and Denmark, 1850–1950. In *The Shaping of the Swedish Health System,* ed. A. J. Heidenheimer and N. Elvander. London: Croom Helm.

Ivanov, G. 1986. Na chistotu. *Izvestiia,* February 7.

Izvestiia. 1987. Nationwide Discussion of Restructuring Health Care: Do We Need to Pay for Medical Treatment? September 29, p. 2. (In English in *Current Digest of the Soviet Press* 39(41):16.)

Jäättelä, A. 1990. Den privata vårdsektorn. *Nordisk Medicin* 105:232.

James, N. 1989. *Emotional Labour: Skill and Work in the Social Regulation of Feelings. Sociological Review* 37:15–41.

Jamous, H., and B. Peloille. 1970. Changes in the French University-Hospital System. In *Professions and Professionalization,* ed. J. A. Jackson, 111–52. London: Cambridge University Press.

Jarausch, K. H. 1990. *The Unfree Professions: German Lawyers, Teachers, and Engineers, 1900–1950.* New York: Oxford University Press.

Jessop, B. 1979. Corporatism, Parliamentarism and Social Democracy. In *Trends toward Corporatist Intermediation,* ed. P. C. Schmitter and G. Lehmbruch, 185–212. Beverly Hills: Sage.

Jewson, N. D. 1974. Medical Knowledge and the Patronage System in Eighteenth Century England. *Sociology* 8:369–85.

Jobert, B. 1989. The Normative Framework of Public Policy. *Political Studies* 38(3):376–86.

Johnson, T. J. 1972. *Professions and Power*. London: Macmillan.

Johnson, T. J. 1973. Imperialism and the Professions: Notes on the Development of Professional Occupations in Britain's Colonies and the New States. *Sociological Review Monograph* 20:281–309.

Johnson, T. J. 1977. What Is to Be Known: The Structural Determination of Social Class. *Economy and Society* 6(2):194–232.

Johnson, T. J. 1982. The State and the Professions, Peculiarities of the British. In *Social Class and the Division of Labour*, ed. A. Giddens and G. Mackenzie. New York: Cambridge University Press.

Jones, A., ed. 1991. *Professions and the State: Expertise and Autonomy in the Soviet Union and Eastern Europe*. Philadelphia: Temple University Press.

Jones, E., and F. E. Grupp. 1987. *Modernization, Value Change and Fertility in the Soviet Union*. New York: Cambridge University Press.

Kauttu, K., and T. Kosonen. 1985. *Suomen lääkäriliito 1910–1985*. Jyväskylä: Gummerus.

Kemeny, I. 1982. The Unregistered Economy in Hungary. *Soviet Studies* 34:349–66.

Kendall, P. L. 1965. The Relationship between Medical Educators and Medical Practitioners: Sources of Strain and Occasions for Cooperation. *Journal of Medical Education* 40 (Parts 1 and 2):137–245.

Kent, G. D. 1989. Socializing Health Services in Greece. *Journal of Public Health Policy* 10:222–45.

Kindig, D. A., and C. M. Taylor. 1985. Growth in the International Physician Supply. *Journal of the American Medical Association* 253:3129–32.

Kissam, P. C. 1983a. Antitrust Law and Professional Behavior. *Texas Law Review* 62:1–66.

Kissam, P. C. 1983b. Government Policy toward Medical Accreditation and Certification: The Antitrust Laws and Other Procompetitive Strategies. *Wisconsin Law Review*, pp. 1–93.

Klein, R. 1977a. The Conflict between Professionals, Consumers and Bureaucrats. *Journal of the Irish Colleges of Physicians and Surgeons* 6(3):88–91.

Klein, R. 1977b. The Corporate State, the Health Service and the Professions. *New Universities Quarterly* 31:161–80.

Klein, R. 1990. The State and the Profession: The Politics of the Double Bed. *British Medical Journal* 301:700–702.

Knaus, W. A. 1981. *Inside Russian Medicine: An American Doctor's First-Hand Report*. New York: Everest House.

Kock, W., ed. 1963. *Medicinalväsendet i Sverige, 1813–1962*. Stockholm: Nordiska Bokhandelns Förlag.

Korpi, W. 1978. *The Working Class in Welfare Capitalism: Work, Unions and Politics in Sweden*. London: Routledge and Kegan Paul.

Kosarev, I., and A. Sakhno. 1985. Prestizh professii vracha. *Sotsiologicheskie issledovania* 2:116–19.

Kovner, A., and R. M. Sigmond. 1988. A Program to Encourage the Implementation of Community Benefit Standards for Hospitals. Proposal submitted to the W. K. Kellogg Foundation.

Krause, E. A. 1988a. Doctors and the State: An Italian/American Comparison. *Research in the Sociology of Health Care* 7:227–45.

Krause, E. A. 1988*b*. Doctors, Partitocrazia, and the Italian State. *Milbank Quarterly* 66(Suppl. 2):148–66.

Krause E. A. 1991. Professions and the State in the Soviet Union and Eastern Europe: Theoretical Issues. In *Professions and the State: Expertise and Autonomy in the Soviet Union and Eastern Europe,* ed. A. Jones, 3–42. Philadelphia: Temple University Press.

Krug, P. F. 1979. Russian Public Physicians and Revolution: The Pirogov Society, 1917–1920. Ph.D. dissertation, University of Wisconsin.

Lahelma, E., and T. Valkonen. 1990. Health and Social Inequities in Finland and Elsewhere. *Social Science and Medicine* 31:257–65.

Läkartidningen. 1991*a*. Husläkarsystem med fritt läkarval—modell för framtidens primärvård, 88:470–73.

Läkartidningen. 1991*b*. Etableringsfrihet för husläkare—inga nya pengar till sjukvårdeb än, 88:3872–73.

Läkartidningen. 1991*c*. Försäkringslösning ger valfrihet i framtidens läns—och regionsjukvård, 88:3968–69.

Lampton, D. M. 1974. *Health, Conflict, and the Chinese Political System.* Ann Arbor, Mich.: Center for Chinese Studies.

Lampton, D. M. 1977. *The Politics of Medicine in China: The Policy Process, 1949–1977.* Boulder, Colo.: Westview Press.

LaPalombara, J. 1963. The Utility and Limitations of Interest Group Theory in Non-American Field Situations. *Journal of Politics* 22:29–49.

Larkin, G. V. 1983. *Occupational Monopoly and Modern Medicine.* London: Tavistock.

Larkin, G. V. 1988. Medical Dominance in Britain: Image on Historical Reality. *Milbank Quarterly* 66(Suppl. 2):116–32.

Larkin, G. V. 1992. Orthodox and Osteopathic Medicine in the Inter-War Years. In *Alternative Medicine in Britain,* ed. M. Saks. Oxford: Oxford University Press.

Larson, M. S. 1977. *The Rise of Professionalism: A Sociological Analysis.* Berkeley: University of California Press.

Larson, M. S. 1979. Professionalism: Rise and Fall. *International Journal of Health Services* 9:607–27.

Larson, M. S. 1990. In the Matter of Experts and Professionals, or How Impossible It Is to Leave Nothing Unsaid. In *The Formation of Professions: Knowledge, State and Strategy,* ed. R. Torstendahl and M. Burrage, 24–50. London: Sage Publications.

Law, S. A. 1974. *Blue Cross: What Went Wrong?* New Haven: Yale University Press.

Lawson, H. 1985. *Reflexivity: The Post-Modern Predicament.* Peru, Ill.: Open Court.

Legg, K. R. 1969. *Politics in Modern Greece.* Stanford: Stanford University Press.

Leone, R. A. 1986. *Who Profits? Winners, Losers, and Government Regulations.* New York: Basic Books.

Light, D. W. 1983. The Development of Professional Schools in America. In *The Transformation of Higher Learning, 1860–1930,* ed. K. H. Jarausch, 345–66. Chicago: University of Chicago Press.

Light, D. W. 1988. Turf Battles and the Theory of Professional Dominance. *Research in the Sociology of Health Care* 7:203–25.

Light, D. W. 1989. Social Control and the American Health Care System. In *Handbook of Medical Sociology,* ed. H. E. Freeman and S. Levine, 456–74. Englewood Cliffs, N.J.: Prentice-Hall.

Light, D. W. 1990. Bending the Rules. *Health Services Journal* 100(5222):1513–15.

Light, D. W. 1991*a*. Professionalism as a Countervailing Power. *Journal of Health Politics, Policy and Law* 16:499–506.

Light, D. W. 1991*b*. The Restructuring of American Health Care. In *Health Politics and Policy,* 2d ed, ed. T. J. Litman and L. S. Robins, 53–65. New York: Delmar Publication.

Light, D. W. 1991*c*. Embedded Inefficiencies in Health Care. *Lancet* 338(8789):102–104.

Light, D. W., and S. Levine. 1988. The Changing Character of the Medical Profession: A Theoretical Overview. *Milbank Quarterly* 66(Suppl. 2):10–32.

Light, D. W., S. Liebfried, and F. Tennstedt. 1986. Social Medicine vs. Professional Dominance: The German Experience. *American Journal of Public Health* 76(1):78–83.

Light, D. W., and A. Schuller, eds. 1986. *Political Values and Health Care: The German Experience.* Cambridge: MIT Press.

Liu, Z. X., and X. C. Yu. 1984. Shilun Weisheng Jihua Gongzuo Gaige (Discussion of the reform of health planning work). Paper presented at Zhongguo Weisheng Yanjiuhui (China health research conference), China.

Llewellyn, K. 1960. *The Bramble Bush.* New York: Oceana Publications.

Lorber, J. 1984. *Women Physicians.* London: Tavistock.

Lorber, J. 1991. Can Women Physicians Ever Be True Equals in the American Medical Professions? *Current Research on Occupations and Professions* 6:25–37.

Lucas, A. 1982. *Chinese Medical Modernization: Comparative Policy Continuities, 1930s–1980s.* New York: Praeger Publishers.

Lundberg, G. D. 1991. National Health Care Reform: An Aura of Inevitability Is Upon Us. *Journal of the American Medical Association* 265:2566–67.

Lundberg, O. 1991. Causal Explanations for Class Inequality in Health—an Empirical Analysis. *Social Science and Medicine* 32:385–93.

Macridis, R. C., ed. 1983. *Modern Political Systems: Europe,* 5th ed. Englewood Cliffs, N.J.: Prentice-Hall.

Madison, D. L., and T. R. Konrad. 1988. Large Medical Group Practice Organizations and Employed Physicians: A Relationship in Transition. *Milbank Quarterly* 66(2):240–82.

Makeyenko, P., and L. Mariukan. 1987. Should We Pay for Medical Treatment? National Discussion. *Izvestiia,* Sept. 24, p. 3. (In Russian. An English translation is available in the *Current Digest of the Soviet Press* 39(27):22, 1987.)

Makovicky, E. et al. 1981. *Socialne lekarstvo a organizacia zdravotnictva: Kompendium,* 2d ed. Martin: Osveta.

Marmor, T. R. 1983. *Political Analysis and American Medical Care.* New York: Cambridge University Press.

Marmor, T. R., and J. B. Christianson. 1982. *Health Care Policy: A Political Economy Approach.* Beverly Hills: Sage.

Marmor, T. R., M. Schlesinger, and R. W. Smithey. 1987. Nonprofit Organizations and Health Care. In *The Nonprofit Sector: A Research Handbook,* ed. W. W. Powell, 221–39. New Haven: Yale University Press.

Martin, R. M. 1987. *The Meaning of Language.* Cambridge: MIT Press.

McKinlay, J. B. 1973. On the Professional Regulation of Change. *Sociological Review Monographs* 20:61–84.

McKinlay, J. B. 1977. The Business of Good Doctoring or Doctoring as Good Business: Reflections on Freidson's View of the Medical Game. *International Journal of Health Services* 7(30):459.

McKinlay, J. B. 1980. Evaluating Medical Technology in the Context of a Fiscal Crisis: The Case of New Zealand. *Milbank Memorial Fund Quarterly (Health and Society)* 58:217–67.

McKinlay, J. B. 1982. Toward the Proletarianization of Physicians. In *Professionals as Workers: Mental Labor in Advanced Capitalism,* ed. C. Derber, 37–62. Boston: G. K. Hall.

McKinlay, J. B. 1986. Proletarianization and the Social Transformation of Doctoring. Paper presented at the annual meeting of the American Sociological Association, New York, August.

McKinlay, J. B. 1988. Introduction. *Milbank Quarterly* 66 (Suppl. 2):1–9.

McKinlay, J. B., and J. Arches. 1985. Toward the Proletarianization of Physicians. *International Journal of Health Services* 15(2):161–95.

McKinlay, J. B., and J. Arches. 1986. Historical Changes in Doctoring: A Reply to Milton Roemer. *International Journal of Health Services* 16:473–77.

McKinlay, J. B., and S. J. McKinlay. 1977. Questionable Contribution of Medical Measures to the Decline of Mortality in the United States in the Twentieth Century. *Milbank Memorial Fund Quarterly (Health and Society)* 55(3):405–28.

McKinlay, J. B., S. J. McKinlay, and R. Beaglehole. 1989. A Review of the Evidence Concerning the Impact of Medical Measures on Recent Mortality and Morbidity in the United States. *International Journal of Health Services* 19(2):181–208.

McKinlay, J. B., and J. D. Stoeckle. 1987. Corporatization and the Social Transformation of Doctoring. *Finnish Journal of Social Medicine* 24:73–84.

McKinlay, J. B., and J. D. Stoeckle. 1988. Corporatization and the Social Transformation of Doctoring. *International Journal of Health Services* 18(2):191–205.

McLeod, G. K. 1975. Critical Commentary on Consumerism in Denmark and the U.S. In *Health Care in Scandinavia,* 25–29. Washington, D.C.: U.S. Department of Health, Education and Welfare.

Mechanic, D. 1975. The Comparative Study of Health Care Delivery Systems. *Annual Review of Sociology* 1:43–65.

Mechanic, D. 1991. Sources of Countervailing Power in Medicine. *Journal of Health Politics, Policy and Law* 16:485–98.

Medical Board of Victoria. 1988. *Medical Workforce Statistics.* Melbourne.

Meditsinskie kadri i zarplata. 1986. *Meditsinskaya Gazeta.* October 22:3.

Mehlman, M. J. 1990. Fiduciary Contracting: Limitations on Bargaining between Patients and Health Care Providers. *University of Pittsburgh Law Review* 51:365–417.

Mejía, A. 1987. Health Manpower out of Balance. *World Health Statistical Quarterly* 40:335–48.

Merrington, J. 1968. Theory and Practice in Gramsci's Marxism. In *Socialist Register,* ed. R. Miliband and J. Saville, 145–76. New York: Monthly Review Press.

Merton, R. K., and E. Barber, eds. 1976. Sociological Ambivalence. In *Sociological Ambivalence and Other Essays.* New York: Free Press.

Meyer, J. W. 1980. The World Polity and the Authority of the Nation-State. In *Studies of the Modern World-System,* ed. A. Bergesen, 109–37. New York: Academic Press.

Meyer, J. W., J. Boli-Bennett, and C. Chase-Dunn. 1975. Convergence and Divergence in Development. *Annual Review of Sociology* 1:223–46.

Millard, F. L. 1981. The Health of the Polish Health Services: Critique. In *Reproduction, Medicine and the Socialist State,* ed. A. Hertlinger, 101. New York: St. Martin's Press.

Mills, C. W. 1956. *The Power Elite.* New York: Oxford University Press.

Ministry of Health and Social Affairs, Czech Republic, Working Group for the Reform. 1990. *Reform of Health Care in the Czech Republic.* Prague.

Ministry of Health, Czech Republic. 1990. *Reform of Health Care in the Czech Republic.* Version II. Draft of a new system of health care. Prague.

Ministry of Health, Welfare and Social Insurance (Greece). 1991. Statistics.

Mirowski, P. 1989. *More Heat Than Light: Economics as Social Physics, Physics as Nature's Economics*. New York: Cambridge University Press.

Mooney, G., and U. J. Jensen. 1990. Changing Values and Changing Policy. In *Changing Values in Medical and Health Care Decision Making*, ed. U. J. Jensen and G. Mooney, 179–87. Chichester: John Wiley.

Mozny, I. 1990. *Moderni rodina—myty a skutecnost*. Brno: Blok.

Muller, C., and J. Kapr. 1984. Psychosocialni a moralni aspekty vykonu lekarskeho povolani. *Prakticky lekar* 64:161–63.

Murray, R. H., and A. J. Rubel. 1992. Physicians and Healers—Unwitting Partners in Health Care. *New England Journal of Medicine* 326(1):61–64.

Mushtum. 1985. 24:4.

Muthumala, D., and C. G. McKendry. 1991. *Health Expenditure Trends in New Zealand*. Wellington: Department of Health.

Najman, J., and M. Bampton. 1991. An ASCO Based Occupational Status Hierarchy for Australia: A Research Note. *Australian and New Zealand Journal of Sociology* 27(2):218–32.

Navarro, V. 1977. *Social Security and Medicine in the USSR: A Marxist Critique*. Lexington, Mass.: Lexington Books.

Navarro, V. 1988. Professional Dominance or Proletarianization? Neither. *Milbank Quarterly* 66(Suppl. 2):57–75.

New York Times. 1991. Text of Rights Adopted by the Soviet Congress. September 7.

Niakas, D., G. Skoutelis, and J. Kryiopoulos. 1990. Private Consumption and Underground Economy in Health Sector in Greece: A First Approach. *Epitheorisi Hygeias* (September–October).

Nordic Medical Statistical Commission (NOMESKO). 1980. *Health Statistics in the Nordic Countries*. Copenhagen: Eloni Tryck.

Nordic Statistical Secretariat. 1990. *Social Security in the Nordic Countries: Scope, Expenditure and Financing*. Copenhagen: Statistical Reports of the Nordic Countries.

Nordisk Medicin. 1984. Växande läkaröverskott i Norden redan 1985. 99:164, 169.

Nordisk Medicin. 1991. Ledarskapstvist ledde till läkarkonflikt i Helsingfors. 106:29.

Northwestern University Law Review. 1988. Symposium: Law and Social Theory. *Northwestern University Law Review* 83:1–472.

Oakes, G. 1988. *Weber and Rickert: Concept Formation in the Cultural Sciences*. Cambridge: MIT Press.

Observer. 1991. NHS Surgeons in Open Revolt over Market Changes. July 14.

Offe, C. 1984. *Contradictions of the Welfare State*. London: Hutchinson.

Official Statistics of Finland. 1962. *Allmän hälso- och sjukvård 1960* (XI:63). Helsinki.

Ontario. 1991. *Regulated Health Professions Act. Bill 43 and Bills 44 to 64*. Toronto: Queen's Printer.

Oppenheimer, M. 1973. The Proletarianization of the Professional. *Sociological Review Monograph* 20:213–27.

Organization for Economic Cooperation and Development. 1991. *OECD in Figures* (Supplement to OECD Observer) 170 (June–July).

Otter, von, C., and R. B. Saltman. 1991. Towards a Swedish Health Policy for the 1990s: Planned Markets and Public Firms. *Social Science and Medicine* 32:473–81.

Our Dialogue: The Science of Health. 1987. *Sovetskaia Rossia* July 5, p. 1. (In Russian. Also available in English in the *Current Digest of the Soviet Press* 39(27):22, 1987.)

Parsons, T., ed. 1947. Introduction to *The Theory of Social and Economic Organization*, 3–86. New York: Oxford University Press.

Parsons, T. 1951. *The Social System*. New York: Free Press.

Parsons, T. 1958. Definition of Health and Illness in the Light of American Values and Social Structure. In *Patients, Physicians and Illness*, ed. E. Gartley Jaco. New York: Free Press.

Parsons, T. 1963. Social Change and Medical Organization in the United States: A Sociological Perspective. *Annals of the American Academy of Political and Social Sciences* 346:21–33.

Parsons, T. 1975. The Sick Role and the Role of the Physician Reconsidered. *Milbank Memorial Fund Quarterly* 53:257–78.

Parsons, T., and G. M. Platt. 1973. *The American University*. Cambridge: Harvard University Press.

Patterson, D. M. 1989. Wittgenstein and the Code: A Theory of Good Faith Performance and Enforcement under Article Nine. *University of Pennsylvania Law Review* 137:335–429.

Patterson, D. M. 1990. Law's Pragmatism: A Theory of Law as Practice and Narrative. *Virginia Law Review* 75:937–96.

Patterson, D. M. 1991. A Fable from the Seventh Circuit: Frank Easterbrook on Good Faith. *Iowa Law Review* 76:503–33.

Patterson, D. M. 1993. Why Habermas's Theory of Law Must Fail. *Indian Socio-Legal Journal*. (Forthcoming.)

Pederson, A. P., et al. 1988. *Coordinating Healthy Public Policy: An Analytic Literature Review*. Cat. No. H39-139. Ottawa: Health and Welfare Canada.

Pehe, J. 1990. *Changes in the Health Care System*. Report on Eastern Europe, Radio Free Europe.

Pekkarinen, T. 1990*a*. Helsingin johtosääntö ja Lääkäriliiton hakusaarto. *Suomen lääkärilehti* 45:2776–78.

Pekkarinen, T. 1990*b*. Opettaako Helsingin johtosäänjtökiista mitään? *Suomen lääkärilehti* 45:2999–3000.

Pensabene, T. 1980. *The Rise of the Medical Practitioner in Victoria*. Canberra: Australian National University.

Pesonen, N. 1980. *Terveyden puolesta- sairautta vastaan. Terveyden- ja sairaanhoito Suomessa 1800–1900-Luvulla*. Porvoo: WSOY.

Petro, M. 1980. *Cesta k socialistickemu zdravotnictvi̇̈*. Praha: Avicenum.

Piri, P., and I. Vohlonen. 1987. Työtyytyväisyys avosairaanhoidon henkilökunnan keskuudessa. *Sosiaalilääketieteellinen Aikakauslehti* 24:287–296.

Potter, D. A., J. B. McKinlay, and R. B. D'Agostino. 1991. *Understanding How Social Factors Affect Medical Decision Making: Application of a Factorial Experiment*. Watertown, Mass.: New England Research Institute.

Potter, D. A., J. B. McKinlay, R. B. D'Agostino, R. Eder, and K. Gear. 1990. Increasing Response Rates in Surveys of Physicians: Reaching Practitioners in Modern Health Care Organizations. Unpublished manuscript.

Powell, D. E. n.d. The Entrepreneurial Spirit and Soviet Medicine. Unpublished manuscript.

Pracovni skupina MZSV CR pro reformu. 1990*a*. *Navrh reformy pece o j zdravi*. Praha.

Pracovni skupina MZSV CR pro reformu z dravotictvi. 1990*b*. *Souhrn predbeznych nametu pro okamzita opatreni ve zdravotnictvi*. Praha.

Pravda. 1987*a*. Diagnoz samomu sebe-zametki c zasedania Kollegii Minzdrava USSR. February 15.

Pravda. 1987*b*. In the USSR Council of Ministers. January 4:2. (In Russian. Available in English in the *Current Digest of the Soviet Press* 39(1):19, 1987.)

Pravda. 1987c. On the Most Vital Question in the Social Sphere: Formula for Health, April 13:3.

Prochazkova, P. 1990. Iluze bezplatneho zdravotnictvi. *Lidove noviny.*

Proekt T. 1987. Oshovnie napravleniia razvitiia zdorovia naseleniia i perestroikii zdravookhraneniia SSSR v dvenatsatoi piatileke i na period do 2000 goda. *Pravda,* August 15.

Programova komise Obcanskeho fora zdravotniku. 1990. Teze k programu zdravi. *Zdravotnicke noviny, no. 4.*

Räty, T. 1991. Naisten näkyvyys tieteessä paranemassa? *Naistutkimustiedote* 11(3):10–30.

Relman A. 1980. The New Medical Industrial Complex. *New England Journal of Medicine* 303:963–70.

Renaud, M. 1987. Reform or Illusion: An Analysis of the Quebec State Intervention in Health. In *Health and Canadian Society: Sociological Perspectives,* 2d ed., ed. D. Coburn et al. Toronto: Fitzhenry and Whiteside.

Rhode, T., and P. F. Hjort. 1986. Privat og offentlig innsats i Nordens helsevesen. *Nordisk Medicin* 101:206–7.

Rice, T., J. Gabel, and S. Mick. 1989. *PPOS: Bigger, Not Better.* Washington, D.C.: HIAA Research Bulletin.

Riska, E. 1988. The Professional Status of Physicians in the Nordic Countries. *Milbank Quarterly* 66(Suppl. 2):133–47.

Roback, G., L. Randolph, and B. Seidman. 1990. *Physician Characteristics and Distribution in the U.S.* Chicago: American Medical Association.

Robb, J. H. 1975. Power, Profession and Administration: An Aspect of Change in English Hospitals. *Social Science and Medicine* 9:373–82.

Rodwin, M. A. 1982. Can Bargaining and Negotiation Change the Administrative Process? *Environmental Impact Assessment Review* 3:373–86.

Roemer, M. I. 1976. *Health Care Systems in World Perspective.* Ann Arbor, Mich.: Health Administration Press.

Roemer, M. I. 1986. Proletarianization of Physicians or Organization of Health Services? *International Journal of Health Services* 16:469–71.

Romøren, T. I. 1989. Kommunehelsetjenestens fem første år. In sosialdepartementet: St. meld. nr. 36 (1989–90). *Røynsler med lova om helsetenesta i kommunane,* 167–223. Oslo: Sosialdepartementet.

Rørbye, B. 1976. Den illegale sygdomsbehandling som folkloristisk problem: Birdrag til en sociokulturel oversight for Danmark. In *Fataburen: Nordiska museets och Skansens årsbok 1976.* Lund: Berlingska Boktryckeriet.

Rosen, R. E. 1989a. Ethical Soap: L.A. Law and the Privileging of Character. *University of Miami Law Review* 43:1229–61.

Rosen, R. E. 1989b. The Inside Counsel Movement, Professional Judgment and Organizational Representation. *Indiana Law Journal* 64:479–553.

Rosenblatt, R. E. 1981. Health Care, Markets, and Democratic Values. *Vanderbilt Law Review* 34:1067–1115.

Rosenthal, M. M. 1989. Physician Surplus and the Growth of Private Practice: The Case of Sweden. *Scandinavian Studies* 61:169–84.

Rosenthal, M. M., I. Butter, and M. G. Field. 1990. Setting the Context. In *The Political Dynamics of Physician Manpower Policy,* ed. M. Rosenthal, I. Butter, and M. G. Field, 1–5. Amsterdam: Elsevier.

Rossiiskoe zdravookhranenie. 1991. *Meditsinskala gazeta* 37 (Sept. 13):7.

Rouse, J. 1987. *Knowledge and Power: Toward a Political Philosophy of Science.* Ithaca: Cornell University Press.

Rust, I., et al. v Louis W. Sullivan. 1991. Secretary of Health and Human Services, 111 S. Ct. 1759.

Ryan, M. 1990. *Doctors and the State in the Soviet Union*. New York: St. Martin's Press.

Saks, M. 1983. Removing the Blinkers? A Critique of Recent Contributions to the Sociology of Professions. *Sociological Review* 31:1–21.

Salive, M. E., J. A. Mayfield, and N. W. Weissman. 1990. Patient Outcomes Research Teams and the Agency for Health Care Policy Research. *Health Services Research* 25:697–708.

Saltman, R. B. 1987. Management Control in a Publicly Planned Health System: A Case Study from Finland. *Health Policy* 8:283–98.

Saltman, R. B. 1991. Emerging Trends in the Swedish Health System. *International Journal of Health Services* 21:615–23.

Saltman, R. B., and C. von Otter. 1987. Re-vitalizing Public Health Care Systems: A Proposal for Public Competition in Sweden. *Health Policy* 7:21–40.

Saltman, R. B., and C. von Otter. 1989a. Public Competition Versus Mixed Markets: An Analytic Comparison. *Health Policy* 11:43–56.

Saltman, R. B., and C. von Otter. 1989b. Voice, Choice and the Question of Civil Democracy in the Swedish Welfare State. *Health Policy* 10:195–209.

Schmidt, S. W., L. Guasti, C. H. Landé, and J. C. Scott, eds. 1977. *Friends, Followers, and Factions: A Reader in Political Clientele*. Berkeley: University of California Press.

Schmitter, P. C. 1979. Still the Century of Corporatisms? In *Trends toward Corporatist Intermediation,* ed. P.C. Schmitter and G. Lehmbruch, 7–52. Beverly Hills: Sage.

Sciulli, D., and P. Jenkins. 1990. Professional by Form and Quality: Professions and the Direction of Social Change. Paper presented at the annual meeting of the American Sociological Association, Washington, D.C.

Scott, C., G. Fougere, and J. Marwick. 1986. *Choices for Health Care*. Wellington: Government Printer.

Seay, J. D., and R. M. Sigmond. 1983. Community Benefit Standards for Hospitals: Perceptions and Performance. *Frontiers Health Services Management* 5:3–39.

Secretaries of State for Health, Wales, Northern Ireland, and Scotland. 1989. *Working for Patients*. London: Her Majesty's Stationery Office.

Secretary of State for Health. 1991. *The Health of the Nation*. Cm 1523. London: Her Majesty's Stationery Office.

Sharlet, R. 1978. *The New Soviet Constitution of 1977*. Brunswick, Ohio: King's Court Communication.

Shchepin, O. P., G. I. Tsaregorodtsev, and B. G. Erokhin. 1983. *Meditsina i obshestvo*. Moscow: Meditsina.

Shils, E. 1982. Great Britain and the United States: Legislators, Bureaucrats and the Universities. In *Universities, Politicians and Bureaucrats: Europe and the United States,* ed. H. Daalder and E. Shils, 437–87. New York: Cambridge University Press.

Shipler, D. K. 1983. *Russia: Broken Idols, Silent Dreams*. New York: New York Times Books.

Sidel, V. W., and R. Sidel. 1973. *Serve the People: Observations on Medicine in the People's Republic of China*. Boulder, Colo.: Westview Press.

Sigerist, H. E. 1943. From Bismarck to Beveridge: Development and Trends in Social Security Legislation. *Bulletin of the History of Medicine* 8:365–88.

SNAPS (Samnordisk arbetsgrupp för prognos- och specialistutbildningfrågor). 1986. *Den Framtida Läkararbetsmarknaden i Norden*.

Soberón, G., J. Frenk, and J. Sepulveda. 1986. The Health Care Reform in Mexico: Before and after the 1985 Earthquakes. *American Journal of Public Health* 76:673–80.

Sosialdepartementet. 1987–1988. *Nasjonal Helseplan. Helsepolitikken mot år 2000.* St. meld. nr. 41. Oslo: Sosialdepartementet.

Southern California Law Review. 1985. Interpretation Symposium. 58:1–725.

Sovetskaia Rossia. 1987. Our Dialogue: The Science of Health (Interview with Evgeny Ivanovich Chazov, USSR Health Minister), July 5:1. (In Russian. Available in English in the *Current Digest of the Soviet Press* 39(27):22, 1987.)

Starr, P. 1978. Medicine and the Waning of Professional Sovereignty. *Daedalus* 107:175–93.

Starr, P. 1982. *The Social Transformation of American Medicine: The Rise of a Sovereign Profession and the Making of a Vast Industry.* New York: Basic Books.

Starr, P., and T. Marmor. 1984. The United States: A Theoretical Forecast. In *The End of an Illusion: The Future of Health Policy in Western Industrialized Nations,* ed. J. deKervasdoue, J. R. Kimberly, and V. G. Rodwin, 234–54. Berkeley: University of California Press.

Statistical Abstract of the United States. 1989. Washington, D.C.: Department of Commerce.

Statistical Yearbook of Finland 1972. 1973. Helsinki: Central Statistical Office of Finland.

Stavrou, N. A. 1970. Pressure Groups in the Greek Political Setting. Ph.D. dissertation, George Washington University.

Steiner, P. O. 1977. The Public Sector and the Public Interest. In *Public Expenditure and Policy Analysis,* ed. R. H. Haveman and J. Margolis, 27–66. Chicago: Rand McNally.

Steuart, J. 1767. *Inquiry into the Principles of Political Economy,* vol. 1. London: A. Miller and T. Cadwell.

Stevens, R. 1971. *American Medicine and the Public Interest.* New Haven: Yale University Press.

Stevens, R. 1989. Cultural Values and Norwegian Health Services: Dominant Themes and Recurring Dilemmas. *Scandinavian Studies* 61:199–212.

Stinchcombe, A. L. 1959. Bureaucratic and Craft Administration of Production: A Comparative Study. *Administration Science Quarterly* 4:168–87.

Stoeckle, J. D. 1988. Reflections on Modern Doctoring. *Milbank Quarterly* 66:76–89.

Stone, D. A. 1988. *Policy Paradox and Political Reason.* Glenview, Ill.: Scott, Foresman.

Stone, D. A. 1991. German Unification: East Meets West in the Doctor's Office. *Journal of Health Politics, Policy and Law* 16(2):401–12.

Strid, L., et al. 1988. Lääkärin työolot ja stressi. *Suomen Lääkärilehti* 43:1277–81.

Strong, P., and J. Robinson. 1990. *The N.H.S. under New Management.* Philadelphia: Open University Press.

Sullivan, C., and T. Rice. 1991. The Health Insurance Picture in 1990. *Health Affairs* 10(2):104–15.

Swartz, D. 1977. The Politics of Reform: Conflict and Accommodation in Canadian Health Policy. In *The Canadian State: Political Economy and Political Power,* ed. L. Panitch. Toronto: University of Toronto Press.

Syrova, L. 1990. Presumpce viny. *Svobodny zitrek.*

Taylor, M. G. 1960. The Role of the Medical Profession in the Formulation and Execution of Public Policy. *Canadian Journal of Economics and Political Science* 25(1):108–27.

Taylor, M. G. 1978. *Health Insurance and Canadian Public Policy.* Montreal: McGill–Queen's University Press.

Teliukov, A. 1991. A Concept of Health Financing Reform in the Soviet Union. *International Journal of Health Services* 3:493–504.

Terris, M. 1978. The Three World Systems of Medical Care: Trends and Prospects. *American Journal of Public Health* 68:1125–31.

Teubner, G. 1989. How the Law Thinks: Toward a Constructivist Epistemology of Law. *Law and Society Review* 23:727–57.

Thane, P. 1982. *The Foundation of the Welfare State*. London: Longman.

Tierney, J. T. 1987. Organized Interests in Health Politics and Policy-Making. *Medical Care Review* 44(1):89–118.

Tilly, C. 1975. *The Formation of National States in Western Europe*. Princeton, N.J.: Princeton University Press.

Todd, J. S., S. V. Seekins, J. A. Krichbaum, and L. K. Harvey. 1991. Health Access America—Strengthening the U.S. Health Care System. *Journal of the American Medical Association* 265:2503–6.

Tomashevskii, I. 1986. Bumazhnaia likhoradka. *Izvestiia*, January 7.

Toren, N. 1975. Deprofessionalization and Its Sources: A Preliminary Analysis. *Sociology of Work and Occupations* 2:323–37.

Torrance, G. 1987. Hospitals as "Health Factories." In *Health and Canadian Society,* 2d ed., ed. D. Coburn, G. Torrance, C. D'Arcy, and P. New. Toronto: Fitzhenry and Whiteside.

Torstendahl, R., and M. Burrage, eds. 1990. *The Formation of Professions: Knowledge, State and Strategy*. London: Sage Publications.

Trehub, A. 1986. Quality of Soviet Health Care under Attack. *Radio Liberty Research,* July 28.

Trehub, A. 1987. Social and Economic Rights in the Soviet Union. *Survey* 29(4):13–24.

Tri kroky ke zdravi. Hovorime s ministrem zdravotnictvi CR a s predsedou vyboru CNR pro socialni politiku a zdravotnictvi. 1990. *Mlada fronta dnes.*

Truman, D. B. 1971. *The Governmental Process: Political Interests and Public Opinion,* 2d ed. New York: Alfred A. Kopf.

Tsalikis, G. 1988. Evaluation of the Socialist Health Policy in Greece. *International Journal of Health Services* 18:543–61.

Tsoukalas, C. 1976. Some Aspects of "Over-Education" in Modern Greece. In *Regional Variation in Modern Greece and Cyprus: Toward a Perspective on the Ethnography of Greece,* ed. M. Dimen and E. Friedl, 419–28. New York: New York Academy of Sciences.

Tsoukalas, C. 1986. *State, Society, and Work in Postwar Greece*. Athens: Themelio. (In Greek)

Tully, J. 1989. Wittgenstein and Political Philosophy: Understanding Practices of Critical Reflection. *Political Theory* 17:172–204.

Tuohy, C. J. 1976. Medical Politics after Medicare: The Ontario Case. *Canadian Public Policy* 2(2):192–210.

Turner, S. P. 1986. *The Search for a Methodology of Social Science: Durkheim, Weber, and the Nineteenth-Century Problem Cause, Probability, and Action*. Boston: D. Reidel.

Ukaz of the USSR Supreme Soviet Presidium. 1988. On the Confirmation of Order on Condition and Procedures for Providing Psychiatric Assistance. January 5, and USSR Ministry of Health Order No. 225. Measures to Further Improve Psychiatric Assistance, March 21.

Unger, R. M. 1984. *Knowledge and Politics*. New York: Free Press.

Unger, R. M. 1987. *Social Theory: Its Situation and Its Task*. New York: Cambridge University Press.

U.S. Congress. 1972. *Abuse of Psychiatry for Political Repression in the Soviet Union*. Washington, D.C.: U.S. Government Printing Office.

U.S. Supreme Court. 1982. Arizona v. Maricopa County Medical Society. *United States Reports* 457:332–67.

U.S. Supreme Court. 1986. Federal Trade Commission v. Indiana Federation of Dentists. *United States Reports* 476:447–66.

U.S. Supreme Court. 1990. Federal Trade Commission v. Superior Court Trial Lawyers Association. *United State Reports* 493:411–54.

Unschuld, P. U. 1979. *Medical Ethics in Imperial China: A Study in Historical Anthropology*. Berkeley: University of California Press.

Upton, S. 1991. *Your Health and the Public Health*. Wellington: GP Print.

Waddington, I. 1990. The Movement towards the Professionalization of Medicine. *British Medical Journal* 301:691–93.

Walder, A. G. 1986. *Communist Neo-Traditionalism: Work Authority in Chinese Industry*. Berkeley: University of California Press.

Wallerstein, I. 1974. *The Modern World-System. I. Capitalist Agriculture and the Origins of the European World-Economy in the Sixteenth Century*. New York: Academic Press.

Wallis, C. 1991. Why New Age Medicine Is Catching On. *Time* 138(18):68–76.

Walsh, P., and G. Fougere. 1989. Fiscal Policy, Public Sector Management and the 1989 Health Sector Strike. *New Zealand Journal of Industrial Relations* 14:219–29.

Walters, V. 1982. State, Capital and Labour: The Introduction of Federal-Provincial Insurance for Physician Care in Canada. *Canadian Review of Sociology and Anthropology* 19:157–72.

Weber, M. 1946a. Bureaucracy. In *From Max Weber: Essays in Sociology,* ed. H. Gerth and C. W. Mills, 196–244. New York: Oxford University Press.

Weber, M. 1946b. Politics as a Vocation. In *From Max Weber: Essays in Sociology,* ed. H. Gerth and C. W. Mills, 77–128. New York: Oxford University Press.

Weber, M. 1947a. Legal Authority with a Bureaucratic Administrative Staff. In *The Theory of Social and Economic Organization,* ed. T. Parsons, 329–41. New York: Oxford University Press.

Weber, M. 1947b. Collegiality and the Separation of Powers. In *The Theory of Social and Economic Organization,* ed. T. Parsons, 392–407. New York: Oxford University Press.

Weber, M. 1977. *Critique of Stammler,* trans. G. Oakes. New York: Free Press.

Weiner, J. P. 1989. Primary Health Care Systems in the United States, Denmark, Finland and Sweden: Can the "Corporatized" Learn from the "Socialized" or Vice Versa? *Scandinavian Studies* 61:199–212.

Weinerman, R. E. 1969. *Social Medicine in Eastern Europe. The Organization of Health Services and Education of Medical Personnel in Czechoslovakia, Hungary and Poland*. Cambridge: Harvard University Press.

Wilk, Chester A., et al. v. American Medical Association et al. 1987. No. 76C 3777, Sept. 25.

Wilensky, H. L. 1964. The Professionalization of Everyone? *American Journal of Sociology* 70:137–58.

Willis, E. 1988. Doctoring in Australia: A View at the Bicentenary. *Milbank Quarterly* 66 (Suppl. 2):167–81.

Willis, E. 1989*a*. *Medical Dominance: The Division of Labour in Australian Health Care.* 2d ed. Sydney: Allen and Unwin.

Willis, E. 1989*b*. Complementary Healers. In *Health and Australian Society: Some Sociological Perspectives,* ed. J. Najman and G. Lupton, 259–79. Melbourne: Macmillan.

Wilsford, D. 1988. Tactical Advantages Versus Administrative Heterogeneity: The Strengths and the Weaknesses of the French State. *Comparative Political Studies* 21(1):126–68.

Wilsford, D. 1989. The Political Economy of the Pharmaceutical Industry in France. Paper presented to the American Political Science Association, Atlanta, August.

Wilsford, D. 1991. *Doctors and the State: The Politics of Health Care in France and the United States.* Durham, N.C.: Duke University Press.

Wittgenstein, L. 1958. *Philosophical Investigations,* 3d ed., ed. G. E. M. Anscombe, R. Rhees, and G. H. von Wright. Oxford: Basil Blackwell.

Wolfe, D. 1984. The Rise and Demise of the Keynesian Era in Canada: Economic Policy, 1930–1982. In *Modern Canada: 1930–1980s,* ed M.S. Cross and G. S. Kealey, 46–78. Toronto: McClelland and Stewart.

Wolinsky, F. D. 1980. *The Sociology of Health: Principles, Professions, and Issues.* Boston: Little, Brown.

Wolinsky, F. D. 1988*a*. The Professional Dominance Perspective, Revisited. *Milbank Quarterly* 66 (Suppl. 2):33–47.

Wolinsky, F. D. 1988*b*. *The Sociology of Health: Principles, Practitioners, and Issues,* 2d ed. Belmont, Calif.: Wadsworth.

Wrong, D. H. 1988. *Power: Its Forms, Bases, and Uses.* Chicago: University of Chicago Press.

Yearbook of Nordic Statistics 1986. 1987. Nordic Statistical Secretariat. Stockholm: Norstedts Tryckeri.

Yearbook of Nordic Statistics 1989/90. 1990. Nordic Statistical Secretariat. Stockholm: Norstedts Tryckeri.

Yearbook of Nordic Statistics 1991. 1991. Nordic Statistical Secretariat. Stockholm: Norstedts Tryckeri.

Yfantopoulos, G. N. 1985. *Health Planning in Greece.* Athens: National Center for Social Research. (In Greek)

Zald, M. N. 1970. Political Economy: A Framework for Comparative Analysis. In *Power in Organizations,* ed. M. N. Zald, 221–69. Nashville, Tenn.: Vanderbilt University Press.

Zald, M. N. 1978. On the Social Control of Industries. *Social Forces* 57:79–102.

Zald, M. N., and F. D. Hair. 1972. The Social Control of General Hospitals. In *Organization Research on Health Institutions,* ed. B. S. Georgopoulos, 51–81. Ann Arbor: Institute for Social Research.

Zdravi zadarmo? 1990. *Respekt,* June 27–July 3.

Zhongguo Weisheng Nianjian 1985, 1987 (China health statistics yearbook 1985 and 1987). Beijing: China Medical Publishing House.

Zola, I. K. 1972. Medicine as an Institution of Social Control. *Sociological Review Monographs* 20:487–504.

Zoldi, D. 1992. What's It Like in Utilization Review. *RN* 55(2):41–44.

BIOGRAPHICAL SKETCHES OF
THE CONTRIBUTORS

Juan Luis Gerardo Durán-Arenas is the Director of Social and Managerial Sciences in the National Institute of Public Health of Mexico. He received his Medical Doctor degree from the National Autonomous University of Mexico in 1981, and his Master's degree in Public Health and his Master in Arts in Sociology from the University of Michigan in 1986. He is currently a doctoral candidate in Health Services Organization and Policy and Sociology at the University of Michigan. His research interests are divided among (a) health manpower research, in particular the study of the determinants of the supply and demand of physicians, the development of the medical profession in Latin American countries, and the power of the medical profession; (b) health management research, in particular the development of integrated health information systems and managerial decision-making tools and methods; and (c) quality of health care research, in particular the design and evaluation of quality improvement interventions. His more recent publications have been in the area of the medical profession.

David Coburn is Professor, Department of Behavioral Science, University of Toronto. He received his Ph.D. (Sociology) from the University of Toronto in 1973. His most recent research has been on the health occupations in Canada in the context of "the rise and fall of medicine." With others, he has analyzed the historical development of medicine, nursing chiropractic, and naturopathy. He is presently carrying out research on the question: After medical dominance—what? He is a co-editor of *Health and Canadian Society: Sociological Perspectives,* 2d. ed. (Fitzhenry and Whiteside, 1987).

John Colombotos, Ph.D., is on the faculty of the Division of Sociomedical Sciences, Columbia University School of Public Health, where he teaches and conducts research on the health professions and the social organization of health care. He is the author (with Corrine Kirchner) of *Physicians and Social Change* (Oxford University Press, 1986). He is currently conducting a national study of physicians' and nurses' responses to the AIDS epidemic.

Nikos P. Fakiolas, Ph.D., is a research associate at the National Center for Social Research in Athens, Greece. He holds a doctorate in social studies from the University of Athens. His research interests include specialty choices of physicians (his doctoral dissertation) and other aspects of health care delivery in Greece, the social implications of tourism in Greece, and other social issues in the areas of education, youth, and drugs.

Mark G. Field, Ph.D., is Emeritus Professor of Sociology at Boston University, Adjunct Professor at the Harvard School of Public Health, and a fellow in the Russian Research Center at Harvard. He is also Assistant Sociologist, Department of Psychiatry, Massachusetts General Hospital. The author, co-author or editor of eight books and over 120 articles in the professional literature, his major area of interest is the sociology of medicine, particularly health and health care in the former Soviet Union. His present interests include comparative health systems and the medicalization of deviance, with specific reference to the use/misuse of psychiatry for political purposes in the former Soviet Union.

Geoff Fougere, Ph.D., teaches sociology at the University of Canterbury, Christchurch, New Zealand, and has published extensively on aspects of the New Zealand health system. His current health-related research focuses on the development of processes of "managed competition" and the working of "quasi-markets" in health care.

David M. Frankford, J.D., is Associate Professor of Law at Rutgers University School of Law–Camden. He has taught seminars regarding the legal regulation of health care; conceptions of professions and professionalism in philosophy, sociology, and economics; the work of Talcott Parsons and Jürgen Habermas as they relate to law and the professions; and the work of Michel Foucault as it relates to the problems of knowledge and freedom. He has written on the relationships between health care law and health care economics, between law and medical sociology, and between law and the professions. He is currently working on a number of projects concerning reimbursement and coverage in national health care systems, and he is writing a book on neoclassical health economics.

Eliot Freidson, Ph.D., is Professor of Sociology in the School of Arts and Science of New York University. He is presently completing a book that establishes a theoretical foundation for the study of professions and uses it to compare and analyze the positions of five professions in five nations. He is collecting material for a future study of intellectual property.

Julio Frenk, M.D., Ph.D., recently finished his term as the founding Director General of the National Institute of Public Health of Mexico and is presently Senior Researcher at that institute as well as Visiting Professor at the Harvard Center for Population and Development Studies. He has also been designated a National Researcher in Mexico. A member of the World Health Organization Expert Advisory Panel on Human Resources for Health, he has carried out several research projects on the dynamics of the medical labor market and the comparative processes of professionalization in different types of countries. At the request of one of the leading Mexican university presses, he has recently completed a compilation, in book form, of his most important writings on these topics during the last decade. He is presently working on the broad area of health transition and is writing a book on the policy implications of shifts in the dominant patterns of health and disease.

Frederic W. Hafferty, Ph.D., is Associate Professor of Behavioral Sciences, University of Minnesota–Duluth School of Medicine. He is the author of *Into the Valley: Death and the Socialization of Medical Students* (Yale University Press, 1991) and is currently at work on a book, *Trust and Medicine,* that explores the evolution of medicine as a profession and the evolving nature of the physician–patient relationship. Other interests include disability studies and rural health issues.

Alena Heitlinger, Ph.D., is Professor of Sociology, Trent University, Peterborough, Ontario, Canada. Born in Czechoslovakia, she has published on a wide variety of topics including women's issues, health care, the family, population dynamics, and the transition from communism. She is the author of *Women and State Socialism* (Macmillan, 1979), *Reproduction, Medicine and the Socialist State* (St. Martin's Press, 1987), and *Women's Equality, Demography and Public Policies: A Comparative Perspective* (St. Martin's Press, 1993).

Gail Henderson, Ph.D., has been on the faculty of the Department of Social Medicine at the University of North Carolina School of Medicine since 1983. She received her Ph.D. in sociology from the University of Michigan, followed by a Mellon post-doctoral fellowship in public health. She is the author (with M. S. Cohen) of *The Chinese Hospital: A Socialist Work Unit* (Yale University Press, 1984) and a number of articles addressing issues in the modernization of medicine in China. She is currently involved in several research projects in China, including a study of health, nutrition, and economic change, in collaboration with the Chinese Academy of Preventive Medicine.

Rudolf Klein, Ph.D., is Professor of Social Policy and Director of the Centre for the Analysis of Social Policy at the University of Bath, England. His publications include *Complaints Against Doctors* (Charles Knight, 1973) and *The Politics of the NHS,* 2d ed. (Longmans, 1989). His current research interests include the role of regulation in social policy and rationing in health care.

Gerald V. Larkin, Ph.D., has held lectureships in sociology at the Universities of Leeds and Kingston and at present is Professor of the Sociology of Health and Illness and Head of Applied Social Sciences at Sheffield Hallam University, England. He has published on the social and historical development of health care, particularly focusing on the evolution of the medical division of labor and contemporary issues in the development of health professions.

Sol Levine, Ph.D., is Co-Director, Joint Program in Society and Health, New England Medical Center and Harvard School of Public Health; Professor of Health and Social Behavior, and Professor of Health Policy and Management, Harvard University; and Adjunct University Professor and Adjunct Professor of Sociology and Community Medicine at Boston University. He received his B.A. from the City University of New York, Queens College, and his M.A. and Ph.D. from New York University. Dr. Levine's numerous articles and essays have appeared in many outstanding journals. He co-edited and contributed to four editions of the *Handbook of Medical Sociology* (Prentice-Hall, 1989). He edited, with Norman A. Scotch, *Social Stress and The Dying Patient* (Aldine, 1970) and, with Abraham Lilienfeld, *Epidemiology and Health Policy* (Tavistock, 1986). Dr. Levine is studying factors affecting health-related quality of life and is developing a national and international research program in society and health. He was elected to the Institute of Medicine, National Academy of Sciences. He is the recipient of the Leo G. Reeder Award from the American Sociological Association's Council of Medical Sociology.

Donald W. Light, Ph.D., is Professor at the University of Medicine and Dentistry of New Jersey and serves on the graduate faculty of Rutgers University. He has written about the medical profession for many years and is currently the senior adviser to the Carnegie Foundation in its second review (since the Flexner Report) of medical education. His works include a review of field studies of medical education, theoretical essays on the profession's relation to society, and research on professional socialization.

John B. McKinlay, Ph.D., is Vice-President and Director of the New England Research Institute (NERI), an independent research organization in Watertown, Massachusetts. He is Director of Boston University's Center for Health and Advanced Policy Studies (CHAPS) and a Professor of Sociology and Research Professor of Medicine. He is also Professor of Epidemiology and Biostatistics at Boston University's School of Public Health. He is internationally respected for his work on professionalization, health policy, health services research, and epidemiology. He is the author, co-author, or editor of 17 books and over 150 professional articles. Several of his papers have been cited as classics in the field of medical sociology.

Elianne Riska received her Ph.D. from the State University of New York at Stony Brook. She is Professor of Sociology at Abo Akademi University, Finland, and also serves as the

Director of the Institute of Women's Studies there. Her research has focused on changes in the status and composition of the medical profession in the United States and in the Nordic countries.

Evan Willis, Ph.D., is Senior Lecturer and Convenor of the Health Sociology Research Group in the Department of Sociology at La Trobe University in Melbourne, Australia. His interests include the division of labor in health care and the social relations of medical technology.

David Wilsford, Ph.D., is Associate Professor of International Affairs at the Georgia Institute of Technology in Atlanta, Georgia. He is the author of *Doctors and the State* (Duke University Press, 1991) and is currently at work on a book, *The Fiscal Imperative in Health Care,* that compares health policy in the advanced, industrial democracies.

Fredric D. Wolinsky, Ph.D., is Professor of Medicine in the Division of General Internal Medicine of the Department of Medicine at Indiana University School of Medicine. His principal responsibilities there involve the continuation of his long-standing research program on the use of health services by older Americans. Funded by a prestigious MERIT award from the National Institute on Aging, this research focuses on the developmental course of health and health behavior among the elderly. Using panel data from the Longitudinal Study on Aging, Dr. Wolinsky is specifically addressing such matters as the consistency of health services utilization over time, the interrelationships among the different dimensions of health services utilization, and the role of health services utilization in the risk for institutionalization and death.

INDEX

Abortion: and gag restrictions, 213–14
Absenteeism: in Czechoslovakia, 175
Accountability: in U.S., 72
Affirmative action: 60–61
Agency for Health Care Policy Research (AHCPR), 18
Agricultural Insurance Organization (Greece), 139–40
AHCPR. *See* Agency for Health Care Policy Research (AHCPR)
Allied health care workers: emergence of, 14; regulation of in U.K., 86–87, 89. *See also* Paraprofessionals
Allied Signal, 79
Allopathic medicine: predominance of, 199; in U.S., 184
Alternative medicine: public interest in, 3; in U.K., 88
AMA. *See* American Medical Associaton
Ambulatory care: in Nordic countries, 156, 157; in U.K., 34
American College of Physicians: on national health insurance, 23
American Medical Association (AMA), 13, 18; advertising campaign by, 23; antitrust law court case, 19–20; dominance of, 138, 203, 220–21; medical ethics principles, 20; on national health insurance, 23
Antitrust law, 11, 19–22. *See also* Trust
Associations. *See* Professional associations
Australia, 104–14, 198, 215; autonomy in, 104–5, 106, 108, 113; corporatization in, 111–13, 114; deprofessionalization in, 104–5; financial and industrial capital, 111–13; historical background of health services, 106–8; intraoccupational changes, 109; professional dominance in, 106, 107, 108, 110, 111, 114; proletarianization in, 105–6; sovereignty in, 106, 111; state-profession relationship, 107, 110–11
Australian Medical Association, 110, 112
Authority: of knowledge, 58, 62; of linguistic practices, 47; of medical profession in Australia, 110; of physicians in New Zealand,
116; principles of, 30. *See also* Cultural authority; Social authority
Automated retrieval systems: and access to knowledge, 14
Autonomy: achieving as two-stage process, 12; of associations, 60; conferral of, 12, 19; definitions of, 26; and discretion, 26; and dominance, 41; and economic capital, 62; and expert knowledge, 32; of individuals, 14; as legal process, 12; of medical profession, 3, 12, 13, 14, 22, 26, 207, 210; and political power, 203–4; and production of services, 27; of professions, 11–12, 22, 26; and self-regulation, 13, 30, 32; of state, 31; and trust, 218; and uncertainty, 32. *See also* Self-regulation; Sovereignty; specific countries

Baxter-Travenol, 79
Belgrave, Michael: on New Zealand health policy, 116
Black Report, 205
Blue Cross/Blue Shield, 40
Board of Registration for Medical Auxiliaries (U.K.): founding of, 86
Britain. *See* United Kingdom
British Medical Association: vs. AMA, 84; and Australian medical profession, 107; and policymaking, 203; and regulation of health occupations, 86–87, 89; on state intervention, 85
British National Health Service. *See* National Health Service (U.K.)
Bureaucracy: and autonomy, 207–8; in Canada, 97; centralism of, 41, 90; in Commonwealth of Independent States, 165–67; and compatibility/incompatibility perspectives, 29–30; as complex organization, 29; conflict with, 30; defined, 29; ethic of service within, 30; and expertise, 29; ideal-typical, 30; and professions, 29–30; and state, 30–31; in U.K., 88, 90, 207

Caisse nationale de l'assurance maladie des travailleurs salariés (CNAMTS), 125–27

253